THE COMPREHENSIVE
NCLEX-RN
REVIEW
2000

NINTH EDITION

PATRICIA A. HOEFLER, R.N., M.S.N.

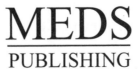

MEDS
PUBLISHING

MEDICAL EDUCATION DEVELOPMENT SERVICES, INC.

12120 PLUM ORCHARD DRIVE, SUITE H

SILVER SPRING, MARYLAND 20904

(301) 572-8080

Senior Editor: Joan Fishburn

Cover Design: Ann C. Hoefler, Director of Marketing

Graphic Designers: Cyndi Pena, Eve Kingsley Booth

Illustrators: Marie Hannah Fitzgerald, Joseph Boquiren, Eve Kingsley Booth

NINTH EDITION 1998

Previously Published as *The Comprehensive NCLEX-RN Review*

The authors and the publisher have prepared this work for student nurses and for graduate nurses preparing for licensing examinations. Care has been taken to confirm the accuracy of the information presented and to describe generally-accepted practices. Nevertheless, it is difficult to ensure that all the information presented is entirely accurate for all circumstances, and the authors and the publisher cannot accept any responsibility for any errors or omissions. The authors and the publisher make no warranty, express or implied, with respect to this work, and disclaim any liability, loss or damage as a consequence, directly or indirectly, of the use and application of any of the contents of this work.

Copies of this book may be obtained from:

MEDICAL EDUCATION DEVELOPMENT SERVICES, INC.

12120 Plum Orchard Drive, Suite H
Silver Spring, Maryland 20904
(301) 572-8080

ISBN 156533-032-3
Printed in the United States of America

CONTRIBUTING
AUTHORS

**CONTRIBUTING AUTHORS
EIGHTH EDITION**

Elizabeth Kassel, R.N., M.S.N.
Associate Professor

Marian Kovatchitch, R.N., M.S.N.
Associate Professor

Laura McQueen, R.N., M.S.N., C.S.
Clinical Specialist

Karyn Plante, R.N., M.S.N.
Associate Professor

CONTRIBUTORS TO PREVIOUS EDITIONS

Jennifer Burks, M.S.N., R.N.
Consultant

Michele Michael, Ph.D., R.N.
Professor of Nursing

Eleanor Walker, Ph.D., R.N.
Professor

Lois Walker, Ph.D., R.N.
Psychotherapist

Carol Jernigan, M.S.N., R.N.
Clinical Nurse Specialist

May Phillips, Ph.D., R.N.
Professor

Sandra Schuler, M.S.N., R.N.
Professor

TABLE
OF CONTENTS

LIST OF TABLES/CHARTS

INTRODUCTION TO
THE NINTH EDITION

WELCOME TO *THE COMPREHENSIVE NCLEX-RN REVIEW 2000!* MEDS Publishing is a professional organization direct-ed by nurse educators and dedicated to excellence in nursing education. MEDS Publishing was the first to offer review courses for the NCLEX-RN, and to introduce unique test-taking strategies and original methods for reviewing nursing information.

If you are now beginning a MEDS Publishing on-site NCLEX review course at your nursing program or one of the MEDS' open enrollment review courses, you are in good company! Students reviewing with MEDS Publishing have experienced a 99% passing rate. MEDS Publishing is the leader in NCLEX-RN reviews.

This MEDS Publishing Review outline, previously available only to students enrolled in the 4-Day Review Course, is now being offered independently "by popular demand." This eighth edition features:

✓ Critical information on the new NCLEX-RN computerized format
✓ Expanded and updated outlines for each of the five clinical areas
✓ An outline of MEDS Publishing's unique test-taking strategies
✓ Easy to understand charts and graphs
✓ Expanded appendices covering the areas of calculations and conversions, nutrition, and pharmacology
✓ An updated easy-to-use pharmacology guide

We hope this outline will facilitate your review of nursing information for the NCLEX-RN Exam. You have our best wishes for success on the exam, and for success and fulfillment in your career as a professional nurse.

ATTENTION, ALL NCLEX-RN CANDIDATES!

For a more in-depth presentation of the MEDS' powerful test-taking strategies outlined in this book, plus an exten-sive set of high-level practice questions with complete rationales, we recommend the MEDS' test-taking book, *Successful Problem Solving & Test Taking for Nursing and the NCLEX-RN Exams*, and computer tutorial, NCLEX-RN Test Taking 2000. MEDS Publishing's *Complete Q&A for the NCLEX-RN* features over 1,000 test questions with complete rationales and a companion computer disk.

To complete your review of nursing content, MEDS publishes a superb series of video tapes, The Comprehensive NCLEX-RN Video Review. These tapes are affordable and can be purchased individually, as well as in sets. Also, MEDS' best-selling audio tape review series offers another alternative for a comprehensive review of nursing content.

See page 363 for a list of many of MEDS Publishing's products for nursing students. For more information about MEDS' books, tapes, and innovative computer tutorials, contact MEDS Publishing at (301) 572-8080. We are always pleased to assist you.

UNIT ONE
REVIEW OF TEST-TAKING STRATEGIES FOR THE NCLEX-RN EXAM

UNIT CONTENT

SYMBOLS		
Key Points	**Nursing Interventions**	**Points to Remember**

SECTION I
PREPARING FOR THE EXAM

A. What You Should Know About the NCLEX-RN Exam

1. General information
   a. The first integrated exam was given in July 1982.
   b. The purpose of the exam is to determine that a candidate is prepared to practice nursing safely.
   c. The exam is designed to test essential knowledge of nursing and a candidate's ability to apply that knowledge to clinical situations.
   d. The purpose of the new test plan is to bring the exam in line with current nursing behaviors (the nursing process and decision making).
   e. Exam is "pass/fail," and no other score is given.

2. Computerized Adaptive Testing
   a. Computer program continuously scores answers and selects questions suitable for each candidate's competency level, for a more precise measurement of competency.
   b. A higher weight is assigned to difficult questions, so a passing score can be obtained by answering a lot of easier questions—or a smaller number of more difficult questions.
   c. Special screen design is used (see SCREEN DESIGN below).
   d. Two color-coded computer keys are used: the space bar to move the cursor, and the enter (or return) key to indicate the selection. If another key is touched accidentally, nothing happens.

SCREEN DESIGN

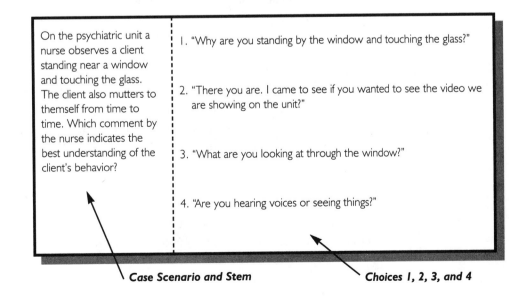

On the psychiatric unit a nurse observes a client standing near a window and touching the glass. The client also mutters to themself from time to time. Which comment by the nurse indicates the best understanding of the client's behavior?

1. "Why are you standing by the window and touching the glass?"

2. "There you are. I came to see if you wanted to see the video we are showing on the unit?"

3. "What are you looking at through the window?"

4. "Are you hearing voices or seeing things?"

Case Scenario and Stem   *Choices 1, 2, 3, and 4*

COMPUTER KEYS

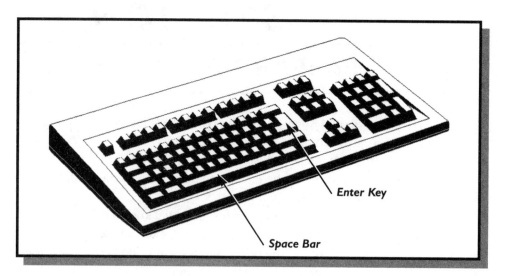

Enter Key

Space Bar

3. Exam schedule
   a. Given year-round
   b. May only take a single exam in one day
   c. Retake policy: not more than once in a three month period, with a maximum of four times in one year
4. Number of questions and time allowed
   a. No minimum amount of time; however, a candidate must answer a minimum of 75 test questions.
   b. Maximum time is five hours, with a maximum of 265 test questions.
   c. About one out of three candidates completes the exam in less than two hours; one in three will use the complete five hours.
   d. The computer will automatically stop as soon as one of the following occurs:
      1) Candidate's measure of competency is determined to be above or below the passing standard.
      2) Candidate has answered all 265 test questions.
      3) Maximum amount of time (five hours) has expired.
5. A candidate will pass by either:
   a. Answering 75 to 265 questions above the passing standard (the required weighted score) for all questions answered, within the time allowed; or
   b. Answering at least 75 questions within the time allowed and achieving the passing standard for the last 60 questions answered.
6. Types of questions
   a. All questions are multiple choice.
      1) Each question has four options.
      2) The best option is the only correct answer.
   b. Exam includes 15 unmarked experimental or "try-out" questions.

7. Exam procedure:
   a. Look for the BEST answer to each question.
   b. It is not possible to skip questions or return to previous questions.
   c. Mandatory 10-minute break after first two hours and after another one-and-one-half hours.
   d. Scratch paper provided for calculations must be returned at end of exam.

8. Structure of the test plan *
   a. **Safe, Effective Care Environment**
      1) Management of Care   17–13%
      2) Safety and Infection Control   5-11%
   b. **Health Promotion and Maintenance**
      1) Growth and Development Through the Life Span   17–13%
      2) Prevention and Early Detection of Disease   5–11%
   c. **Psychosocial Integrity**
      1) Coping and Adaptation   5–11%
      2) Physiological Adaptation   5–11%
   d. **Psychosocial Integrity**
      1) Basic Care and Comfort   7–13%
      2) Pharmacological and Parenteral Therapies   5–11%
      3) Reduction of Risk Potential   12–18%
      4) Physiological Adaptation   12–18%

B. Schedule Your Study Time
1. The minimum time for preparation is two hours a day for six to eight weeks.
   a. Spend 1/3 of your time reviewing content.
   b. Spend 2/3 of your time answering test questions.
2. For content review, use an NCLEX-RN exam review book such as this one, which outlines content.
3. Begin with areas that are most difficult for you, or the areas that are least familiar.
4. For more detailed information on your difficult or less familiar areas, use a good nursing reference manual.
5. Review medical/surgical, pediatric, maternal/child, and psychiatric nursing.
6. Use a body systems approach for medical/surgical, and pediatric nursing areas.

7. When studying body systems and the associated diseases, remember to:
   a. Define the disease in terms of the pathophysiological process that is occurring.
   b. Identify the client's early and late manifestations.
   c. Identify the most important or life threatening complications.
   d. Define the medical treatment.
   e. Identify the nursing interventions associated with early and late manifestations.
   f. Identify what the nurse teaches client/family to prevent or adapt to disease.
8. To schedule your study time:
   a. List the areas you need to review.
   b. Count the number of days you have available to study.
   c. Estimate the amount of time needed for each area.
   d. On your calendar, write the area to review, the number of questions to answer, and the amount of time needed for each study day.

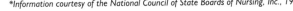

*Information courtesy of the National Council of State Boards of Nursing, Inc., 1997.

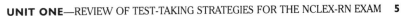

C. Answer Many Questions

1. Answering questions will develop your test-taking skills.
2. Use questions similar to those on the NCLEX-RN exam.
3. Answer a minimum of 3,000 test questions.
4. Include answering test questions in your study plan. For example, answer 100 questions each day for a month.
5. If you are at high risk, answer 5,000 test questions.

6. Use at least three different question-and-answer books, including MEDS Publishing's *Complete Q&A for the NCLEX-RN* with computer disk.
7. Using a variety of books provides a more comprehensive preparation.

D. Assess Your Progress

1. Each time you answer questions, check the number of questions you answered correctly.
   a. If you answer less than 65% correctly, this is a warning signal! Spend lots of time reviewing content and answering more questions in this area of nursing.
   b. If you answer 65 to 75% correctly, your performance is average. Success in this area is uncertain. Continue working with this content until your score is above 75%. Work on building your confidence by answering more questions in this area.
   c. If you answer 75 to 85% correctly, your performance is very good. Only return to this area after you have at least 75% in all other areas. Feel confident.
   d. If you answer 85 to 95% correctly, your performance is superior. Don't waste time on this. Feel very confident.
2. For each wrong answer, identify why you answered wrong.
   a. You may have answered a question wrong because you did not know the facts or got confused about the information.
      1) Identify this as a content weakness.
      2) Review the content again.
   b. You may have answered a question wrong because you misread the question, did not understand what it was asking, or did not know how to select the best answer.
      1) Identify this as a test-taking deficiency.

      2) If you have a problem with test-taking deficiencies, we recommend MEDS's test-taking book, *Successful Problem Solving & Test Taking for Nursing and NCLEX-RN Exams*. We also recommend MEDS's computer tutorial, *NCLEX-RN Test Taking 2000*, which may be available in your bookstore or purchased through MEDS Publishing. See the catalog at the end of this book for a list of more products by MEDS Publishing.
3. Check the number of questions that you identified as difficult and went back to answer later. See how many of them you answered correctly.

SECTION II
ANSWERING QUESTIONS

A. Identify the Critical Elements in the Question

1. Identify the **issue** in the question.
    a. The issue is the problem about which the question is asking.
    b. The issue may be a:
        1) Drug (e.g., digoxin *[Lanoxin]*, hydrodiuril *[Lasix]*)
        2) Nursing problem (e.g., alteration in comfort, potential for infection)
        3) Behavior (e.g., restlessness, agitation)
        4) Disorder (e.g., diabetes mellitus, ulcerative colitis)
        5) Procedure (e.g., glucose tolerance test, cardiac catheterization)
2. Identify the **client** in the question.
    a. The client in the question is usually the person with the health problem.
    b. The client in a test question may also be a relative or significant other or another member of the health care team with whom the nurse is interacting.
    c. The correct answer to the question must relate to the client in the question.
3. Look for the **key words**.
    a. Key words focus attention on what is important.
    b. Key words may appear in bold print.
    c. Examples:
        1) During the **early** period, which of the following nursing procedures would be best?
        2) The nurse would expect to find which of the following characteristics in an **adult** diabetic?
        3) Which of the following nursing actions is **vital?**
        4) Which of the following nursing actions would be best **initially?**
4. Identify what the stem is asking, and determine whether the question has a **true response stem or false response stem.**
    a. Be clear about what the stem is asking before you look at the options.
    b. If the question is not clear to you, rephrase it using your own words.
    c. Determine whether the question has a true response stem or a false response stem.
        1) True response stem
            a) Definition: A true response stem requires an answer that is a true statement.
            b) Examples:
                (1) Which of these interpretations is most justifiable?
                (2) The nurse would demonstrate best judgment by taking which of the following actions?
                (3) The chief purpose of the drug is to:

(4) The nurse should give immediate consideration to which of the following findings?

2) False response stem

   a) Definition: A false response stem requires an answer that is a false statement.

   b) Examples:

     (1) Which of the following nursing actions would be inappropriate?

     (2) Which of the following statements by the client would indicate a need for further instruction?

     (3) Which of the following describes incorrect placement of the hands during CPR?

     (4) Which of the following actions would place the client at risk?

B. Use a Selection Procedure to Eliminate Incorrect Options

1. Each NCLEX question has four options. The correct answer is the BEST answer. The other three options are "distractors."

2. Distractors are options made to look like correct answers. They are intended to distract you from answering correctly.

3. As you read each of the four options, make a decision about it.

   a. This option is true (+).

   b. This option is false (–).

   c. I am not sure about this option (?).

4. If the stem is a true response stem:

   a. An option that is true (+) might be the correct answer.

   b. An option that is false (–) is a distractor. Eliminate this option.

   c. An option that you are not sure about (?) is possibly the correct answer.

5. If the stem is a false response stem:

   a. An option that is true (+) is a distractor. Eliminate this option.

   b. An option that is false (–) may be the correct answer.

   c. An option that you are not sure about (?) is possibly the correct answer.

6. Do not return to options you have eliminated.

7. If you are left with one option, that is your answer.

8. If you are left with one (+) option and one (?) option, select the (+) option as your answer.

9. If you are left with two (+) options, use strategies to select the best answer.

C. Use Test-Taking Strategies When You Are Unable to Select the Best Option

1. The Global Response Strategy

   a. A global response is a general statement that may include ideas of other options within it.

   b. Look for a global response when more than one option appears to be correct.

   c. The global response option will probably be the correct answer.

2. The Similar Distractors Strategy

   a. Similar distractors say basically the same thing using different words.

   b. Since there is only one correct answer in a question, similar distractors must be wrong.

   c. Eliminate similar distractors. Select for your answer an option that is different.

3. The Similar Word or Phrase Strategy
   a. When more than one option appears to be correct, look for a similar word or phrase in the stem of the question and in one of the four options.
   b. The option that contains the similar word or phrase may be the correct answer.
   c. Use this strategy after you have tried to identify a global response option and eliminated similar distractors.

D. **Answering Communication Questions**
   1. The NCLEX-RN exam includes many communication questions because the ability to communicate therapeutically is essential for safe practice.
   2. Identify the critical elements as in all questions. Pay particular attention to identification of the client in the question. Remember that the answer must relate to the client.
   3. Learn to identify communication tools that enhance communication.
      a. Being silent: Nonverbal communication
      b. Offering self: "Let me sit with you."
      c. Showing empathy: "You are upset."
      d. Focusing: "You say that . . ."
      e. Restatement: "You feel anxious?"
      f. Validation/clarification: "What you are saying is . . .?"
      g. Giving information: "Your room is 423."
      h. Dealing with the here and now: "At this time, the problem is . . ."
   4. Learn to identify non-therapeutic communication blocks.
      a. Giving advice: "If I were you, I would . . ."
      b. Showing approval/disapproval: "You did the right thing."
      c. Using cliches and false reassurances: "Don't worry. It will be all right."
      d. Requesting an explanation: "Why did you do that?"
      e. Devaluing client feelings: "Don't be concerned. It's not a problem."
      f. Being defensive: "Every nurse on this unit is exceptional."
      g. Focusing on inappropriate issues or persons: "Have I said something wrong?"
      h. Placing the client's issues "on hold": "Talk to your doctor about that."

   5. When answering communication questions, select an option that illustrates a therapeutic communication tool. Eliminate options that illustrate non-therapeutic communication blocks.

E. **Answering Questions that Focus on Setting Priorities**
   1. Priority-setting questions ask the test taker to identify either what comes first, is most important, or gets the highest priority.
   2. Examples:
      a. What is the nurse's **initial** response?
      b. The nurse should give **immediate** consideration to which of the following?
      c. Which nursing action receives the **highest** priority?
      d. What should the nurse do **first?**

3. Use guidelines to help you to answer priority setting questions.
   a. Maslow's Hierarchy of Needs indicates that physiological needs come first.
   b. Maslow's Hierarchy of Needs indicates that when no physiological need is identified, safety needs come first.
   c. Nursing Process indicates that assessment comes first.
   d. Communication Theory indicates focusing on feelings first.
   e. Teaching/Learning Theory indicates focusing on motivation first.

SECTION III
PREPARING FOR EXAM TIME

A. Plan for Everything
   1. Assemble everything you will need for the exam the night before:
      a. Identification: two IDs with signatures, including one with recent photograph.
      b. Watch.
      c. Several sharpened pencils (with erasers) for calculations.
   2. Plan to arrive at the test site early.
      a. Know the route to the exam site.
      b. Know how long it will take to get there.
      c. Know where you will park and if you will need coins for a parking meter.
   3. Pay close attention to your own physiological needs.
      a. Dress in layers.
      b. Get a good night's sleep the night before the exam.
      c. Eat a good breakfast.
      d. Avoid stimulants and depressants.
      e. Use the bathroom just before the exam.
   4. During the exam:
      a. Listen to the instructions.
      b. Pace yourself; don't spend too long on any one question.
      c. Don't let yourself become distracted. Focus your attention on answering the questions.
    d. Go with your first choice. Use test-taking strategies only when you cannot decide between close options.
      e. Keep your thoughts positive!

B. Manage Your Anxiety Level

1. Moderate levels of anxiety increase your effectiveness.
2. Don't cram the night before the exam.
3. Do something enjoyable and relaxing the night before the exam.
4. Learn and practice measures to manage your anxiety level during the exam as needed.
   a. Take a few deep breaths.
   b. Tense and relax muscles.
   c. Tell yourself positive affirmations.
   d. Visualize a peaceful scene.
   e. Visualize your success.

C. Test-Taking Tips

1. **Prepare comprehensively** and be sure to be well rested for the exam.
2. **Read each question carefully,** identifying the critical elements. Each question must be answered in sequence, and you **may not skip or go back** to change your answers to any questions.
3. **Don't panic** if the computer stops after a short time! It does not mean that you failed. The computer stops when the exam is able to determine with at least 95% certainty that you have demonstrated the ability, or inability, to practice safely at the minimal level of nursing competency.
4. It is helpful to know that **most students pass by answering a maximum of 119 questions.** However, you can still pass the exam even if you answered all 265 questions.
5. If you are having difficulty choosing between the best two options, **use the three test-taking strategies you learned in this review:** 1) look for the global response option; 2) eliminate similar distractors; and 3) look for similar words in the question and one of the options.
6. You should anticipate that the **test questions will increase in difficulty.**
7. **Use your scratch paper wisely.** Since you cannot review earlier questions to help recall previous facts, use the scratch paper provided for calculations to remember facts from previous questions. **Sometimes, information from one question is helpful in answering another question.**
8. **Don't panic if someone finishes before you!** The test adapts to each candidate's level of ability, and it means that you may take longer to prove that you are capable of practicing competently at the beginning level of nursing.
9. **Keep a positive attitude!** Remember that you have learned a great amount of nursing knowledge, and the exam is only designed to determine whether you are able to practice safely at the entry level.

UNIT TWO
MEDICAL/SURGICAL NURSING

UNIT CONTENT

SYMBOLS

 Key Points
 Nursing Interventions
 Points to Remember

SECTION I

REVIEW OF FLUIDS AND ELECTROLYTES, ACID-BASE BALANCE

Fluids and Electrolytes

A. Body Fluids
1. Adults
   a. Women: 50–55% body weight is water
   b. Men: 60–70% body weight is water
   c. Elderly: 47% body weight is water
2. Infant: 75–80% body weight is water
3. Intracellular: 80% of total body water
4. Extracellular: 20% of total body water
   a. Interstitial
   b. Intravascular (plasma)
   c. Other: cerebrospinal fluid, intraocular fluid, bone water, gastrointestinal secretions

B. Electrolytes
1. Extracellular
   a. Na^+ 135–145 mEq/l
   b. K^+ 3.5–5.5 mEq/l
   c. Cl^- 85–115 mEq/l
   d. HCO_3 22–29 mEq/l
2. Intracellular
   a. K^+
   b. HPO_4
3. Function
   a. Promote neuromuscular irritability
   b. Maintain fluid volume
   c. Distribute water between fluid compartments
   d. Regulate acid-base balance

C. Movement of Fluids and Electrolytes

1. Diffusion: molecules move from an area of higher concentration to an area of lower concentration
2. Osmosis: water moves from an area of lower concentration of particles to an area of higher concentration
3. Filtration: movement of water and dissolved substances from an area of greater hydrostatic pressure to an area of lower hydrostatic pressure
4. Types of solution
   a. Isotonic   0.9% NaCl
   b. Hypertonic 3.0% NaCl
   c. Hypotonic   0.45% NaCl
5. Types of pressures
   a. Osmotic
   b. Hydrostatic

D. Mechanisms of Fluid Balance

1. Kidneys: control fluids and electrolytes, secrete renin
2. Lungs: control CO_2 levels, water vapor
3. Skin: fluid losses
4. Hormonal control
   a. ADH
   b. Aldosterone

E. Assessment of Fluid and Electrolyte Balance/Imbalance

1. Fluid volume deficit: water and electrolytes lost in same proportion
   a. Causes
      1) Fever
      2) Vomiting
      3) Diarrhea
      4) Increased urine output (diuretics)
      5) Increased respirations
      6) Insufficient IV fluid replacement
      7) Excessive tap water enema
      8) Draining fistulas
      9) Ileostomy, colostomy: third spacing—burns, ascites
   b. Manifestations
      1) Weight loss
      2) Poor skin turgor
      3) Urine: decrease in volume, dark, odorous, increased specific gravity
      4) Decreased central venous pressure (CVP)
      5) Increased respirations
      6) Increased hematocrit
      7) Dry mucous membrane
      8) Increased heart rate

2. Fluid volume excess
   a. Causes
      1) Too many IV fluids
      2) Decreased kidney function, congestive heart failure (CHF), cirrhosis
      3) Excessive ingestion of table salt
   b. Manifestations
      1) Cough, dyspnea, rales, tachypnea
      2) Increased blood pressure, pulse
      3) Increased CVP
      4) Neck vein distention
      5) Tachycardia
      6) Flushed skin
      7) Headache
      8) Pitting edema
      9) Decreased hematocrit
      10) Weight gain

3. Electrolyte imbalances: (see Table II-1. Major Electrolytes: Imbalance/Interventions)

F. Regulation of Body pH
   1. Normal value is 7.35–7.45
   2. Mechanisms regulating pH
      a. Chemical buffers: bicarbonate, protein molecules, phosphate
      b. Lungs: control carbon dioxide levels
      c. Kidneys

TABLE II-1.
MAJOR ELECTROLYTES: IMBALANCE/INTERVENTIONS

ELECTROLYTE	NORM. VALUE	SOURCES	LOW/CAUSES	MANIFES-TATIONS	NURSING INTERVEN.	EXCESS CAUSES	MANIFES-TATIONS	NURSING INVERVEN.
1. Potassium: (K$^+$)	3.5mEq/L 5.5mEq/L	**Fruits:** bananas, figs, peaches, melons, prunes, raisins, apricots. **Juices:** tomato, orange, grape. Nuts & Veg.	**Hypokalemia** associated with renal loss, diuretics, burns, massive trauma, colitis, uncontrolled **diabetes,** diarrhea, excessive perspiration, decreased intake, vomiting, gastric suction	Muscle cramping, muscle weakness, weak pulse, dyspnea, mental changes, loquacious, hallucinations, depression, EKG changes (sensitivity to digitalis), respiratory arrest	**Keep I&O** Observe for ECG changes **Potassium supplements:** Never give bolus injection IV or P.O **Check renal** function before giving **Dilute and mix** well before adm. Not greater than 40 mEq/L.	**Hyperkalemia, Renal failure,** Cell damage, Addison's disease, acidosis	**CNS stimulation, listlessness, weakness,** flaccid paralysis, abdominal cramps, **arrhythmias, muscle weakness**	**Monitor IV glucose** and insulin (promote entry of K into cells) **Give fluids** to increase urinary output. Kayexalate—exchanges Na+ for K+ ion
2. Sodium: (Na$^+$)	135–145 mEq/L	Common Table Salt	**Hyponatremia,** increased perspiration, drinking water, gastrointestinal suction, irrigation of tube with plain water, adrenal insufficiency, potent diuretics	Lethargy, hypotension, cramps, vomiting, oliguria, apprehension, muscular weakness, headache, convulsions	Use normal saline (not distilled water) for irrigation Avoid tap water enemas **Drink juices** and bouillon	**Hypernatremia,** decreased water intake, **diarrhea, impaired renal function,** acute tracheo bronchitis, unconsiousness, base bicarbonate deficit	Edema, hypertonicity, dry sticky mucous membranes, elevated temperature, flushed skin, thirst	D/5/W Give water between tube feedings **Elderly clients to drink 8-10 glasses** Check humidifier water level
3. Calcium: (Ca^{++})	8.5–10.5 mg/dl or 4.5–5.5 mEq/L	Milk, Cheese, Sardines, Salmon	**Hypocalemia, massive infection, burns,** administration of citrated blood, hypoparathyroidism, surgical removal of parathyroids	**Tetanycramps, tingling, numbness** hyperactive reflexes, **Cardiac arrhythmias**	Teach proper use of antacids/laxatives Importance of **adequate milk intake** Keep 10% calcium gluconate on hand for use, start after thyroid surgery	**Hypercalcemia,** excessive Vit. D milk ingestion, **hyperparathyroid,** multiple myeloma, **Prolonged bedrest,** Renal disease	**Renal calculi,** nausea, anorexia, weight loss, deep bone pain, flank pain, lethargy, anoxemia, muscle weakness, **pathological fractures**	Increase mobility Avoid large doses of Vit. D supplementation Adequate hydration
4. Magnesium: (mg^{++})	1.7 mEq/L 2.3 mEq/L or 2–7mg/ 100ml	Fruit, Peas, Beans, Nuts	**Hypomagnesemia, vomiting, diarrhea,** chronic alcoholism, impaired GI absorption, enterostomy drainage. Use of diuretics	Disorientation, convulsion, hyperactive deep reflexes, tremors, positive response to magnesium		**Hypermagnesemia,** hypotension, respiratory, paralysis Associated with renal failure, DM, dehydration		

Metabolic/Respiratory Imbalance—Acidosis/Alkalosis

A. **Acid-Base Imbalance**
  1. Metabolic acidosis
     a. Definition: base bicarbonate deficit; increase in hydrogen ion concentration
     b. Causes
        1) Starvation, malnutrition
        2) Systemic infections
        3) Renal failure
        4) Diabetic acidosis
        5) Ketogenic diet (high-fat)
        6) Diarrhea
        7) Excessive exercise
     c. Manifestations
        1) Headache
        2) Confusion, stupor
        3) Loss of consciousness
        4) pH below 7.35
        5) HCO_3^- below 22
        6) Urine pH below 6
        7) Hyperpnea (increased respirations) or Kussmaul's respirations

     d. **NURSING INTERVENTIONS**
        1) Treat underlying cause
        2) Promote good air exchange
        3) Give sodium bicarbonate
        4) Monitor K^+ level
  2. Metabolic alkalosis
     a. Definition: base bicarbonate excess; decreased hydrogen ion concentration
     b. Causes
        1) Vomiting (excessive loss of chloride)
        2) Gastric suction
        3) Alkali ingestion (excessive bicarbonate)
        4) Long-term diuretic therapy
     c. Manifestations
        1) CNS symptoms: confusion, irritability, agitation, coma
        2) Shallow respirations
        3) Hypertonic muscles
        4) Tetany
        5) pH above 7.45
        6) HCO_3^- above 26

     d. **NURSING INTERVENTION**: restore fluid volume

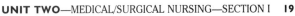

3. Respiratory acidosis
   a. Definition: excess H^+, excess carbonic acid
   b. Causes
      1) Acute: respiratory suppression or obstruction due to pulmonary edema, over-sedation, pneumonia
      2) Chronic: chronic airflow limitation (CAL) or COPD
   c. Manifestations
      1) Acute
         a) Confusion
         b) Coma
         c) Weakness
         d) Restlessness
         e) Headache
         f) pH below 7.35
         g) HCO_3^- below 22
      2) Chronic
         a) Pco_2 above 45 mm Hg
         b) tachypnea
         c) dyspnea
         d) weight loss

   d. **NURSING INTERVENTIONS**
      1) Administer sodium bicarbonate
      2) Good respiratory exchange
      3) Bronchodilators
      4) Monitor arterial blood gases (ABGs)

4. Respiratory alkalosis
   a. Definition: carbonic acid deficit
   b. Causes
      1) Hyperventilation (secondary to pain, anxiety, thyroid toxicosis)
      2) Decreased O_2 (pneumonia, pulmonary edema)
      3) Elevated body temperature
      4) Salicylate intoxication
   c. Manifestations
      1) Unconsciousness
      2) Circumoral numbness
      3) Pco_2 below 35 mm Hg

   d. **NURSING INTERVENTIONS**
      1) Breathe into paper bag
      2) Breathe into cupped hands
      3) Oxygen if hypoxic

TABLE II-2.
ACIDOSIS/ALKALOSIS

ACIDOSIS		ALKALOSIS
Respiratory:	Pco_2 (52) pH (7.32) HCO_3^- Normal (compensation)	(32) (7.51) Normal or (compensation)
Metabolic:	HCO_3^- (16) pH (7.3) CO_2 (compensation)	(38) (7.56) (compensation)
Norms:	Pco_2 : 35–45 HCO_3^- : 22–26 pH: 7.35–7.45 H_2CO_3 : HCO_3^- 1 : 20	

B. Blood Gases

1. ABGs
   a. Most accurate means of assessing respiratory function
   b. Must be sterile, anaerobic
   c. Drawn into heparinized syringe
   d. Keep on ice and transport to lab immediately
   e. Document whether receiving oxygen, temperature
   f. Apply pressure to site for 5–10 minutes

2. Components

   pH   measure of acidity or alkalinity of blood
   $\qquad$ N = 7.35–7.45

   pco_2 partial pressure of carbon dioxide respiratory parameter influenced by
   $\qquad$ lungs only
   $\qquad$ N = 35–45, remember this by taking the seven away from pH

Hypoventilation results in hypercapnia; hyperventilation results in hypocapnia

   pO_2 partial pressure of oxygen
   $\qquad$ measure of amount of oxygen delivered to the lungs
   $\qquad$ N = 80–100

   HCO_3^- bicarbonate, metabolic parameter influenced only by metabolic factors
   $\qquad$ N = 22–26

POINTS TO REMEMBER:

Pco_2 inversely associated to pH

HCO_3^- directly associated with the pH

Regardless of the pO_2, delivery of oxygen to the tissues is affected by the pH and temperature

3.   Examples:

RESPIRATORY ACIDOSIS	RESPIRATORY ALKALOSIS
pH 7.32 Pco_2 48 HCO_3^- 24 pO_2 90	pH 7.48 Pco_2 33 HCO_3^- 24 pO_2 90
METABOLIC ACIDOSIS	**METABOLIC ALKALOSIS**
pH 7.32 Pco_2 40 HCO_3^- 20 pO_2 90	pH 7.48 Pco_2 38 HCO_3^- 28 pO_2 90

POINTS TO REMEMBER:

1.   Clients with low sodium will present with acute onset of confusion
2.   Never give K^+ to a client who is not voiding: no "P," no "K"
3.   When patient has high calcium levels, phosphorus levels will be low and vice versa; works like a see-saw

SECTION II

REVIEW OF RESPIRATORY SYSTEM DISORDERS

Anatomy and Physiology

A. Function of the Lungs
1. Respiration: overall process by which exchange takes place between the atmosphere and the cells of the body. Normal respiratory rate: 12–20 breaths per minute
2. Ventilation: movement of air in and out of the airways, intermittently replenishing the oxygen and removing the carbon dioxide from the lungs

B. Thoracic Cavity—Lined by Visceral and Parietal Pleura
1. Right pulmonary space
2. Left pulmonary space
3. Pericardial space
4. Mediastinal space contains the esophagus, trachea, great vessels and heart

C. Subdivisions of the Lungs
1. Right: 3 lobes, 10 segments
2. Left: 2 lobes, 8 segments
3. Alveoli: tiny distal air sacs where gas exchange takes place; produce surfactant, which is a phospholipid secretion of the alveoli (Type II cells) that reduces the surface tension of fluid lining the alveoli; allowing expansion to take place; without surfactant, the lungs would collapse; oxygen is required for surfactant production

D. Factors Affecting Airflow
1. Obstructive disorders: COPD, bronchiectasis, allergy
2. Restrictive disorders: kyphoscoliosis, abdominal distension, edema
3. Trauma: stab wound, surgery
4. Secretions: infections, irritations

Diagnostic Tests

A. Chest X-ray: noninvasive procedure with no special preparation; lead shield for women of child-bearing age

B. Mantoux Test

C. Sputum Examination: first morning specimen preferable, approximately 15 ml required

D. Thoracentesis: aspiration of pleural fluid and/or air from the pleural space
   1. Preparation
      a. Consent and explanation
      b. Position sitting on side of bed with feet on chair, leaning over bedside table
      c. No more than 1,200 ml should be removed at one time
   2. Post-procedure
      a. Apply pressure to puncture site
      b. Semi-Fowler's position or puncture site up
      c. Monitor for shock, pneumothorax, respiratory arrest, subcutaneous emphysema

E. Bronchoscopy: examination of tracheobronchial tree using a bronchoscope
   1. Preparation
      a. Consent and explanation
      b. NPO after midnight
      c. ABG, oxygen administration
   2. Post procedure
      a. NPO until gag reflex returns
      b. Vital signs until stable
      c. Assess respiratory distress
      d. Warm saline gargles
      e. Semi-Fowler's position

Management of Clients with Respiratory System Disorders

A. Chronic Airflow Limitation (CAL); formerly called Chronic Obstructive Pulmonary Disease (COPD)
   1. Definition: a group of chronic lung diseases including pulmonary emphysema, chronic bronchitis and bronchial asthma; diseases are not truly "obstructive," therefore chronic airflow limitations (CAL) may be a more accurate description
   2. Major diseases
      a. Pulmonary emphysema
         1) Definition: destruction of alveoli, narrowing of small airways (bronchioles) and the trapping of air resulting in loss of lung elasticity

2) Etiology: cigarette smoking, deficiency of alpha anti-trypsin (enzyme that blocks the action of proteolytic enzymes that are destructive to elastin and other substances in the alveolar walls)

3) Manifestations
   a) Shortness of breath
   b) Difficult exhalation
   c) Pursed lip breathing
   d) Wheezing, rales
   e) Barrel chest
   f) Shallow, rapid respirations
   g) Anorexia, weight loss
   h) Hypoxia
   i) Productive cough
   j) Chronic respiratory acidosis

4) **NURSING INTERVENTIONS**
   a) Position sitting up, leaning forward
   b) Pulmonary toilet
   c) Frequent rest periods
   d) Nebulization
   e) Use intermittent positive pressure breathing (IPPB)
   f) Oxygen at low flow

5) Teaching
   a) Avoid crowds
   b) Diaphragmatic breathing
   c) Pursed lip breathing
   d) Report first sign of upper respiratory infection (URI)
   e) Home care
      (1) Dust with wet cloth
      (2) Avoid powerful odors
      (3) Avoid extremes of temperature
      (4) No fireplace
      (5) No pets
      (6) No feather pillows

b. Chronic bronchitis (blue bloater)
   1) Definition: excessive mucus secretions within the airways, and recurrent cough
   2) Etiology: heavy cigarette smoking, pollution, infection
   3) Manifestations
      a) Cough (copious sputum)
      b) Dyspnea on exertion, later at rest
      c) Hypoxemia resulting in polycythemia
      d) Rales, rhonchi
      e) Pulmonary hypertension leading to cor pulmonale and peripheral edema

4) **NURSING INTERVENTIONS**
   a) Prevent exposure to irritants
   b) Reduce irritants
   c) Increase humidity
   d) Relieve bronchospasm
   e) Provide chest physiotherapy
   f) Provide postural drainage
   g) Promote breathing techniques

c. Asthma
   1) Definition: condition of abnormal bronchial hyperreactivity to certain substances
   2) Etiology
      a) Extrinsic: antigen-antibody reaction triggered by food, drugs or inhaled particles
      b) Intrinsic: pathophysiologic conditions within the respiratory tract, non-allergic form
   3) Manifestations
      a) Severe, sudden dyspnea
      b) Use of accessory muscles
      c) Sitting up
      d) Diaphoresis
      e) Anxiety, apprehension
      f) Wheezing
      g) Cyanosis

   4) **NURSING INTERVENTIONS**
      a) Remain with client
      b) High-Fowler's position
      c) Emotional support
      d) Monitor respiratory status, ABGs
      e) Promote hydration
      f) Administer epinephrine subcutaneously
      g) Administer aminophylline IV
      h) Provide bronchodilators, nebulization
      i) Monitor oxygen therapy, lowest liter flow possible
      j) Corticosteroids
   5) Status asthmaticus: attack lasting more than 24 hours; medical emergency
      a) High-Fowler's position
      b) Monitor vital signs
      c) Monitor respiratory status
      d) Aminophylline IV
      e) Emotional support

B. Complications of CAL (COPD)
   1. Cor pulmonale
      a. Definition: right ventricular hypertrophy secondary to disease of the lungs; may or may not be accompanied by heart failure

b. Etiology
    1) Decrease in the size of the pulmonary vascular bed from destruction of the pulmonary capillaries
    2) Increased resistance of pulmonary vascular bed
    3) Shunting of unaerated blood across collapsed alveoli

c. Manifestations
    1) Dyspnea
    2) Cyanosis
    3) Cough
    4) Substernal pain
    5) Syncope on exertion
    6) Precordial systolic lift
    7) Heart failure: orthopnea, peripheral edema, jugular vein distension

d. **NURSING INTERVENTIONS**
    1) Promote bedrest
    2) Monitor oxygen therapy
    3) Maintain low sodium diet
    4) Monitor for side effects of digitalis and diuretics

2. Carbon dioxide narcosis/oxygen toxicity
  a. Definition: near comatose state secondary to increased CO_2 due to chronic retention
  b. Etiology: carbon dioxide retention, often secondary to excess O_2 delivery
  c. Manifestations
    1) Drowsy
    2) Irritable
    3) Hallucinations
    4) Coma
    5) Paralysis
    6) Convulsions
    7) Tachycardia
    8) Arrhythmias
    9) Poor ventilation

d. **NURSING INTERVENTIONS**
    1) Avoid high concentrations of oxygen
    2) Monitor response to oxygen therapy

3. Pneumothorax
  a. Definition: collection of air or fluid in the pleural space
  b. Etiology
    1) Trauma
    2) Thoracic surgery
    3) Positive pressure ventilation
    4) Iatrogenic, adverse effects of
      a) Thoracentesis
      b) Central venous pressure line insertion

c. Types
  1) Spontaneous
  2) Tension
d. Manifestations
  1) Spontaneous
    a) Sudden, sharp chest pain
    b) Sudden shortness of breath with violent attempts to breathe
    c) Hypotension
    d) Tachycardia
    e) Hyperresonance and decreased breath sounds over the affected lung
    f) Anxiety, diaphoresis, restlessness
  2) Tension
    a) Subcutaneous emphysema, dyspnea
    b) Cyanosis
    c) Acute chest pain
    d) Tympany on percussion
  3) Mediastinal shift: contents of mediastinum pushed to unaffected side
    a) Cyanosis
    b) Tracheal deviation—away from injured side
    c) Change in point of maximum impulse (PMI)

e. **NURSING INTERVENTIONS**
  1) Remain with client and remain calm
  2) Position in high-Fowler's
  3) Assess vital signs
  4) Notify physician of any changes in condition
  5) Provide chest x-ray
  6) Provide thoracentesis tray
  7) Monitor ABGs
  8) Monitor for shock
  9) Assist with insertion of chest tubes
    a) At the bedside or in operating room by physician
    b) Aseptic technique
    c) Local anesthetic, stab wound
      (1) Upper for evacuation of air
      (2) Lower for evacuation of fluid
    d) Occlusive dressing

C. **Closed Chest Drainage**
  1. Purposes
    a. Remove fluid and/or air from the pleural space
    b. Re-establish normal negative pressure in the pleural space
    c. Promote re-expansion of the lung
    d. Prevent reflux of air/fluid into pleural space from the drainage apparatus

2. Types
   a. One-bottle system
      1) Water seal and drainage in same bottle
      2) Observe for: intermittent bubbling fluctuation of fluid with each respiration air vent open to the air
      3) Uses: empyema
   b. Two-bottle system
      1) Air and fluid into first bottle water; seal in second bottle
      2) Observe for intermittent bubbling and fluctuation of fluid with each respiration in the water-seal bottle
      3) Uses: after thoracic surgery; pneumothorax
   c. Disposable chest tube systems (Pleur-evac, Thora-seal)
      (see illustration below)
      1) Replace two- and three-bottle systems, made of molded plastic to form three chambers
         a) Suction control chamber (closest to suction)
         b) Water seal chamber is middle seal
         c) Drainage collection (closest to chest tube)
      2) Suction is controlled by the amount of water in the suction control chamber
      3) Observe for: intermittent bubbling and fluctuation with each respiration in the water-seal chamber; continuous bubbling in the suction-control chamber
      4) Uses: after thoracic surgery; pneumothorax

PLEUR-EVAC DRAINAGE SYSTEM

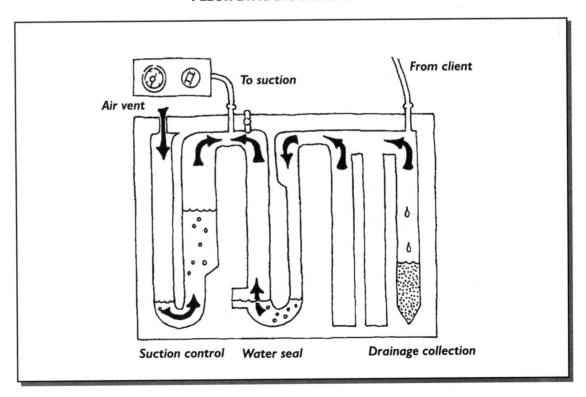

Suction control   Water seal   Drainage collection

3. **NURSING INTERVENTIONS**
    a. Know the purpose for the system
    b. Be sure a chest x-ray is done to assess placement
    c. Check for bubbling and fluctuation
    d. Assess respiratory status
    e. Turn client; ask client to cough, deep breathe
    f. Mark the amount of drainage at the beginning of each shift
    g. Note character of drainage
    h. Be sure tubing is without kinks, coiled on the bed
    i. Keep bottles below level of heart
    j. Maintain water seal
    k. Maintain dry, sterile, occlusive dressing
    l. Do not strip tubes, avoid milking
4. Removal of chest tubes: done by physician
    a. Equipment: suture removal kit, sterile gauze, petroleum gauze, adhesive tape
    b. Semi-Fowler's or high-Fowler's position
    c. Removal of tubes during expiration or at end of full inspiration
    d. Apply air-occlusive dressing
    e. Chest x-ray
    f. Assess complications: subcutaneous emphysema; respiratory distress

POINTS TO REMEMBER

1. Problem: Continuous, rapid bubbling in water-seal bottle/chamber
   Solution: Locate leak in the system; repair or replace

2. Problem: No fluctuation in water-seal chamber with respirations
   Solution: Check for kinks in the tubing
                 Listen for breath sounds
                 Lung may have re-expanded

3. Problem: No bubbling in suction-control bottle/chamber
   Solution: Turn up suction until gentle continuous suctioning

4. Problem: Broken bottle
   Solution: Insert tubing into sterile water until the bottle can be replaced

D. Infectious Pulmonary Diseases
    1. Tuberculosis
        a. Reportable, communicable, infectious, inflammatory disease that can occur in any part of the body
        b. Etiology: mycobacterium tuberculosis (nonmotile, aerobic, killed by heat and ultra-violet light); droplet nuclei spread by laughing, sneezing

c.   Risk factors
1) Overcrowded, poor living conditions
2) Poor nutritional status
3) Virulence of the organism
4) Previous infection
5) Alcohol abuse
6) Inadequate treatment of primary infection
7) Close contact with infected person
8) Immune dysfunction or HIV
9) Long-term care facilities, prisons

d.   Manifestations
1) Productive cough
2) Rales
3) Dyspnea
4) Hemoptysis
5) Malaise
6) Night sweats, low-grade fever
7) Weight loss
8) Anorexia, vomiting
9) Indigestion, pallor

e.   Diagnostic tests
1) Skin test such as Mantoux test
   a) Upper 1/3 of inner surface of left arm
   b) Intracutaneous injection of 0.1 ml of purified protein derivative (PPD)
   c) Needle with bevel up
   d) Read in 48–72 hours
   e) Palpate and measure induration: 10mm = positive
2) Sputum for acid-fast bacillus, x3
3) Chest x-ray
4) History and physical exam

f.   Treatment
1) Chemotherapy
   a) Ethambutol *(Myambutol):* impairs RNA synthesis; side effects: optic neuritis, skin rash
   b) Rifampicin *(Rifadin):* impairs RNA synthesis; side effects: red-orange color to urine and feces; negates birth control pill; nausea, vomiting, thrombocytopenia
   c) Isoniazid *(INH):* interferes with DNA synthesis used in prophylactic treatment; side effects: peripheral neuritis, hepatotoxicity, GI upset
   d) Pyridoxine *(B_6):* counteracts the effects of (INH)
   e) Streptomycin; side effects: 8th nerve damage, use with caution in renal disease

2) **NURSING INTERVENTIONS**
   a) Teaching plan includes
      (1) Knowledge that TB can be controlled
      (2) Drugs must be taken in combination to avoid bacterial resistance
      (3) Drugs should be taken either once each day or 2-3 timers per week, but always at the same time of day and on an empty stomach
      (4) Drugs must be taken for 6–12 months
      (5) Preventive measures to avoid catching viral infections
      (6) Maintaining adequate nutritional status
      (7) Promoting yearly checkups
   b) Hospital care
      (1) Prevent spread of infection
      (2) Provide psychological support
      (3) Observe for/prevent complications
      (4) Teaching: hand washing, cover nose and mouth when sneezing, coughing
      (5) Wear special particulate respirator mask when in the client's room
      (6) Isolation room ventilated to outside; discontinued when client no longer considered infectious

POINTS TO REMEMBER
1. Obtain sputum specimens before drug therapy is initiated
2. Multiple drug therapy is necessary to prevent the development of resistant organisms
3. New drugs should be introduced in combination
4. Give drugs in a single daily dose
5. Drug therapy must be continued for 6–12 months even though the x-ray, sputum specimens and manifestations are within normal limits
6. Drug therapy must be long term and uninterrupted
7. Client is generally considered noninfectious after 1–2 weeks of continuous drug therapy
8. Avoid use of alcohol during drug therapy to reduce risk of hepatotoxicity

2. Pneumonia
   a. Definition: inflammation of the lung parenchyma caused by infectious agents
   b. Etiology: classified as community acquired or hospital acquired (nosocomial)
      1) Community acquired
         a) Streptococcus pneumoniae or pneumococcal
         b) Haemophilus influenzae
         c) Legionella pneumonia
         d) Mycoplasma pneumoniae (atypical pneumonia)
      2) Hospital acquired
         a) Staphylococcus aureus
         b) Klebsiella pneumoniae
         c) Pseudomonas pneumoniae
         d) Fungi (various types, i.e., histoplasmosis)

c. Persons at risk
  1) Elderly
  2) Infants
  3) Alcohol abusers
  4) Cigarette smokers
  5) Postoperative clients
  6) Clients with chronic airway limitation (CAL), chronic illnesses
  7) Clients with viral infections
  8) Clients with AIDS (Pneumocystis carinii pneumonia [PCP])
  9) Clients on prolonged bedrest or immobility
d. Common manifestations
  1) Sudden onset of chills, fever
  2) Cough: dry and painful at first, later produces rusty colored sputum
  3) Dyspnea
  4) Flushed cheeks
  5) Pallor, cyanosis
  6) Pleuritic pain that increases with respiration
  7) Tachypnea, tachycardia

e. **NURSING INTERVENTIONS**
  1) Administer drug therapy
    a) Cough suppressants, expectorants
    b) Bronchodilators
    c) Penicillin
    d) Cephalosporin
    e) Tetracycline
    f) Erythromycin
    g) Mild analgesic
  2) Bedrest to ambulation after first day
  3) Oral hygiene
  4) Maintain fluid and electrolyte balance
  5) Pulmonary toilet
  6) Assess for sputum thickness, color
  7) Oxygen to maintain oxygen saturations >92%
  8) Isolate as necessary
  9) Small frequent meals, increase fluid intake
  10) Health teaching, teach MDI use

POINTS TO REMEMBER
1. Most pneumonias have a sudden onset
2. Penicillin remains the drug of choice for pneumococcal pneumonias
3. Antibiotics must be given on time to maintain blood levels
4. Watch for side effects of penicillin therapy
5. Prevention is the best therapy; monitor carefully those clients who are at risk

5. Cancer of the lung
   a. Definition: primary or secondary (metastatic from a primary site) malignant tumor located in lung or bronchi
   b. Types:
      1) Epidermoid (squamous cell)
      2) Oat cell (small cell)
      3) Adenocarcinoma
      4) Large cell (anaplastic)
   c. Etiology: cigarette smoking, exposure to asbestos and other carcinogens (coal dust, uranium, nickel)
   d. Asymptomatic in early states
   e. Later stages
      1) Coughing
      2) Wheezing
      3) Dyspnea
      4) Hemoptysis
      5) Weight loss
      6) Anorexia
      7) Fever

   f. **NURSING INTERVENTIONS**
      1) Support cessation of smoking
      2) Postoperative care for lung excision (see illustration below)
         a) Pneumonectomy: removal of an entire lung (reasons: cancer, abscess); postop: dorsal recumbent or semi-Fowler's position on AFFECTED side; range of motion to affected shoulder; NO CHEST TUBE
         b) Lobectomy: removal of a lobe for TB or abscess; postop: chest tube
         c) Segmentectomy: removal of a lobe (reason: infection in localized area); postop: chest tube
         d) Wedge resection: removal of a small portion of lung tissue (reason: small localized area of disease near the surface of the lung); postop: chest tube

LUNG EXCISION TYPES

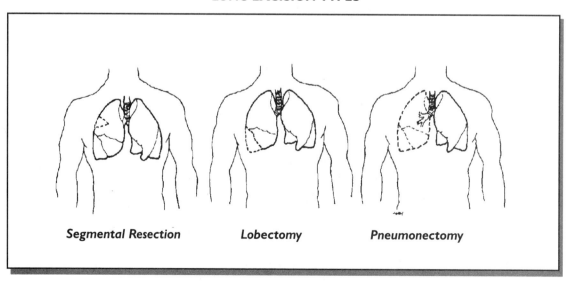

Segmental Resection   *Lobectomy*   *Pneumonectomy*

E. **Disorders of the Pleural Space**

1. Pleural effusion

   a. Definition: accumulation of nonpurulent fluid in the pleural cavity

   b. Etiology

      1) Blood vessels exudate

      2) Tissue surfaces transudate, associated with leukemias, lymphomas, pulmonary edema, cirrhosis of the liver

2. Empyema

   a. Definition: accumulation of pus in the pleural cavity

   b. Etiology: spread of infection from lungs, chest wall; complication of pneumonia, TB, abscess, bronchiectasis

Pulmonary Therapies

A. **Chest Physiotherapy (Chest PT)**

1. Definition: percussion and vibration over the thorax to loosen secretions in the affected areas of the lung

2. Nursing responsibilities

   a. Keep a layer of material (gown or pajamas) between your hands and the client's skin

   b. Stop if pain occurs

   c. Dispose of sputum properly

   d. Provide mouth care after procedure; best time is in the morning upon arising, 1 hour before meals or 2–3 hours after meals

3. Contraindications

   a. When bronchospasm is increased by its use

   b. History of pathological fractures

   c. Obesity

   d. Rib fractures

   e. Incisions

B. **Postural Drainage** (see illustration p. 36)

1. Definition: use of gravity to drain secretions from segments of the lung; may be combined with chest PT

2. **NURSING INTERVENTIONS**

   a. Proper positioning (lung segment to be drained is uppermost)

   b. Stop if cyanosis or exhaustion is increased

   c. Dispose of sputum properly

   d. Provide mouth care after procedure; best time is in the morning upon arising, 1 hour before meals or 2–3 hours after meals

   e. Maintain position 5–20 minutes

3. Contraindications

   a. Unstable vital signs

   b. Increased intracranial pressure

POSITIONS FOR POSTURAL DRAINAGE

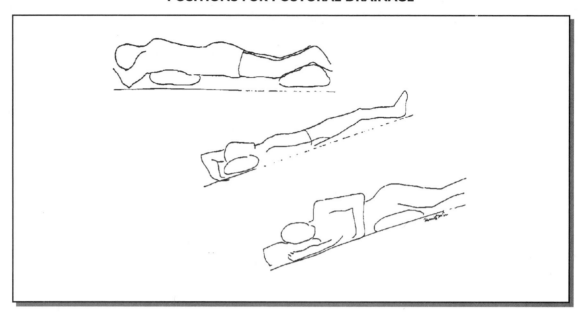

C. **Pulmonary Toilet**
1. Cough
2. Breathe deeply
3. Chest PT
4. Turn and position

D. **Intermittent Positive Pressure Breathing (IPPB)**
1. Definition: delivery of aerosolized medications to the respiratory tree by positive pressure
2. Adverse effects
   a. Dizziness
   b. Headache
   c. Anxiety
   d. Cardiac arrhythmias
   e. Pneumothorax

E. Bronchodilators

1. Types of Bronchodilators

Drug	Nebulization Dose	Inhaler Dose	Side Effects
albuterol (Proventil)	2.5mg, 3–4/daily	2 puffs q 4–6h	tachycardia
isoetharine (Bronkosol)	0.25–05ml q 1% diluted to 1:3 q4h	1–2 puffs q 4h	headache tachycardia
isoproterenol (Isuprel)	0.25 ml q 1% diluted to 2.5–5ml	1–2 puffs q 4h	tachycardia arrhythmias
terbutaline (Brethine)		2 puffs q 4–6h	tachycardia

2. Using inhalers (metered dose inhalers); teach client procedure
   a. Shake the inhaler
   b. Remove the cap from the inhaler
   c. Breathe deeply in and out through the mouth
   d. Insert the mouth piece into the mouth and form a tight seal with the lips
   e. With the index finger on top of the canister, depress the top while inhaling slowly
   f. Remove the inhaler and hold breath for as long as possible
   g. Exhale
   h. Wait 1–2 minutes before the next dose

F. Suctioning

1. Indications: client is unable to raise secretions after coughing or chest PT; to obtain a sputum sample
2. Procedure
   a. Aseptic technique
   b. Lubricate catheter before insertion
   c. Oxygenate client
   d. Advance catheter during inspiration
   e. Pull catheter back 2–3 cm after reaching the bronchial bifurcation
   f. Withdraw catheter while applying intermittent suction and rotating catheter between thumb and index finger
   g. Oxygenate client
   h. Rinse catheter and discard with gloves
   i. Document client response, character and volume of sputum
3. Adverse effects
   a. Hypoxia
   b. Arrhythmia
   c. Bronchospasm
   d. Infection

SECTION III

REVIEW OF GENERAL PREOPERATIVE AND POSTOPERATIVE CARE

Preoperative Care

A. Purpose
1. Ensure the client is in the best physical and psychological condition for surgery
2. Eliminate or reduce postoperative discomfort and complications

B. General Preoperative Care
1. Psychological support
2. Client teaching
   a. Coughing and deep breathing
   b. Supporting the wound
   c. Leg exercises
   d. Turning
   e. Getting out of bed
   f. Analgesics
   g. Recovery room procedures
   h. Other postoperative expectations: type of dressing, NGT, drains, IV
3. Informed consent
4. Physical care
   a. Vital signs
   b. Nutritional support
   c. Skin preparation
   d. Oral hygiene
   e. Enema
5. Preoperative drugs
   a. Purpose
      1) Reduce anxiety
      2) Decrease secretions
      3) Reduce amount of general anesthesia
      4) Control nausea and vomiting
   b. Common preoperative drugs
      1) Meperidine *(Demerol)*, morphine sulfate *(Roxanol)*
      2) Hydroxyzine *(Vistaril)*, promethazine *(Phenergan)*
      3) Atropine, scopolamine
      4) Pentobarbital sodium *(Nembutal)*, secobarbital sodium *(Seconal)*

c. Anesthetics
   1) General
      a) Inhalation
      b) Intravenous
   2) Local
      a) Topical
      b) Spinal
         (1) Lumbar space three to four or four to five
         (2) Side effects: hypotension, nausea, vomiting, headache

General Postoperative Care

A. Immediate Assessment
1. Pulmonary
  a. Airway
  b. Breath sounds
  c. Coughing, deep breathing
2. Neurological
  a. Level of consciousness
  b. Reflexes
3. Circulatory
  a. Vital signs
  b. Peripheral perfusion
  c. IVs
  d. Dressing
  e. Drainage tubes
4. Gastrointestinal
  a. Bowel sounds
  b. NGT
  c. Distention
5. Genitourinary
  a. Urinary output
  b. Intake and output

B. NURSING INTERVENTIONS
1. Assess for complications
  a. Take vital signs frequently
  b. NPO until alert
  c. Suction p.r.n.
  d. Medicate p.r.n.
  e. Turn client; have client cough and breathe deeply
  f. Monitor intake and output
  g. Increase fluids for spinal anesthesia
2. Positioning
  a. Head to side, chin forward if unconscious
  b. Lateral Sims, semiprone

DEEP BREATHING EXERCISES

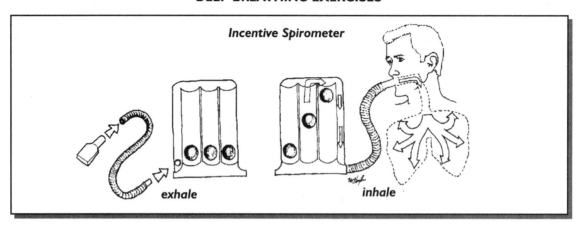

Incentive Spirometer

exhale   inhale

TABLE II-3.
COMMON POSTOPERATIVE COMPLICATIONS

COMPLICATION	COMMON CAUSES	OCCURRENCE	MANIFESTATIONS
EARLY COMPLICATIONS			
Atelectasis	Shallow respirations	First 48 hours postop	Fever, increased pulse and respiration
Hypostatic pneumonia	Shallow respirations	> 48 hours postop	Fever, increased pulse and respiration
Hypoxia	Respiratory depressants	First 48 hours	Increased blood pressure
Nausea	Reaction to anesthesia	First 48 hours	Nausea
Shock	Loss of fluids and and electrolytes	Immediately or later	Drop in blood pressure
Urinary retention	Medications, local edema	2–3 days	Inability to void, restlessness, bladder distention
Wound hemorrhage	Slipping of suture, wound evisceration	Immediately or later	Drop in blood pressure
LATER COMPLICATIONS			
Thrombophlebitis	Venous stasis, irritation from IV	7–14 days	Skin warm to touch
Wound infection	Poor technique, obesity, debilitation	4–5 days	Skin warm to touch
Wound dehiscence	Old age, malnutrition	4–15 days	
Wound evisceration	Old age, malnutrition	4–15 days	Wound dehiscence; "pink lemonade" drainage
Urinary tract	Indwelling catheter	5–8 days	Dysuria, hematuria, urgency, frequency

SECTION IV

REVIEW OF GASTROINTESTINAL, HEPATIC AND PANCREATIC DISORDERS

Nursing Assessment

A. Client's Chief Complaint

B. Appearance—thin, emaciated, obese, skin turgor

C. Nausea and Vomiting—what precipitates it, what relieves it

D. Abdominal Pain—location, what precipitates it, what relieves it, radiation

E. Swallowing and Food Intake—difficulty swallowing, increased or decreased intake

F. Nutrition—assess likes, dislikes, calories, vitamins, other nutrients

G. Elimination—pattern, consistency of stool, use of laxatives

H. Examination of Abdomen—inspection, auscultation, percussion, palpation

I. Associated Symptoms—flatus, eructation, heartburn, pain

Diagnostic Procedures

A. Upper GI
1. Method: barium swallow
2. Purpose: assessment of esophagus and stomach
3. NPO 6–8 hours before procedure
4. Laxative after procedure
5. Follow-up x-ray 6 hours after procedure

B. Lower GI
1. Method: barium enema
2. Purpose: assessment of large colon
3. Liquid diet before procedure
4. Laxative before and after procedure

C. **Endoscopy (Gastroscopy, Esophagogastric Duodenoscopy, Colonoscopy)**
1. Method: visualization of the inside of the body by means of a lighted tube
2. Purpose: assessment of esophagus, stomach, and colon
3. Gag reflex inactivated
4. NPO 6–8 hours before procedure
5. Resume diet after gag reflex returns

D. **Sigmoidoscopy**
1. Method: endoscope inserted through the anus
2. Purpose: assessment of sigmoid colon
3. Administer enema before
4. Monitor for complications: perforation, bleeding

E. **Analysis of Secretions**
1. Gastric analysis
    a. Method: contents of stomach analyzed
    b. Purpose: assessment of ulcers
    c. Purpose: rule out pernicious anemia
    d. NPO 8–10 hours before procedure, no smoking, no anticholinergics
2. Tubeless gastric analysis
    a. Method: ingestion of dye that is displaced by acid and excreted
    b. Purpose: determines the amount of free HCl in stomach

F. **Analysis of Stools**
1. Method: culture, fat analysis, guaiac (no ASA, NSAID, red meat, Vitamin C for 3 days before)
2. Purpose: assessment for bacteria, virus, malabsorption, blood

G. **Biopsy and Cytology**
1. Method: examination of tissue or cells
2. Purpose: assessment for malignancy, inflammation

H. **Radionuclide Uptake**
1. Method: use of isotopes
2. Purpose: assessment for hepatoma, abscess

I. **Cholecystogram (Gallbladder Series)**
1. Method: dye conjugated in the liver and excreted into the bile that outlines the gallbladder
2. Purpose: assessment of gallstones, proper gallbladder function
3. Check for allergy to iodine or seafood
4. Telepaque tablets 12 hours before test
5. Low-fat diet
6. NPO after midnight

J. Cholangiogram
1. Method: bile ducts visualized
2. Check for allergy to iodine or seafood

K. Liver Biopsy (see illustration below)
1. Method: removal of liver tissue
2. Purpose: to rule out liver disease
3. Obtain consent and results of hemostasis tests before the test
4. NPO after midnight
5. Position on left side during biopsy
6. Position on right side after biopsy for two hours
7. Bedrest for 24 hours after biopsy
8. Observe for complications (bleeding, pneumothorax)

L. Paracentesis
1. Temporary removal of fluid accumulated in the peritoneum
2. Indicated when ventilation is impaired, abdominal discomfort
3. Void immediately prior to procedure
4. During procedure: sitting up with feet resting on stool
5. Fluid should be removed slowly over 30–90 minutes, generally <1500cc
6. Bedrest after the procedure
7. Observe for complications
8. Indications
   a. Therapeutic: to relieve shortness of breath when ventilation is impaired
   b. Diagnostic: to examine contents of peritoneal fluid

LIVER BIOPSY

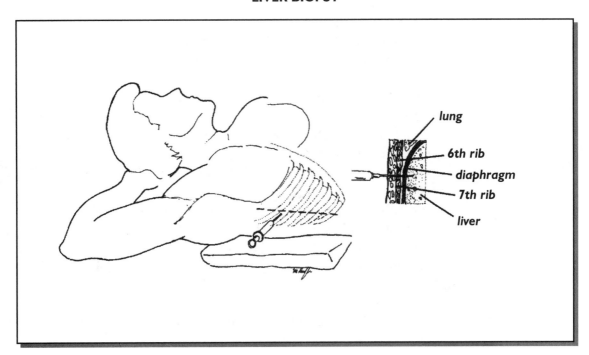

M. **Liver Function Tests**
   1. Pigment studies: assess bilirubin levels
   2. Dye clearance: assess liver's ability to detoxify substances
   3. Protein studies: assess synthesis of protein by the liver
   4. Alkaline phosphatase
      a. Enzyme found in liver tissue
      b. Released during liver damage
      c. Elevated in cardiac disorder, bone disease, biliary obstruction
   5. Prothrombin time
      a. Assess extrinsic clotting process
      b. Value is prolonged with liver damage
   6. Blood ammonia: assess liver's ability to deaminate protein byproducts
   7. Serum transaminase studies
      a. Elevated in liver disease
      b. Also elevated in heart disease and muscle trauma
      c. SGOT, SGPT, LDH, AST, ALT
   8. Cholesterol
      a. Produced by the liver
      b. Increased in bile duct obstruction
      c. Decreased with liver damage

Gastrointestinal Intubation

A. **Types**
   1. Levin (nasogastric tube): decompression of stomach
   2. Salem sump: for continuous suction
   3. Miller-Abbot: intestinal suction
   4. Harris: intestinal suction
   5. Cantor: intestinal suction
   6. Ewald: removal of secretions through the mouth
   7. Sengstaken-Blakemore: for treatment of esophageal varices

B. **Nasal Gastric Tube Feeding/Irrigation**
   1. **NURSING INTERVENTIONS**
      a. Assess placement before each feeding and every 4 hours with continuous feeding
      b. Semi-Fowler's position
      c. Check for residual
      d. Nose and mouth care
      e. Assess secretions
      f. Use correct solution for irrigation
      g. Hold for aspirates of >100cc, recheck in one hour
      h. Aspirated contents replaced to prevent metabolic acidosis

C. **Gastrostomy Tube**
   1. Anterior wall of the stomach is sutured to the abdominal wall and the tube is sutured in place; skin care is important

C. NURSING INTERVENTIONS
1. Relieve pain (meperidine *[Demerol]*)
2. Maintain fluid and electrolytes balance
3. Administer antibiotic, antiemetic
4. Maintain low-fat diet
5. Administration of bile acid (chenodeoxycholic acid)

D. Cholecystectomy: Postoperative
1. Nursing care same as any abdominal surgery
2. Penrose drain in gallbladder
3. T-tube to gravity after cholecystostomy and choledochostomy
   a. To prevent total loss of bile drainage, tube may be elevated above level of abdomen
   b. Use drains only if pressure develops in duct
   c. Clamp 1 hour ac and pc
   d. Discontinue in 7–14 days
4. Low-fat, high-carbohydrate and high-protein diet

Pancreatitis

A. Definition: inflammation brought about by the digestion of this organ by the very enzymes it produces

B. Manifestations
1. Extreme upper abdominal pain radiating into back
2. Persistent vomiting
3. Abdominal distention
4. Weight loss
5. Steatorrhea: bulky, pale, foul smelling stools
6. Elevated serum amylase

C. NURSING INTERVENTIONS
1. Assess for complications
2. Withhold oral intake, provide IV fluids
3. Administer anticholinergics, antacids, pancreatic extracts: pancrelipase *(Viokase)*
4. Provide meperidine *(Demerol)* for pain relief
5. Maintain low-fat diet; avoid alcohol and caffeine
6. Encourage fat soluble vitamins
7. Give fluid and electrolyte replacement

BILIARY SYSTEM

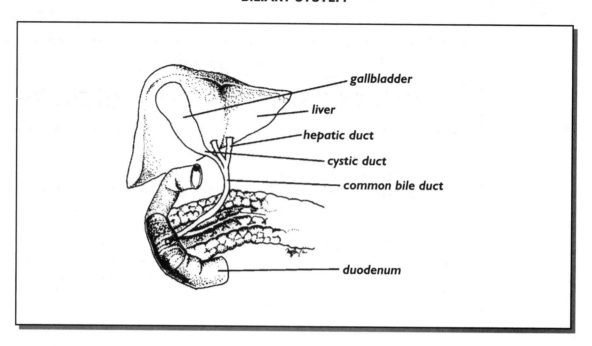

- gallbladder
- liver
- hepatic duct
- cystic duct
- common bile duct
- duodenum

TABLE II-8.
TYPES OF INTESTINAL OSTOMIES

	Ileostomy	Ileal Loop (Urinary Conduit)	Transverse Colostomy	Decending or Sigmoid Colostomy
Intestinal segment involved	End of ileum	Pouch is made from loop of ileum into which ureters are transplanted for urine drainage	Transverse colon	Descending or sigmoid colon
Consistency of excretion	Liquid	Urine only	Semiformed to soft	Formed
Appliance worn	Open-ended pouch, no appliance if Kock's (continent) ileostomy	Open-ended pouch	Open-ended pouch	If controlled, no appliance

REVIEW OF MUSCULOSKELETAL DISORDERS

Rheumatoid Arthritis and Osteoarthritis

TABLE II-9.
COMPARISON OF RHEUMATOID ARTHRITIS AND OSTEOARTHRITIS

	Rheumatoid Arthritis	**Osteoarthritis**
Onset:	20–50 years	Middle to older age
Sex:	Women 3:1	Women 20:1
Defined:	Chronic systemic disease of unknown cause, with recurrent inflammation involving the synovium or lining of the joints	Degeneration of the articular cartilage in the joints caused by prolonged wear and tear of joint surfaces
Joints involved:	Any finger joint, cervical, spine; systemic disease can involve heart, lung, etc.	Distal interphalangeal joints (Heberden's nodes); weight bearing joints: hips, knees, spine
Joints appearance:	Bilateral involvement; tenderness, swelling, warm, redness, subcutaneous nodules; every bone prominence; remission and exacerbation; increased symptoms in morning, decreasing with moderate activity	Normal on exam; grating (crepitus) during movement; pain and stiffness worsen after inactivity or after exercise
Other symptoms:	Low-grade temperature, malaise, fatigue stiffness	
Treatment:	Rest with joints extended; emotional support, heat: warm baths, paraffin baths; daily exercise program; drugs: ASA, NSAIDs, Phenylbutazone *(Butazolidin)*, gold salts *(Myochrysine)*, steroids (P.O. or into joints); other rheumatoid drugs not effective	Normal amount of rest; rest affected joint; avoid over-activity, emotional support; heat: hot packs, warm soaks, paraffin baths exercise: ROM; drugs: ASA, steriods in joints only; phenylbutazone *(Butazolidin)*, indomethacin *(Indocin)*;
Nursing interventions:	Position joints in extension; maintain body alignment; balance rest with exercise; nutritious diet	

Fractures

A. **Definition:** break in the continuity of bone

B. **First Aid**
1. Maintain airway
2. Prevent shock
3. Splint limb
4. Monitor for fat embolism 12–72 hours after long bone fractures

C. **Traction**
1. Types
   a. Skin
      1) Buck's extension
      2) Pelvic
   b. Skeletal
      1) Thomas splint with Pearson attachment
      2) Crutchfield tongs

2. **NURSING INTERVENTIONS**
   a. Skin
      1) Detection of pressure points
      2) Provide daily rewrapping
      3) Maintain positioning
      4) Maintain weights hanging freely
      5) Maintain countertraction
      6) Monitor for vascular occlusion
   b. Skeletal
      1) Inspection
         a) Dressing
         b) Traction apparatus (maintain alignment)
         c) Skin
      2) Prevent complications of bed rest
   c. Muscles
      1) Strengthening exercises for upper extremities
      2) Strengthening exercises for lower extremities
      3) Preparation for crutch walking
   d. Vascular occlusion (the five P's)
      1) Pain
      2) Pallor
      3) Pulselessness
      4) Paresthesia
      5) Paralysis

D. Casts

    1. Applied to maintain immobilization while the fracture heals

    2. **NURSING INTERVENTIONS**

        a. Handle wet cast with palms of hands, not fingers

        b. Cast should be allowed to air dry

        c. Elevate the cast on one to two pillows during drying

        d. Adhesive tape petals reduce irritation at cast edges

        e. Assess for vascular occlusion

        f. Prevent complications of immobility

E. Hip Fractures

    1. Classification

        a. Fracture of the neck of femur (intracapsular)

        b. Fracture of trochanteric region of femur (extracapsular)

        c. Subtrochanteric fracture

    2. Treatment

        a. Skin traction for immobilization (preop)

        b. Trochanter roll

        c. Open reduction and internal fixation

        d. Total hip replacement (THR)

    3. **NURSING INTERVENTIONS**

        a. Preoperative care

            1) Immobilization

            2) Anticoagulation therapy

            3) Assess for complications

                a) Skin breakdowns

                b) Thromboembolisms

                c) Respiratory congestion

                d) Senile dementia

        b. Postoperative care

            1) Turning and positioning

            2) Exercise

            3) Observation for complications

                a) Thromboembolisms

                b) Pneumonia

                c) Fat embolism

            4) Crutch walking

                a) Measure for crutches in walking shoes

                b) Avoid leaning on crutches

                c) Good leg first going upstairs, "bad" leg first when going down

            5) THR postoperative care

                a) Avoid adduction, flexion, and external rotation

                b) Abductor pillow

                c) Drain/dressing care

F. **Pelvic Fractures**

1. **NURSING INTERVENTIONS**
   a. Major assessments
      1) Bladder injuries
      2) Bowel injuries
      3) Bleeding
   b. Immobilization
      1) Bed rest
      2) Pelvic sling

Amputation

A. **Preoperative Care**
   1. Psychological adjustment
   2. Physical
      a. Assessment
         1) Circulation
         2) Infection
         3) Nutritional status
      b. Physical conditioning

B. **Surgical Approaches**
   1. Closed
   2. Opened
   3. Immediate post-surgical prosthesis
      a. Improved position sense
      b. Early ambulation

C. **Postoperative Care**
   1. Positioning
      a. Extended position
      b. Elevated
   2. Complications
      a. Hemorrhage
      b. Infection
      c. Phantom limb

D. **Rehabilitation**
   1. Major problems
      a. Flexion deformities
      b. Nonshrinkage of stump
      c. Abduction deformities of hip
   2. Exercise
      a. Stretching of flexor muscles
      b. ROM

3. Stump conditioning (see illustration below)
    a. Stump shrinking
    b. Stump "toughening"

Gout

A. Definition: inflammatory type of arthritis caused by deposits of urate crystals in and around the joints; there is an hereditary error in purine metabolism that results in excessive uric acid production

B. Manifestations
  1. Severe pain, usually in great toe
  2. Monarticular or polyarticular
  3. Large accumulations of crystals in the joints (tophi)
  4. Joints are red, warm, painful, and swollen
  5. Joint damage and deformity increase with each attack
  6. Hyperuricemia

C. Treatment
  1. Indomethacin *(Indocin)*
  2. Probenecid *(Benemid)*
  3. Allopurinol *(Zyloprim)*

  4. **NURSING INTERVENTIONS**
    a. Bed rest during acute attacks
    b. Keep covers away from affected joints
    c. Applications of heat or cold
    d. Fluid intake
    e. Limit intake of high purine foods (glandular and red meats)
    f. Limit alcohol intake

DRESSING A STUMP

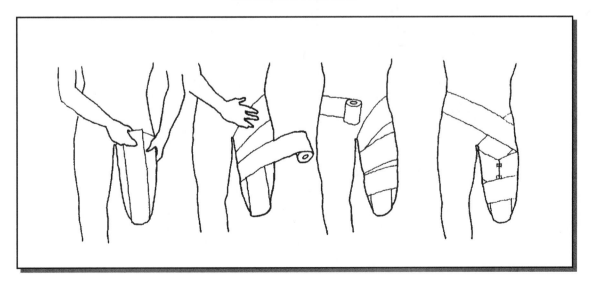

Systemic Lupus Erythematosus

A. Definition: chronic inflammatory disease that involves the vascular and connective tissue of multiple organs; cause is unknown, may be autoimmune

B. Manifestations
1. Insidious onset
2. Characterized by remissions and exacerbations
3. Erythematous "butterfly rash" on both cheeks and across the bridge of the nose; rash worsens on exposure to sunlight
4. Polyarthralgia
5. Normochromic, normocytic anemias
6. Fever, malaise, weight loss
7. Positive for antinuclear antibodies (ANA)
8. Raynaud's phenomenon

C. NURSING INTERVENTIONS
1. Supportive, depends on organs involved
2. Teaching
    a. Avoid the sun (wear large brimmed hats, sunscreen)
    b. Avoid stressful situations
    c. Adequate rest, exercise
    d. Regular, nutritious meals
    e. Follow treatment regimen
    f. Oral contraceptives can precipitate an acute exacerbation
    g. No intrauterine devices
    h. Salicylates, NSAIDs, steroids

KEY INFORMATION

NOTE: Lupus nephritis occurs early in the disease
    1) Manifestations
        a) Microscopic hematuria
        b) Proteinuria
        c) Red cell casts
    2) Treatment
        a) Symptomatic
        b) Salicylates, steroids
        c) Dialysis
    3) Prognosis: variable

SECTION VI

REVIEW OF ENDOCRINE SYSTEM FUNCTIONS AND DISORDERS

Pituitary Gland

TABLE II-10.
PITUITARY GLAND: HORMONES PRODUCED AND FUNCTIONS

Endocrine Gland	Hormones Produced	Function
Pituitary gland		Controlled primarily by the hypothalamus; termed "master gland" as it directly affects the function of other endocrine glands
Anterior lobe	Adrenocorticotropic hormone (ACTH)	Concerned with growth and secretory activity of adrenal cortex, which produces steroids
	Thyrotropic hormone (TSH)	For growth and secretory activity of thyroid; controls release rate of thyroxine, which controls rate of most chemical reactions in the body; target is thyroid gland
	Somatotropic hormones (STH or GH)	Promote growth of body tissue
	Gonadotropic hormones and estrogen secretion; stimulates	Stimulate development of ovarian follicles
(FHS)		seminiferous tubules and sperm maturation
	Luteinizing hormone (LH)	Works with FSH in final maturation of follicles; promotes ovulation and progesterone secretion
	Prolactin secretion	Maintains corpus luteum and progesterone
	Melanocyte stimulating hormone (MSH)	Produces the characteristic skin darkening
Posterior lobe	Vasopressin (ADH)	Influences water absorption by kidney
	Oxytocin	Influences the menstrual cycle, labor and lactation

Endocrine System Disorders

A. **Disorders of Anterior Pituitary**
1. Acromegaly (see illustration below)
   a. Definition: hypersecretion of GH that occurs in adulthood; commonly associated with benign pituitary tumors
   b. Manifestations
      1) Enlargement of skeletal extremities (e.g., nose, jaw, hands, feet)
      2) Protrusion of the jaw and orbital ridges
      3) Course features
      4) Visual problems, blindness
      5) Hyperglycemia, insulin resistance
      6) Hypercalcemia
   c. Treatment
      1) Irradiation of pituitary
      2) Transphenoidal hypophysectomy: removal of pituitary gland
         a) Assess for signs of increased cranial pressure—signs of adrenal insufficiency, hypothyroidism, and temporary diabetes insipidus
         b) Elevate head of bed 30 degrees
         c) Avoid coughing, sneezing, blowing nose
      3) Bromocriptine *(Parlodel)* with surgery or radiation

   d. **NURSING INTERVENTIONS**
      1) Provide emotional support
      2) Directed toward symptomatic care

ACROMEGALY

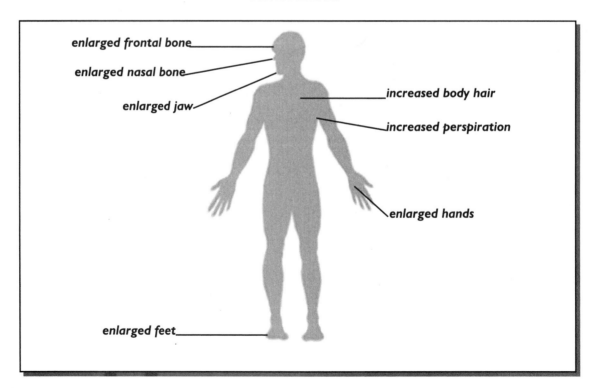

enlarged frontal bone

enlarged nasal bone

enlarged jaw

increased body hair

increased perspiration

enlarged hands

enlarged feet

2. Gigantism
   a. Definition: hypersecretion of GH that occurs in childhood
   b. Manifestations
      1) Proportional overgrowth in all body tissue
      2) Overgrowth of long bones—height in childhood may reach 8 or 9 feet
   c. Treatment (see acromegaly)
   d. Nursing responsibilities (see acromegaly)
3. Dwarfism
   a. Definition: hyposecretion of GH during childhood
   b. Manifestations
      1) Retarded symmetrical physical growth
      2) Premature body aging processes
      3) Slow intellectual development
   c. Treatment
      1) Removal of the causative factor, e.g., tumors
      2) Human growth hormone injections (HGH)
   d. Nursing responsibilities (see acromegaly)

B. Disorder of Posterior Pituitary
   1. Diabetes insipidus
      a. Definition: hyposecretion of ADH, due to a tumor or damage of the posterior lobe of the pituitary; may be idiopathic; may be genetic
      b. Manifestations
         1) Polyuria/polydipsia
         2) Dehydration
      c. Treatment
         1) Desmopressin acetate *(DDAVP)* nasal spray
         2) Vasopressin tannate *(Pitressin Tannate)* in Oil (IM for chronic severe cases)
         3) Lypressin *(Diapid)* nasal spray

      d. **NURSING INTERVENTIONS**
         1) Maintain adequate fluids
         2) Avoid foods with diuretic-type action
         3) Monitor intake and output
         4) Teach self-injection techniques
         5) Daily weights
         6) Specific gravity
   2. Syndrome of inappropriate secretion of antidiuretic hormone (SIADH)
      a. Definition: inappropriate, continued release of antidiuretic hormone resulting in water intoxication; caused by neoplastic tumors, respiratory disorders, drugs

b. Manifestations
   1) Hyponatremia
   2) Mental confusion
   3) Personality changes
   4) Lethargy
   5) Weakness
   6) Headache
   7) Weight gain
   8) Abdominal cramping
   9) Anorexia, nausea
   10) Vomiting
c. Treatment
   1) Fluid restriction (less than 500 cc/24 hours)
   2) Treat underlying cause (surgery, radiation, chemotherapy)
   3) Demeclocycline HCL *(Declomycin)*
   4) Lithium carbonate *(Lithium Citrate)*
   5) Butorphanol tartrate *(Stadol)*

Adrenal Gland

TABLE II-11.
ADRENAL GLAND: HORMONES PRODUCED AND FUNCTIONS

Hormone Produced	Function
Cortex:	

Glucocorticoids
    Cortisol
    Cortisone
    Corticosterone
	Affect carbohydrate, fat, and protein metabolism; affect stress reactions and the inhibition of the inflammatory process

Mineralocorticoids
    Aldosterone
    Corticosterone
    Deoxycorticosterone
	Regulate sodium and electrolyte balance

Sex Hormones
    Androgens
    Estrogens
	Influence the development of sexual characteristics

Medulla:	
Epinephrine Norepinephrine	Stimulate "fight or flight" response to danger

A. Disorders of Adrenal Cortex

1. Addison's disease

    a. Definition: hyposecretion of adrenal cortex hormones, (insufficency of cortisol, aldosterone and androgens)

    b. Manifestations

        1) Slow, insidious onset

        2) Malaise and generalized weakness

        3) Hypotension, hypovolemia

        4) Increase pigmentation of the skin

        5) Anorexia, nausea, vomiting

        6) Electrolyte imbalance (hyponatremia, hyperkalemia)

        7) Weight loss

        8) Loss of libido

        9) Hypoglycemia

        10) Personality changes

    c. Treatment

        1) Lifelong steroid replacement: hydrocortisone *(Florinef)*

        2) High-protein, high-carbohydrate diet, may increase Na$^+$ intake

    d. **NURSING INTERVENTIONS**

        1) Observe for addisonian crisis secondary to stress caused by infection, trauma, surgery

        2) Observe for side effects of hormone replacement

        3) Provide emotional support

        4) Teaching (lifelong medications, prompt treatment of infection, illness, stress management)

        5) Monitor fluid and electrolyte balance

2. Cushing's syndrome (see illustration, p. 66)

    a. Definition: hypersecretion of the glucocorticoids

    b. Manifestations

        1) Central-type obesity, moon face, buffalo hump and obese trunk with thin extremities

        2) Mood swings

        3) Malaise and muscular weakness

        4) Masculine characteristics in females (hirsutism)

        5) Hypokalemia

        6) Hyperglycemia

        7) Hypertension

        8) Acne

        9) Amenorrhea

        10) Osteoporosis

    c. Treatment

        1) Adrenalectomy: unilateral or bilateral

        2) Chemotherapy: bromocriptine *(Parlodel)*

        3) High-protein, low-carbohydrate, low-sodium diet with potassium supplement

d. **NURSING INTERVENTIONS**
   1) Protect from infection
   2) Protect from accidents
   3) Client education concerning self-administration of hormone replacement

e. Steroid replacement
   1) Purpose
      a) Anti-inflammatory and antiallergy reaction
      b) Enables one to tolerate high degree of stress
   2) Used in
      a) Crisis (e.g., shock, bronchial obstruction)
      b) Long-term therapy (e.g., post-adrenalectomy, arthritis, leukemia)
   3) Side effects due to prolonged use
      a) Moon face
      b) Abnormal distribution of body fat, weight gain
      c) Causes peptic ulcers, hyperglycemia and osteoporosis
      d) Mass infections
      e) Euphoric effect
   4) Dosage schedule
      a) Large dosages should be given at 8:00 a.m. (2/3 morning, 1/3 night)
      b) Should be taken same time every day
      c) Withdraw steroids by tapered dosages
      d) Can be given with antacids to minimize GI upset and ulceration

CUSHING'S SYNDROME

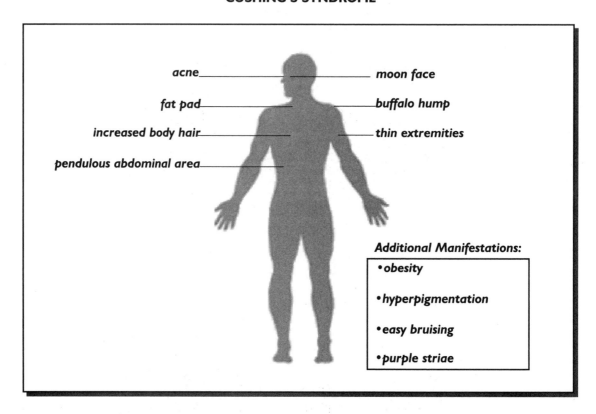

acne   moon face

fat pad   buffalo hump

increased body hair   thin extremities

pendulous abdominal area

Additional Manifestations:
- *obesity*
- *hyperpigmentation*
- *easy bruising*
- *purple striae*

3. Aldosteronism (Conn's syndrome)
    a. Definition: hypersecretion of aldosterone from adrenal cortex
    b. Manifestations
        1) Hypokalemia
        2) Hypertension
    c. Treatment
        1) Surgical removal of tumors
        2) Potassium replacement
        3) Anti-hypertensive drugs

    d. **NURSING INTERVENTIONS**
        1) Provide quiet environment
        2) Monitor BP

B. Disorders of Adrenal Medulla
1. Pheochromocytoma
    a. Definition: hypersecretion of the hormones of adrenal medulla
    b. Manifestations
        1) Hypertension
        2) Sudden attacks resemble manifestatinos of over-stimulation of sympathetic nervous system
            a) Sweating
            b) Apprehension
            c) Palpitations
            d) Nausea
            e) Vomiting
            f) Orthostatic hypotension
            g) Headache
            h) Tachycardia
        3) Hyperglycemia
    c. Treatment
        1) Surgical excision of tumor
        2) Symptomatic if surgery not feasible

    d. **NURSING INTERVENTIONS**
        1) Provide high-calorie, nutritious diet
        2) Promote rest
        3) Preoperative: control hypertension

Thyroid Gland

TABLE II-12.
THYROID GLAND: HORMONES PRODUCED AND FUNCTIONS

Hormones Produced	Function
Thyroxine (T4)	Acts as a catalyst; influences metabolic rate, growth and development
Triiodothyronine (T3)	Controls rate of body metabolism, growth, and nutrition
Thyrocalcitonin	Assists in control of calcium levels; decreases reabsorption of bone

A. **Disorders of Thyroid Gland**
   1. Cretinism
      a. Definition: hyposecretion of the thyroid hormones in the fetus or soon after birth
      b. Manifestations
         1) Severe physical and mental retardation
         2) Dry skin, coarse dry hair
         3) Constipation
         4) Poor appetite
         5) Sensitivity to cold
      c. Treatment
         1) Hormone drug replacement
   2. Myxedema
      a. Definition: hyposecretion of thyroid hormone in adulthood
      b. Manifestations
         1) Slow rate of body metabolism
         2) Personality changes (depression)
         3) Anorexia and constipation
         4) Intolerance to cold
         5) Decreased sweating
         6) Hypersensitivity to barbiturates and narcotics
         7) Generalized interstitial edema
         8) Coarse, dry skin
         9) Generalized weakness
         10) Goiter
         11) Weight gain
         12) Puffy appearance
      c. Treatment
         1) Levothyroxine *(Synthroid)*
         2) Desiccated thyroid *(Thyrar)*
            a) Thyroid replacement hormones should be taken on an empty stomach
            b) Monitor heart rate: fewer than 100 beats per minute is desirable

d. **NURSING INTERVENTIONS**
   1) Directed toward manifestations of decreased metabolism
      a) Provide warm environment
      b) Low-calorie, low-cholesterol, low-saturated-fat diet
      c) Increase roughage
      d) Promote fluids
      e) Avoid sedatives
      f) Plan rest periods
   2) Observe for overdosage manifestations of thyroid preparations (tachycardia, nervousness)
   3) Assess for effectiveness of drug therapy
   4) Teaching

3. Hyperthyroidism (Graves' disease, diffuse toxic goiter)
   a. Definition: hypersecretion of thyroid hormone
   b. Manifestations
      1) Increased rate of body metabolism
      2) Personality changes
      3) Enlargement of the thyroid gland
      4) Exophthalmos
      5) Cardiac arrhythmias
      6) Increased appetite
      7) Weight loss
      8) Diarrhea
      9) Heat intolerance
      10) Diaphoresis
      11) Easy fatigability
      12) Muscle weakness
      13) Hypertension
      14) Anxiety
      15) Insomnia
   c. Treatment
      1) Drug therapy
         a) Methimazole *(Tapazole):* blocks thyroid hormone production
         b) Propylthiouracil *(Propyl-Thyracil):* blocks thyroid hormone production
         c) Iodides: decrease vascularity; inhibit release of thyroid hormones
            (1) Lugol's solution
            (2) Saturated solution of potassium iodide (SSKI)
         d) Propranolol *(Inderal):* relief of tachycardia, palpitations
      2) Radioiodine therapy: slowly destroys hyper-functioning thyroid tissue
      3) Thyroidectomy: subtotal or total

d. **NURSING INTERVENTIONS**
   1) Provide adequate rest
   2) Provide cool, quiet environment
   3) Provide high caloric, protein, carbohydrate, vitamin diet without stimulants, extra fluids
   4) Weigh client daily
   5) Provide emotional support
   6) Provide eye protection: ophthalmic medicine, tape eyes at night
   7) Elevate head of bed
   8) Be alert for complications
      a) Corneal abrasion
      b) Heart disease
      c) Thyroid storm

e. Thyroidectomy
   1) Definition: removal of the thyroid gland, either total or partial
   2) Preoperative goals (see illustration, p. 63)
      a) Thyroid function in normal range: Lugol's solution, saturated solution of potassium iodide (SSKI)
      b) Signs of thyrotoxicosis are diminished
      c) Weight and nutritional status normal

   3) **NURSING INTERVENTIONS** (postoperative care)
      a) Semi-Fowler's position
      b) Check dressing: especially back of neck
      c) Observe for respiratory distress: tracheostomy tray, oxygen, and suction apparatus at bedside
      d) Be alert for signs of hemorrhage
      e) Talking limited, note any hoarseness; may indicate injury to laryngeal nerve
      f) Observe for signs of tetany: Chvostek's sign and Trousseau's sign
      g) Calcium gluconate IV at bedside
      h) Observe for thyroid storm (life threatening)
         (1) Fever
         (2) Tachycardia
         (3) Delirium
         (4) Irritability
      i) Gradually increase range of motion to neck

Parathyroid Gland

TABLE II-13.
PARATHYROID GLAND: HORMONES PRODUCED AND FUNCTIONS

Hormones Produced	Function
Parathyroid hormone (PTH)	Controls calcium and phosphate metabolism

A. Disorders of Parathyroid Gland

1. Hypoparathyroidism
   a. Definition: hyposecretion of the parathyroid hormone
   b. Manifestations
      1) Acute: increased neuromuscular irritability
      2) Chronic
         a) Poor development of tooth enamel
         b) Lethargic
         c) Mental retardation
   c. Treatment
      1) Acute: IV calcium gluconate
      2) Chronic
         a) Oral calcium salts
         b) Vitamin D
         c) High-calcium, low-phosphorous diet

   d. **NURSING INTERVENTIONS**
      1) Provide quiet room, no stimulus
      2) Assess for increased signs of neuromuscular irritability

2. Hyperparathyroidism
   a. Definition: hypersecretion of parathyroid hormone
   b. Manifestations
      1) Bone deformities, susceptible to fractures
      2) Calcium deposits in various body organs
      3) Gastric ulcers and GI disturbances
      4) Apathy, fatigue, weakness
      5) Nausea, vomiting
      6) Constipation
   c. Treatment
      1) Subtotal surgical resection of parathyroid gland

   d. **NURSING INTERVENTIONS**
      1) Force fluids
      2) Provide a low-calcium diet
      3) Prevent constipation and fecal impaction
      4) Strain all urine

Pancreas

TABLE II-14.
PANCREAS: HORMONES PRODUCED AND FUNCTIONS

Hormones Produced	Functions
Insulin	Decreases blood sugar by:
	• Stimulating active transport of glucose into muscle and adipose tissue
	• Promoting the conversion of glucose to glycogen for storage
	• Promoting conversion of fatty acids into fat
	• Stimulating protein synthesis
Glucagon	Increases blood sugar by promoting conversion of glycogen to glucose

A. **Disorder of the Pancreas**
　1. Diabetes mellitus
　　a. Definition: chronic disorder of carbohydrate metabolism characterized by an imbalance between insulin supply and demand; either a subnormal amount of insulin is produced or the body requires abnormally high amounts
　　　1) IDDM: insulin dependent diabetes mellitus (Type I)
　　　2) NIDDM: non-insulin dependent diabetes mellitus (Type II)
　　b. Manifestations
　　　1) Polyuria
　　　2) Polydipsia
　　　3) Weight loss
　　　4) Polyphagia

　　c. **NURSING INTERVENTIONS**
　　　1) Administer insulin therapy

	ONSET	PEAK	DURATION
Rapid acting: Regular *(Semilente)*	1/2–1 hr	2–4 hrs	6–8 hrs
Intermediate: *(NPH, Lente)*	1–2 hrs	7–12 hrs	24–30 hrs
Long acting: Protamine Zinc *(Ultralente)*	4–6 hrs	18+ hrs	30–36 hrs
Mixing insulins: draw up regular first, then NPH			

2) Administer hypoglycemics
   a) Tolbutamide *(Orinase)*
   b) Chlorpropamide *(Diabinase)*
   c) Glyburide *(Micronase)*
3) Maintain diet therapy
   a) Goal is to provide the body with adequate nutrients for cell growth and function
   b) Caloric requirements prescribed by physician
4) Monitor for complications
   a) Hypoglycemia
      (1) Causes: decreased dietary intake, excess insulin
      (2) Manifestations
         (a) Tachycardia
         (b) Diaphoresis
         (c) Tremors
         (d) Weakness, fatigue
         (e) Irritability, anxiety
         (f) Confusion
      (3) **NURSING INTERVENTIONS**
         (a) Give hard candy
         (b) Apple juice
         (c) Soft drinks
         (d) Follow with meal or carbohydrates within 1/2 hour
   b) Ketoacidosis (hyperglycemia)
      (1) Causes: lack of insulin; infection, stress
      (2) Manifestations
         (a) Three P's (polyuria, polydipsia, polyphagia)
         (b) Nausea
         (c) Vomiting
         (d) Dry mucous membranes
         (e) Kussmaul respirations
         (f) Coma
      (3) **NURSING INTERVENTION:** give regular insulin
   c) Lipodystrophy: indurated areas of subcutaneous tissue secondary to injecting cold insulin or not rotating sites
   d) Hyperglycemic hyperosmolar nonketotic coma (HHNK)
      (1) Extremely high glucose levels
      (2) No ketosis
5) Insulin pump
   a) External device that provides a basal dose of regular insulin with a bolus dose before meals
   b) Needles are inserted into subcutaneous abdominal tissue (changed q 48h)
   c) Complications
      (1) Insulin overdosage
      (2) Continued insulin injections during hypoglycemia

6) Health teaching
   a) Foot care: daily cleanse feet in warm soapy water; rinse and dry carefully; inspect, don't break blisters; trim nails to follow natural curve of toe; always wear shoes
   b) Injection techniques (intrasite rotation)
   c) Dietary management
   d) Quit smoking
   e) Complications

THYROID GLAND

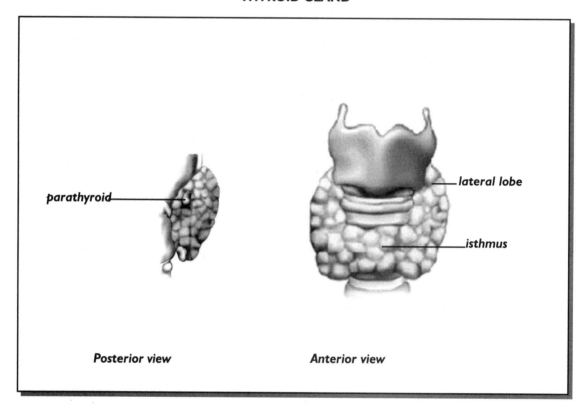

parathyroid

lateral lobe

isthmus

Posterior view   *Anterior view*

SECTION VII

REVIEW OF BLOOD DISORDERS

Anemia

A. Definition: a deficiency of red blood cells that is characterized by a decreased red blood cell count and a below-normal hemoglobin and hematocrit

Normal values:	RBC: female 4.2–5.4 million per cu. mm; male 4.6–6.2
	Hgb: female 12–16 gm/dl, male 13–18
	Hct: female 37%–48%, male 45%–52%
	WBC: 4.5–11/cu mm

B. Causes
1. Acute or chronic blood loss
2. Greater than normal destruction of red blood cells
3. Abnormal bone marrow function
4. Decreased erythropoietin
5. Inadequate maturation of red blood cells

C. Manifestations
1. Fatigue
2. Weakness
3. Dizziness
4. Pallor
5. Decreased Hgb, Hct, RBC

D. Classifications
1. Hypoproliferation anemia bone marrow is unable to produce adequate numbers of cells
   a. Anemia secondary to renal disease (lack of erythropoietin)
   b. Iron deficiency anemia
      1) Due to chronic blood loss (e.g., bleeding ulcer)
      2) Due to nutritional deficiency
      3) Common in young adult women, older adults
   c. Aplastic anemia
      1) Lack of precursor cells in the bone marrow with a decrease in all blood producing cells (WBC: leukopenia; platelet: thrombocytopenia) due to drugs, virus, toxins, irradiation

2) Manifestations
   a) Hypoxia
   b) Increased susceptibility to infection
   c) Hemorrhage, ecchymosis
   d) Fatigue

3) **NURSING INTERVENTIONS**
   a) Protective isolation
   b) Psychological support
   c) Monitor for manifestations of infection

4) Medical therapy
   a) Remove cause
   b) Steroids
   c) Splenectomy
   d) Transfusions
   e) Antibiotics
   f) Bone narrow transplant

2. Megaloblastic anemia
  a. Pernicious anemia: a vitamin B_{12} deficiency due to a lack of the intrinsic factor in the gastric juice

KEY INFORMATION

B_{12} combines with intrinsic factor for absorption in the small intestine

  b. Causes
   1) Atrophy of the gastric mucosa
   2) Total gastrectomy
   3) Malabsorption (secondary to Crohn's disease, pancreatitis)
  c. Manifestations
   1) Numbness, tingling of extremities
   2) Paresthesia
   3) Gait disturbances
   4) Behavioral problems

  d. **NURSING INTERVENTIONS**
   1) Protect lower extremities, bed cradle
   2) Rest in quiet, non-stimulating environment
   3) Patience, teach family
   4) Assist with Schilling's test
   5) B_{12} three times a week for two week; two times a week for two weeks; then once a month

KEY INFORMATION

B_{12} is important for RNA production, which is necessary for maintenance of CNS integrity

3. Hemolytic anemia
   a. Sickle cell anemia: defective hemoglobin molecule that assumes a sickle shape when oxygen in venous blood is low; the sickled cells become lodged in the blood vessels (see illustration below)
   b. Manifestations
      1) Severe pain
      2) Swelling
      3) Fever
      4) Jaundice
      5) Susceptibility to infection
      6) Hypoxic damage to organs

   c. **NURSING INTERVENTIONS** (symptomatic)
      1) Refer for genetic counseling
      2) Hydration
      3) Oxygen
      4) Analgesics
      5) Rest

SICKLE CELL ANEMIA

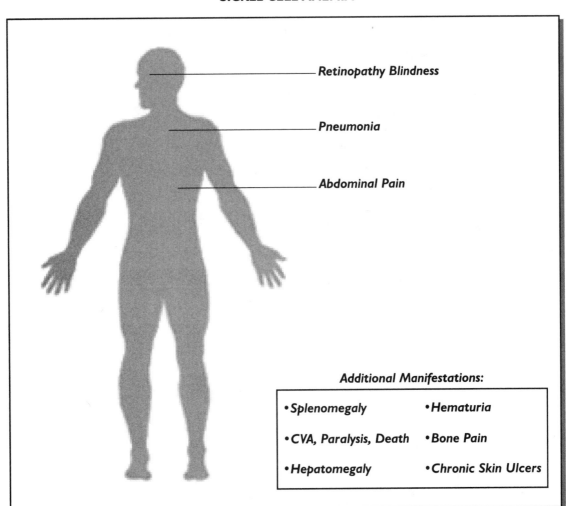

Retinopathy Blindness

Pneumonia

Abdominal Pain

Additional Manifestations:

• Splenomegaly	• Hematuria
• CVA, Paralysis, Death	• Bone Pain
• Hepatomegaly	• Chronic Skin Ulcers

Administration of Iron Preparations

A. Oral
1. Dilute liquid preparations in juice or water and administer with a plastic straw to avoid staining teeth
2. Orange juice facilitates absorption
3. Monitor for constipation, GI upset

B. Intramuscular
1. Use large bore needle (19 gauge)
2. Z-track
3. Do not massage

Blood Transfusions

A. Equipment
1. Y-type tubing with filter
2. Normal saline
3. Blood

B. NURSING INTERVENTIONS
1. Check ID, name, blood type
2. Take baseline vital signs
3. Monitor for transfusion reaction
   a. Allergic (pruritus, respiratory distress, urticaria)
   b. Hemolytic (low back pain, fever, chills)
4. Treat transfusion reaction
   a. Stop blood
   b. Start saline
   c. Take vital signs
   d. Notify physician

SECTION VIII
REVIEW OF CARDIOVASCULAR SYSTEM DISORDERS

Cardiovascular System in Failure

A. Deficits Present in at Least One Area:
1. Adequately pump blood to all parts of the body, thus good working cardiac muscles and conduction system
2. Good circulating blood volume to meet body's needs
3. Peripheral vascular resistance must be sufficient to maintain adequate blood pressure
4. Normal heart rate 60–90 beats per minute

Diagnostic Procedures

A. Laboratory Tests
1. Blood electrolytes (see Table II-1.)
2. Sedimentation rate (0–30)
3. Blood coagulation test
   a. PTT (16–40 seconds)
   b. PT (9–12 seconds); INR
   c. Clotting time (10 min.)
4. BUN (6–20 mg/dl)
5. Serum cholesterol (150–250 mg/dl)
6. Triglycerides 50–250 mg/dl
   a. LDL cholesterol 73–20 mg/dl
   b. HDL cholesterol 32–75mg/dl
7. Blood cultures
8. Enzymes
   a. CPK: men: 55–170; women: 30–135; increase 3–6 hours after MI
   b. LDH: 150–450 u/ml; rises 12 hours after MI
   c. SGOT: 5–40 u/ml

B. Central Venous Pressure (5–10 cm Water)
1. Provides an indication of pressure in the right atrium
2. Trends are more important than values

C. Electrocardiogram (ECG)

1. Interpretation
   a. P wave: atrial depolarization
   b. QRS complex: ventricular depolarization
   c. T wave: ventricular repolarization
   d. PR interval: 0.12–.20 seconds
   e. QRS: .08–.10 seconds

D. Arteriography

1. Definition: injection of contrast medium into the vascular system to outline the heart and blood vessels; usually done with cardiac catheterization
2. Purpose: obtain information regarding coronary anatomy, structural abnormalities of the coronary artery

3. **NURSING INTERVENTIONS**
   a. Before angiogram, keep client NPO, obtain consent, explain, check for iodine allergy
   b. After angiogram
      1) Vital signs q 15 minutes till stable
      2) Check for bleeding at puncture sites
      3) Check distal extremity for color, pulse, temperature, sensation

E. Cardiac Catheterization

1. Definition: a diagnostic procedure; catheter is introduced into the right or left side of the heart
2. Purpose
   a. Measure oxygen concentration, saturation, tension and pressure in various chambers of the heart
   b. Detect shunts
   c. Provide blood samples
   d. Determine cardiac output and pulmonary blood flow
   e. Determine need for cardiac bypass surgery

3. **NURSING INTERVENTIONS**
   a. Before
      1) Know approach: right (venous) or left (arterial)
      2) NPO for 6 hours, consent
      3) Mark distal pulses
      4) Explain procedure to client
      5) Assess allergy to dye
   b. After
      1) Blood pressure and apical pulse q 15 minutes for 2–4 hours
      2) Check peripheral pulses q 15 minutes for 2–4 hours
      3) Check puncture sites for bleeding
      4) Assess for chest pain
      5) Keep extremity extended 4–6 hours
      6) Assess for impaired circulation
      7) Assess femerol site after 6–8 hours bed rest

Disorders

A. Angina

1. Definition: insufficient coronary blood flow, thus inadequate oxygen supply causing intermittent chest pain
2. Manifestations
   a. Location
   b. Character
   c. Duration
   d. Precipitating events

3. **NURSING INTERVENTIONS**
   a. Assess pain
      1) Location
      2) Character
      3) Duration
      4) Precipitating factors
   b. Help client to adjust living style to prevent episode of angina
      1) Avoid excessive activity in cold weather
      2) Avoid overeating
      3) Avoid constipation
      4) Rest after meals
      5) Exercise
   c. Teach client how to cope with an attack: use of nitroglycerin (peripheral vasodilation decreases myocardial oxygen demand; coronary artery vasodilation increases supply of oxygen to myocardium)
      1) When to take
      2) How often
      3) Storage
      4) Side effects
      5) Types: tablets, ointment, patch, spray

B. Myocardial Infarction

1. Definition: process by which myocardium tissue is destroyed due to reduced coronary blood flow
2. Causes
   a. Atherosclerotic heart disease
   b. Coronary artery embolism
3. Manifestations
   a. Heavy (viselike, crushing, squeezing) chest pain that may radiate down left arm, hand, jaw, neck; not relieved by rest, often lasts longer than 15 minutes
   b. Nausea, vomiting
   c. Diaphoresis, dizziness
   d. Drop in blood pressure
   e. ECG changes: inverted T wave, depressed ST segment, ischemic changes, elevated ST segment, infarction
   f. Denial
   g. Increased CPK, LDH isoenzymes

4. **NURSING INTERVENTIONS**
   a. Early
      1) Treat arrhythmias promptly: lidocaine
      2) Give analgesics: morphine
      3) Provide physical rest
      4) Administer oxygen via cannula
      5) Frequent vital signs
      6) Nifedipine *(Procardia)*
      7) Propranolol HCl *(Inderal)*
      8) Emotional support
      9) Nitroglycerine IV
      10) Streptokinase *(Kabikinase)* or tPA ("clot busters") if patient arrives within first 6 hours
   b. Later
      1) Give stool softeners
      2) Provide low-fat, low-cholesterol, low-sodium diet, soft food
      3) Commode
      4) Self-care
      5) Plan for rehabilitation
         a) Exercise program
         b) Stress management
         c) Teach risk factors
            (1) Heredity
            (2) Race
            (3) Age
            (4) Sex
            (5) Obesity
            (6) Stress
            (7) Diet
            (8) Hypertension
            (9) Smoking
            (10) Lack of exercise
            (11) Type A personality
         d) Psychological support
         e) Long-term drug therapy
            (1) Antiarrhythmics: quinidine *(Quinora)*, lidocaine *(Xylocaine)*
            (2) Anticoagulants: heparin *(Hep-Lock)*, aspirin
            (3) Antihypertensives: propranolol *(Inderal)*, chlorathiazide *(Diuril)*

C. Congestive Heart Failure

1. Definition: inability of the heart to meet tissue requirements for oxygen
2. Left ventricular failure: usually appears before right heart failure; inadequate ejection of blood into the systemic circulation, usually associated with MI, hypertension
   a. Manifestations (left sided usually respiratory symptoms)
      1) Dyspnea
      2) Moist cough
      3) Rales, wheezing
      4) Orthopnea
   b. Pulmonary edema results, causing excessive quantity of fluid in pulmonary interstitial spaces or alveoli evidenced by:
      1) Moist rales, frothy sputum
      2) Severe anxiety
      3) Marked dyspnea and cyanosis
      4) Edema
3. Right ventricular failure: congestion due to blood not adequately pumped from systemic system to the lungs; also related to COPD/CAL; (right sided will reveal systemic symptoms)
   a. Manifestations
      1) Peripheral edema
      2) Distended neck veins
      3) Weight gain
      4) Enlarged liver
      5) Elevated CVP
      6) Hypotension
      7) Tachycardia
      8) Rales

   b. **NURSING INTERVENTIONS**
      1) Bronchodilation and relief of anxiety
      2) Improve oxygenation
      3) Reduce congestion
      4) Improve myocardial contraction
   c. Digitalis therapy
      1) Purpose: decrease heart rate, improve ventricular filling, stroke volume and coronary artery perfusion; improve strength of contraction
      2) Manifestations of toxicity
         a) Halo around lights
         b) Anorexia, diarrhea
         c) Nausea and vomiting
         d) Bradycardia, frequent PVCs

      3) **NURSING INTERVENTIONS**
         a) Monitor K levels
         b) Apical heart rate
         c) Client teaching: live within cardiac reserve; report symptoms of CHF

D. Valvular Disorders

1. Definition: results in narrowing of valve that prevents blood flow (stenosis) or impaired closure that allows backward leakage of blood (regurgitation); affects mitral, aortic, or tricuspid: stenosis or insufficiency; rheumatic fever history frequent causative factor

2. Manifestations
   a. Right heart failure (mitral stenosis, mitral regurgitation, tricuspid stenosis)
   b. Left heart failure (aortic stenosis, insufficiency)
   c. Murmurs
   d. Decreased cardiac output

3. **NURSING INTERVENTIONS**
   a. Same as CHF
   b. Antibiotic therapy for damage due to infection

4. Surgical management
   a. Heart valve replacement
   b. Mitral commissurotomy (valvulotomy)

   1) **NURSING INTERVENTIONS** (postoperative care)
      a) Monitor vital signs, ECG q 15 minutes until stable
      b) Provide tissue oxygenation initially on ventilator
      c) Monitor intake and output
      d) Maintain fluid and electrolyte balance
      e) Chest tubes
      f) Relieve client's pain
      g) Neuro checks
      h) Peripheral pulses
      i) TED stockings
   2) **NURSING INTERVENTIONS** (rehabilitation)
      a) Activities
      b) Diet: low-sodium, low-cholesterol
      c) Medications (anticoagulants)
      d) Special needs of clients with valve replacements

E. AV Heart Block

1. Definition: altered transmission of impulse from SA node through AV node
2. First degree
   a. Delayed transmission of impulse through AV node
   b. Prolonged PR interval
   c. No treatment necessary
3. Second degree
   a. Some impulses pass through AV node, some do not
      May be: 2:1, 3:1, or 4:1
   b. Atropine and isoproterenol *(Isuprel)* may be used, but not always helpful
   c. Pacemaker sometimes necessary
4. Third degree
   a. No impulses pass through AV node; atria and ventricles beat independently of each other
   b. Ventricular pacemaker

F. Pacemaker

1. Definition: electronic device that provides repetitive electrical stimuli to the heart muscle to control heart rate
2. Types
   a. Demand
   b. Fixed
   c. Transcutaneous
3. Temporary pacemakers: for emergency situations, external
4. Permanent pacemakers (see illustration, p. 91)
   a. Types
      1) Transvenous (most common)
      2) Myocardial (transthoracic) implantation

   b. **NURSING INTERVENTIONS**
      1) Preoperative teaching
      2) Postoperative care
         a) Monitor ECG and pulse
         b) Check wound for hematoma
         c) Administer analgesics as necessary
         d) Maintain electrically safe environment
         e) Observe for hiccups (pacing diaphragm)
         f) Sterile technique at insertion site
5. Complications after pacemaker insertion
   a. Local infection
   b. Arrhythmias
   c. Dislodging of electrode
   d. Pacemaker malfunction
6. Client teaching
   a. Wear loose fitting clothes
   b. No contact sports
   c. Carry ID information at all times
   d. Stay away from cell phones, arc welders, and electrical generators
   e. Be aware when battery needs charging (lithium batteries last between three and 15 years)
   f. Body image
   g. Resume regular activities in 6 weeks
   h. Telephone transmission of pacer function

G. Arterial Disorders

1. Causes
   a. Arteriosclerosis
   b. Atherosclerosis
2. Classic manifestations
   a. Intermittent claudication
   b. Tingling and numbness of toes
   c. Cool extremities

3. Client teaching
   a. Stop smoking
   b. Avoid stressful situations
   c. Avoid constricting garments
   d. Keep legs in straight plane or dependent
   e. Buerger-Allen exercises
4. Arteriosclerosis obliterans (ASO): usually affects aorta or the arteries of the lower extremities
   a. Characteristics
      1) Commonly associated with diabetes
      2) Occlusion usually proximal to pain zone
      3) Advanced manifestations: pain at rest, commonly at night
   b. Surgical management
      1) Vascular graft
      2) Patch grafts
      3) Endarterectomy

   c. **NURSING INTERVENTIONS** (postoperative)
      1) Frequent checks of extremities for pulses, color and temperature
      2) Observe for paralysis of lower extremities after operation upon thoracic aorta
      3) Ensure adequate circulating blood volume through arterial repair: intake and output; central venous pressure (CVP)
      4) Client teaching: avoid dependent positions, elevate extremities, use of TEDS
      5) Mini doses of heparin
5. Buerger's disease (thromboangiitis obliterans)
   a. Definition: recurring inflammation of the arteries and veins of lower and upper extremities resulting in thrombus and occlusion
   b. Characteristics
      1) Occurs in men ages 20–35 years
      2) Most common manifestations: pain in legs relieved by inactivity, numbness and tingling of toes and fingers in cold weather
      3) Cessation of smoking important; client teaching is same as arteriosclerosis
6. Raynaud's phenomenon
   a. Definition: vasospastic condition of arteries that occurs with exposure to cold or stress and primarily affects the hands
   b. Characteristics
      1) Arteriolar vasoconstriction results in coldness, pain, occasional ulceration of the fingertips; color changes from white to blue to red

   c. **NURSING INTERVENTIONS**
      1) Avoid cold
      2) Stop smoking

H. Vascular Disorders

1. Aortic aneurysm
   a. Definition: local distention of the artery wall, usually thoracic or abdominal
   b. Cause
      1) Infections
      2) Congenital
      3) Atherosclerosis
   c. Manifestations
      1) Thoracic: pain, dyspnea, hoarseness, cough, dysphagia
      2) Abdominal: abdominal pain, persistent or intermittent low back pain; may be asymptomatic; pulsating abdominal mass
   d. Treatment: usually surgery
      1) Preoperative: careful monitoring because of a possible rupture; prepare for abdominal surgery
      2) Postoperative: same as abdominal surgery, careful monitoring of peripheral circulation

2. Hypertension
   a. Definition: persistent BP above 140/systolic and 90/diastolic; called "silent killer"
   b. Essential hypertension
      1) 90% have this kind
      2) Hereditary disease
      3) Cause unknown
      4) Late manifestations: headaches, fatigue, dyspnea, edema, nocturia, blackouts
   c. Secondary hypertension
      1) Due to identifiable problem
      2) Pheochromocytoma

   d. **NURSING INTERVENTIONS**
      1) Correct overweight
      2) Avoid stimulants
      3) Program of regular physical exercise
      4) Promote lifestyle with reduced stress
      5) Maintain salt restricted diet
      6) Teach risk factors
   e. Antihypertensive drugs
      1) Potassium depleting diuretics
         a) Chlorthalidone *(Hygroton)*
         b) Chlorothiazide *(Diuril)*
         c) Hydrochlorothiazide *(Hydrodiuril)*
         d) Quinethazone *(Hydromox)*
         e) Ethacrynic acid *(Edecrin)*
            (1) Potassium supplement may be ordered
            (2) Teach dietary sources of potassium
            (3) Be aware of possible interaction of low K$^+$ and digitalis preparations
      2) Potassium sparing diuretics
         a) Spironolactone *(Aldactone)*
         b) Triamterene *(Dyrenium)*

3) Adrenergic inhibitors
   a) Propranolol HCl *(Inderal):* beta adrenergic blocker
      (1) Bradycardia
      (2) Avoid alcohol, caffeine, smoking
   b) Clonidine *(Catapres):* central acting inhibitor
      (1) Drowsiness
      (2) Sexual dysfunction
      (3) Dry mouth
   c) Methyldopa *(Aldomet)*
      (1) Postural hypotension
4) Vasodilators
   a) Hydralazine *(Apresoline)*
      (1) Postural hypotension
      (2) Vit B_6 deficiency
   b) Minoxidil *(Loniten)*
5) Calcium agonist
   a) Nifedipine *(Procardia)*
      (1) Headache
      (2) Bradycardia
   b) Verapamil *(Calan)*
      (1) Flushing
      (2) Constipation

Venous Disorders

A. **Thrombophlebitis**
   1. Definition: clot in the vein with inflammation of the wall
   2. Precipitating factors
      a. Stasis
      b. Hypercoagulability
      c. Damage to intima of blood vessels
   3. Manifestations
      a. Edema of affected limb
      b. Local swelling, bumpy, knotty
      c. Red, tender, local induration
      d. Positive Homans' sign

   4. **NURSING INTERVENTIONS**
      a. Bed rest
      b. Elevate leg and apply moist warm compresses
      c. Heparin therapy
      d. TED stocking

B. Varicose Veins

1. Precipitating factors
   a. Prolonged standing
   b. Pregnancy
   c. Obesity
2. Manifestations
   a. Enlarged, tortuous veins in lower extremities
   b. Pain
   c. Edema

3. **NURSING INTERVENTIONS**
   a. Elevate legs
   b. TEDS
   c. Avoid constrictive clothing, prolonged sitting or standing
   d. Avoid crossing legs at knee
   e. Postop care for vein stripping and ligation
      1) Monitor circulation
      2) Elevate feet
      3) Stand, lie down

Shock

A. Types

1. Cardiogenic: failure of the heart to pump adequately
2. Hypovolemic: decreased blood volume
3. Distributive (vasogenic)
   a. Neurogenic: increased size of vascular bed due to loss of vascular tone
   b. Anaphylactic: hypersensitivity reaction
   c. Septic: systemic reaction vasodilation due to infection

B. Manifestations

1. Tachycardia
2. Tachypnea
3. Oliguria
4. Cold, moist skin
5. Color ashen: pallor
6. Hypotension, tachycardia

C. NURSING INTERVENTIONS

1. Elevate feet
2. Secure client IV
3. Administer oxygen
4. Record vital signs q 5 minutes

D. **Emergency Drugs**
1. Atropine
2. Dopamine *(Intropin)*
3. Epinephrine HCl *(Adrenalin)*
4. Isoproterenol *(Isuprel)*
5. Lidocaine *(Xylocaine)*
6. Dobutamine *(Dobutrex)*
7. Norepinephrine levanerenol *(Levophed)*
8. Sodium bicarbonate

Cardiopulmonary Resuscitation (CPR)

A. **Indications**
1. Absence of palpable carotid pulse
2. Absence of breath sounds

B. **Purpose**
1. Establish effective circulation and respiration
2. Prevent irreversible cerebral anoxic damage

C. **Procedure**
1. Airway (head tilt/chin lift)
2. Breathing (two breaths)
3. Circulation
4. One rescuer (15:2)
5. Two rescuers (5:1)

D. **Complications**
1. Fractured ribs
2. Punctured lungs
3. Lacerated liver
4. Abdominal distension

E. **Stop CPR When:**
1. Physician pronounces client dead
2. Exhausted
3. Help arrives
4. Heartbeat returns

F. Obstructed Airway

1. Conscious
    a. Establish that victim is choking
    b. Heimlich maneuver
2. Unconscious
    a. Establish unresponsiveness
    b. Attempt to ventilate
    c. Reposition and reventilate
    d. Tongue-jaw lift, fingersweep
    e. Reattempt ventilation
    f. Abdominal thrusts
    g. Repeat steps d through f

PACEMAKERS

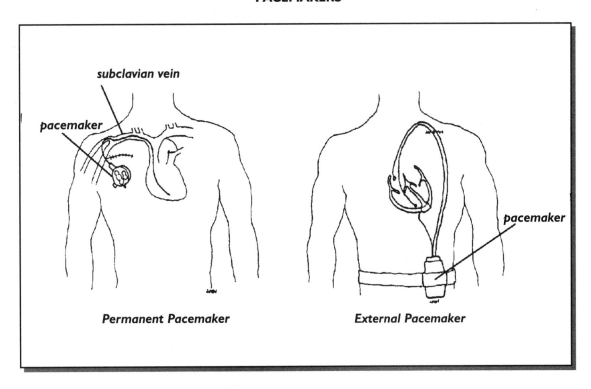

Permanent Pacemaker   **External Pacemaker**

SECTION IX

REVIEW OF GENITOURINARY SYSTEM DISORDERS

Assessment of the Client

A. History
1. Has there been renal disease in the past?
2. Is there a family history of renal disease?

B. Manifestations
1. Pain (usually in acute conditions): flank radiating to upper thigh, testis, or labium
2. Changes in voiding: hematuria, proteinuria, dysuria, frequency, urgency, burning, nocturia, incontinence, polyuria, oliguria, anuria
3. Thirst, fatigue, edema

C. Functions of the Kidney
1. Acid-base balance
2. Excretion of metabolic wastes (creatinine, urea)
3. Blood pressure regulation: renin (stimulated by decreased blood pressure or blood volume) stimulates production of anistensin I, which is converted to angiotensin II in the lungs; angiotensin II is a strong vasoconstrictor and also stimulates aldosterone secretion; vasoconstriction and sodium reabsorption result in increased blood volume and increased blood pressure
4. Secretes erythropoietin
5. Converts vitamin D to its active form for absorption of calcium
6. Excretion of water soluble drugs and drug metabolites

Diagnostic Tests

KEY INFORMATION
A. Urinalysis
1. Specific gravity: 1.001–1.030
2. Color: yellow/amber
3. Negative glucose, protein, red blood cells and white blood cells
4. pH: 5–8
5. First voided morning sample preferred; 15 ml
6. Send to lab or refrigerate

B. Clean Catch
1. Cleanse labia, glans penis
2. Obtain midstream sample

C. Renal Function Tests (several tests over a period of time are necessary)
1. BUN (blood urea nitrogen): 10–20 mg/100 ml
2. Serum creatinine: 0–1 mg/dl
3. Creatinine clearance: 100–120 ml/minute; collect 24 hour urine (refrigerate); blood drawn at start (measures glomerular filtration rate)
4. Uric acid serum: 3.5–7.8 mg/dl
5. Uric acid (urine): 250–750 mg/24 hour;. 24 hour urine
6. Phenolsulfonphthalein (PSP) give fluids 1–1 1/2 hours before the test. PSP given IV; collect urine specimens 15, 30, 60 minutes after PSP given

D. Radiologic Test
1. KUB (x-ray): shows size, shape and position of kidneys, ureters, bladder; no preparation
2. Intravenous pyelography (IVP): visualization of urinary tract
   a. Nursing care
      1) Consent
      2) NPO for 8–10 hours
      3) Laxative to clear bowel
      4) Check for allergies to iodine or shellfish
      5) Flushing, warmth, nausea, salty taste may accompany injection of dye
      6) Have emergency equipment available during procedure
      7) Push fluids after procedure
3. Renal angiography: visualization of renal arterial supply; contrast material injected through a catheter

   a. **NURSING INTERVENTIONS** (before procedure)
      1) Consent
      2) NPO after midnight
      3) Give cathartic or enema
      4) Shave proposed injection sites: groin or ankle
      5) Locate and mark peripheral pulses
      6) Void before procedure
      7) Teach client:procedure takes 1/2 hour to 2 hour; he/she will feel heat along vessel
   b. **NURSING INTERVENTIONS** (after procedure)
      1) Bed rest 4–12 hrs
      2) Take vital signs until stable
      3) Cold compresses to puncture site
      4) Observe for swelling and hematoma
      5) Palpate peripheral pulses
      6) Check color and temp of involved extremity
      7) Monitor urinary output

E. Cystoscopy

1. Diagnostic uses: inspect bladder and urethra; insert catheters into ureters; see configuration and position of urethral orifices
2. Treatment uses: remove calculi from urethra, bladder and ureter; treat lesions of bladder, urethra, prostate

3. **NURSING INTERVENTIONS**
   a. NPO if general anesthesia; liquids if local anesthesia
   b. Consent
   c. Deep breathing exercises to relieve bladder spasms
   d. Monitor for postural hypotension
   e. Pink-tinged or tea-colored urine common; bright red urine or clots should be reported to physician
   f. Back pain and/or abdominal pain may be present
   g. Leg cramps due to lithotomy position
   h. Warm sitz baths comforting
   i. Push fluids
   j. Monitor intake and output

F. Needle Biopsy of Kidney

1. Prebiopsy interventions
   a. Bleeding, clotting and prothrombin times
   b. X-ray of kidney, IVP
   c. Maybe ultrasound
   d. NPO 6–8 hours
   e. Position prone with pillow under abdomen, shoulders on bed

2. **NURSING INTERVENTIONS** (post biopsy)
   a. Client supine, bed rest for 24 hours
   b. Vital signs q 5–15 minutes for 4 hours; then decrease if stable
   c. Pressure to puncture site 20 minutes
   d. Observe for pain, nausea, vomiting, BP changes
   e. Fluids to 3,000 cc
   f. Assess Hct and Hgb 8 hours after
   g. Measure output
   h. Avoid strenuous activity, sports, and heavy lifting for at least 2 weeks

G. Catheterization

1. Purpose: to empty contents of bladder, obtain a sterile specimen, determine residual urine, allow irrigation of bladder, bypass an obstruction.; procedure is sterile

2. **NURSING INTERVENTIONS**
   a. Maintain closed system
   b. Measure each shift
   c. Keep bag below bladder

Specific Disorders and Nursing Intervention

A. Cystitis

1. Definition: inflammation of the urinary bladder
2. Etiology: ascending infection after entry via the urinary meatus; more common in females; acute infections usually E. coli
3. Manifestations
   a. Frequency and urgency
   b. Dysuria
   c. Suprapubic tenderness; pain in region of bladder
   d. Hematuria
   e. Fever
   f. Cloudy, foul-smelling urine

4. **NURSING INTERVENTIONS**
   a. Obtain urine for culture and sensitivity
   b. Give antimicrobial medications
   c. Maintain appropriate urine pH
   d. Force fluids
   e. Give analgesics; heat to perineum
   f. Teaching: good perineal care, cotton underwear, avoid bubble baths, high fluid intake

B. Glomerulonephritis

1. Definition: inflammatory disease involving the renal glomeruli of both kidneys; thought to be an antigen-antibody reaction that damages the glomeruli of the kidney
2. Etiology: group A beta-hemolytic streptococcal infection; usually a history of pharyngitis or tonsillitis 2–3 weeks prior to manifestations
3. Manifestations
   a. Hematuria, proteinuria fever, chills, weakness, nausea, vomiting
   b. Edema
   c. Oliguria
   d. Hypertension
   e. Headache
   f. Increased urea nitrogen
   g. Flank pain
   h. Anemia

4. **NURSING INTERVENTIONS**
   a. Goal: protect kidney; recognize and treat infection
   b. Bed rest
   c. Penicillin for streptococcal infection
   d. Reduce dietary protein if oliguria and elevated BUN
   e. Sodium and fluid restriction
   f. Good prognosis if treated

C. Nephrotic Syndrome

1. Definition: clinical disorder associated with any condition that impairs the glomerulus
2. Etiology: chronic glomerulonephritis, diabetes mellitus, systemic lupus erythematosus, toxins, renal vein thrombosis, primary lipoid nephrosis in children, sickle cell anemia
3. Manifestations
   a. Insidious onset of pitting edema, especially periorbital
   b. Proteinuria
   c. Anemia
   d. Anorexia
   e. Nausea
   f. Diarrhea
   g. Fatigue
   h. Oliguria
   i. Ascites
   j. Hypoalbuminemia
   k. Hyperlipidemia

4. **NURSING INTERVENTIONS**
   a. Goal: preserve renal function
   b. Bed rest
   c. Low-sodium, high-protein, high-calorie diet
   d. Protect client from infection
   e. Monitor intake and output
   f. Weigh client daily
5. Drug therapy
   a. Diuretics
   b. Steroids (prednisone [Deltasone])
   c. Immunosuppressive agents
   d. Anticoagulants (renal vein thrombosis)

D. Urolithiasis

1. Definition: stones in the urinary system
2. Etiology
   a. Obstruction and urinary stasis
   b. Proteus infection
   c. Dehydration
   d. Immobilization
   e. Hypercalcemia
   f. Excessive excretion of uric acid
   g. Vitamin A deficiency
   h. Heredity
   i. More common in men 30–50
   j. Tends to recur
   k. Most stones calcium or magnesium with phosphate or oxalate

3. Manifestations
   a. Pain: renal colic (ureter); dull, aching (kidney)
   b. Nausea, vomiting, diarrhea
   c. Hematuria
   d. Manifestations of urinary tract infection

4. NURSING INTERVENTIONS
   a. Goals: to eradicate the stone, determine stone type and prevent nephron destruction
   b. Force fluids: at least 3,000cc/day
   c. Strain all urine
   d. Give drugs as ordered (depends on type of stone)
   e. Maintain proper urine pH (depends on stone type)
   f. Diet therapy if stone type is known (see Appendix B: Therapeutic Diets)

E. Acute Renal Failure
1. Definition: abrupt reversible cessation of renal function; may be result of trauma, allergic reactions, kidney stones
2. Etiology: any condition that obstructs renal blood flow
   a. Pre-renal: hemorrhage, dehydration, burns
   b. Renal: calculi, acute tubular necrosis
   c. Post-renal: BPH, tumors, strictures
3. Manifestations: three phases
   a. Oliguric phase (8th–14th day): sudden onset, less than 400 cc/24 hours, edema, elevated BUN, creatinine, potassium, decreased specific gravity
   b. Period of diuresis (14th–24th day): dilute urine, 1,000cc/24 hours, BUN and creatinine rise in early stage
   c. Recovery period: up to one year

4. NURSING INTERVENTIONS
   a. Treat/eliminate/prevent cause
   b. Aim is to prevent acidosis by maintaining fluid and electrolyte balance
   c. For increased potassium level, may give Kayexalate (an ion exchange resin given orally or by enema)
   d. IV glucose and insulin or calcium carbonate (causes K^+ to enter cells)
   e. Diet
      1) Oliguric: low-protein, high-carbohydrate, high-fat; restrict K^+ intake
      2) Diuresis: high-protein, high-calorie, restrict fluids as indicated
   f. Phosphate binding gels
   g. Prevent infection
   h. Weigh client daily
   i. Monitor intake and output
   j. Dialysis

F. Chronic Renal Failure
1. Definition: a slower or progressive failure of the kidneys to function that results in death unless hemodialysis or transplant is performed; irreversible

2. Etiology
    a. Chronic glomerulonephritis
    b. Pyelonephritis
    c. Uncontrolled hypertension
    d. Diabetes mellitus
    e. Congenital kidney disease
    f. Renal vascular disease
3. Stages of renal failure
    a. Diminished renal reserve (creatinine 1.6–2.0)
    b. Renal insufficiency (creatinine 2.1–5.0)
    c. Renal failure (creatinine >8.0)
    d. Uremia: end stage (creatinine >12.0)
4. Manifestations
    a. Fatigue
    b. Headache
    c. GI manifestations
    d. Hypertension
    e. Irritability
    f. Convulsions
    g. Anemia
    h. Edema
    i. Hypocalcemia
    j. Pruritus, uremic frost
    k. Peculiary pallid, gray-yellow complexion
    l. Metabolic acidosis
    m. Elevated BUN, creatinine, sodium, potassium
5. **NURSING INTERVENTIONS**
    a. Goal: help the kidneys maintain homeostasis
    b. Bed rest
    c. Diet: low-protein, low-potassium, high-carbohydrate, vitamin & calcium supplements, low-sodium, low-phosphate
    d. Treat hypertension
    e. Watch for signs of cerebral irritation
    f. Prevent water and electrolyte disturbances
    g. Fluid replacement: 500–600cc more than 24-hour urine output
    h. Aluminum hydroxide
    i. No magnesium, phosphorus *(M.O.M., Fleets Phospho-soda)*
    j. Dialysis
        1) Goals
            a) Remove end products of metabolism
            b) Maintain safe concentration of electrolytes
            c) Correct acidosis and restore blood buffers
            d) Remove excess fluid from blood
        2) Types
            a) Hemodialysis
            b) Peritoneal dialysis (intermittent, continuous ambulatory, cyclic, continuous)

k.   Diuretics
    l.   Skin care
    m. Emotional support

6. Hemodialysis
   a. Definition: process of cleansing the blood of accumulated waste products; used for end-stage renal failure and those clients who are acutely ill and require short-term treatment; uses diffusion, osmosis and filtration

   b. **NURSING INTERVENTIONS**
      1) Weigh client before and after procedure
      2) Withhold antihypertensives and sedatives
      3) Continuous monitoring during procedure
      4) Care of access site to prevent clotting and infection
      5) Assess bruit and thrill
      6) Provide adequate nutrition
      7) Observe for psychologic problems: depression, changes in body image, dependency-independence conflict, anxiety, suicidal behavior, denial; be alert for frequently occurring medical problems
         a) Arteriosclerotic cardiovascular disease
         b) Intercurrent infection
         c) Anemia
         d) Bleeding
         e) Disordered calcium metabolism
         f) Chronic ascites
         g) Disequilibrium syndrome from rapid fluid and electrolyte changes (headache, vomiting, convulsions, coma, hyperkalemia, psychiatric problems)
         h) Fatigue after procedure

7. Peritoneal dialysis
   a. Definition: substitute for kidney function during failure that uses the peritoneum as a dialyzing membrane; usually short term; peritoneal catheter inserted by physician
   b. Goals
      1) Removal of the end products of protein metabolism (urea and creatinine) from the blood
      2) Maintenance of a safe concentration of the serum electrolytes
      3) Correction of acidosis and replenishment of the blood's bicarbonate buffer system
      4) Removal of excess fluid from the blood

   c. **NURSING INTERVENTIONS**
      1) Have client void
      2) Weigh client daily
      3) Take vital signs frequently, baseline electrolytes
      4) Maintain asepsis
      5) Keep accurate record of fluid balance

6) Procedure
   a) Warm dialysate (1–2 liters of 1.5%, 2.5% or 4.25% glucose solution)
   b) Allow to flow in by gravity
   c) 5–10 minutes inflow time
   d) 30 minutes of equilibration (dwell time)
   e) 10–30 minutes of drainage (clear yellow)
7) Continued for 24–48 exchanges
8) Monitor for complications: peritonitis, bleeding, respiratory difficulty, abdominal pain, bowel or bladder perforation

G. Continuous Ambulatory Peritoneal Dialysis (CAPD)

1. Definition: dialyzing method involving almost continuous peritoneal contact with a dialysis solution for clients with end-stage renal disease
2. Procedure
   a. Permanent indwelling catheter into peritoneum
   b. Fluid infused by gravity
   c. Dwell time: 4–8 hours
   d. Dialysate drains by gravity: 20–40 minutes
   e. Four to five exchanges daily, 3–7 days a week
3. Complications
   a. Peritonitis (rebound tenderness, fever, cloudy outflow)
   b. Bladder perforation (yellow outflow)
   c. Hypotension
   d. Bowel perforation (brown outflow)
4. Advantages
   a. More independence
   b. Free dietary intake; better nutrition
   c. Easy to use
   d. Satisfactory control of uremia
   e. Least expensive dialysis
   f. Decreased likelihood of transplant rejection
   g. Closely approximates normal renal function

H. Urinary Tract Surgery

1. **NURSING INTERVENTIONS**
   a. Monitor vital signs (hemorrhage and shock are frequent complications)
   b. Provide pain control
   c. Be alert for manifestations of paralytic ileus
   d. Provide adequate fluid replacement
   e. Weigh client daily
   f. Prevent respiratory complications
   g. Ambulate client early
   h. Monitor drainage tubes
   i. Indwelling catheter (dependent position, tape tubing to thigh)
   j. Nephrostomy tube (never clamp, irrigate only with order of 10 cc normal saline)
   k. Change dressings as indicated when profuse drainage

I. **Benign Prostatic Hyperplasia (BPH)**
1. Definition: enlargement of the prostate
2. Etiology: unknown, accompanies aging process in the male
3. Manifestations
    a. Difficulty starting stream
    b. Urinary tract infection
    c. Nocturia, hematuria, dribbling
    d. Decrease in size and force of urinary stream
4. Treatments
    a. Cystoscopy for diagnosis
    b. Urinary antiseptics
    c. Prostatectomy (see illustration, p. 102)

5. **NURSING INTERVENTIONS**
    a. Preoperative
        1) Maintain adequate bladder drainage (catheter)
        2) Antibiotics
        3) Check BP
        4) Ensure adequate hydration
        5) Weigh client daily
    b. Postoperative
        1) Observe for shock and hemorrhage
        2) Promote bladder drainage
        3) Avoid heavy lifting for 6 weeks
        4) Avoid straining at stool
        5) Monitor bladder irrigation (CBI)
        6) Encourage fluid intake
        7) Assess for TUR syndrome (altered mental status, bradycardia, tachycardia and confusion due to absorption of bladder irritant)
        8) Pain control
        9) Urinary control
        10) Avoid strenuous exercise
        11) Avoid sex for six weeks

J. **Prostatitis**
1. Definition: inflammation of the prostate gland
2. Etiology
    a. Bacterial infection from urethra or kidneys
    b. Stress
    c. BPH
    d. Sexual activity
3. Manifestations
    a. Pain in perineum, rectum, lower back, abdomen, and penile head

PROSTATECTOMY TYPES

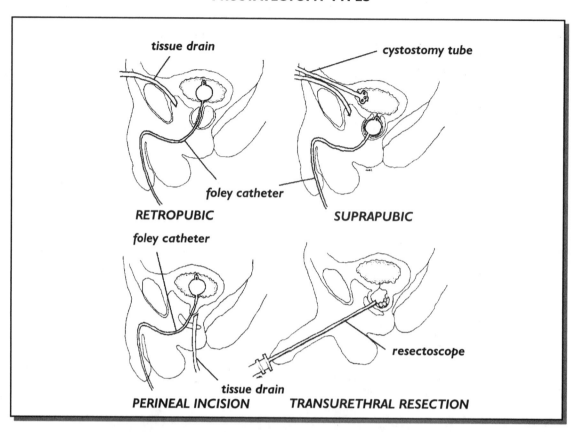

RETROPUBIC   SUPRAPUBIC

PERINEAL INCISION   TRANSURETHRAL RESECTION

4. **NURSING INTERVENTIONS**
   a. Acute: maintain IV antimicrobial
   b. Chronic
      1) Antimicrobial
      2) Bed rest
      3) Antispasmodics
      4) Analgesics
      5) Sitz bath
      6) Stool softeners
      7) Adequate fluid intake
   c. Client education: client should avoid spicy foods, coffee, alcohol, prolonged auto rides, and sexual intercourse during acute inflammation

K. Kidney Transplantation
   1. Indicated for individual with irreversible end-stage renal disease
   2. Requires well-matched donor; best donors are twin or family member
   3. Preoperative management
      a. Regain normal metabolic state
      b. Tissue typing
      c. Immunosuppressive therapy
      d. Hemodialysis within 24 hours
      e. Teaching and emotional support

TABLE II-15.
SURGICAL APPROACHES FOR PROSTATECTOMY

APPROACH	ADVANTAGE	DISADVANTAGE	NURSING INTERVENTION
Transurethral (removal of prostatic tissue by instrument introduced through urethra)	Safer for client at risk; shorter period of hospitalization and convalescence	Not indicated for greatly enlarged prostate	Observe for hemorrhage, stricture, and incontinence
Open Surgical Removal			
Suprapubic	Technically simple	Requires surgical approach through the bladder	Strict aseptic care
Perineal	Offer direct anatomic approach	Impotency and urinary incontinency; use drainage pads to absorb	Avoid rectal tubes, thermometers and enemas after perineal surgery.
Retropubic	Most versatile procedure; affords direct visualization	Cannot treat associated pathology in bladder	Watch for evidence of hemorrhage

4. **NURSING INTERVENTIONS** (postoperative management)
   a. Maintain homeostasis until kidney is functioning
   b. Immunosuppressive drugs: azathioprine *(Imuran)*, cyclosporine *(Sandimmune)*, steroids
   c. Monitor for rejection: oliguria, edema, fever, tenderness over graft, fluid and electrolyte imbalance, hypertension, elevated BUN, creatinine
   d. Monitor for infection
   e. Reverse isolation
   f. Emotional support

SECTION X

REVIEW OF NEUROLOGICAL SYSTEM DISORDERS

Neurological Assessment

A. History

B. Mental Status
1. Level of consciousness (alert, lethargic, obtunded, stupor, coma)
2. Orientation (person, place, time)
3. Appearance
4. Affect
5. Knowledge and vocabulary
6. Judgement and abstraction
7. Mood
8. Language and speech

C. Cranial Nerves (I thru XII)

D. Motor System
1. Muscles
   a. Size
   b. Symmetry
   c. Tone
   d. Strength
2. Coordination
3. Movement
   a. Voluntary control
   b. Tremors
   c. Twitches
   d. Balance and gait

E. Reflexes
1. Babinski
2. Corneal
3. Gag
4. Deep tendon (muscle-stretch)

F. Sensory System
1. Touch
2. Temperature
3. Superficial and deep pain

Diagnostic Procedures

A. Brain Scan
1. Obtain consent
2. Method: IV radioisotope accumulates in area of pathology
3. Explain procedure to client
4. Purpose: detects neoplasms, brain abscess, subdural hematoma

B. Lumbar Puncture (LP)
1. Obtain consent
2. Empty bladder and bowel
3. Position client with back arched during LP
4. Needle inserted L2–S1, subarachnoid space
5. Withdraw cerebrospinal fluid
6. After LP
    a. Position client horizontal
    b. Encourage fluid intake
    c. Check puncture site for redness, swelling, drainage
    d. Assess movement of extremities
7. Normal cerebrospinal fluid (CSF) pressure

C. Cerebral Arteriogram
1. Obtain consent
2. Method: dye injected into artery and vascular system of brain visualized
3. Clear liquids before procedure
4. May have sedative
5. Void before procedure
6. Mark distal peripheral pulses
7. Feeling of warmth in face during procedure
8. **NURSING INTERVENTIONS** (post procedure)

    a. Monitor for altered loss of consciousness, sensory or motor deficits
    b. Check for hematoma
    c. Ice cap to decrease swelling
    d. Check peripheral pulses
    e. Check color and temperature of extremities
    f. Bed rest overnight
    g. Maintain extremity in extension

D. CT Scan (Computed Tomography)

1. **NURSING INTERVENTIONS** (pre-procedure)
   a. Obtain consent
   b. Check for allergies
   c. Explain procedure (noninvasive, must remain still), can eliminate need for angiography
   d. If dye used, NPO 4 hours before
   e. Assess for claustrophobia

E. Myelogram

1. Method: contrast medium or air injected into spinal subarachnoid space by spinal puncture

2. **NURSING INTERVENTIONS** (pre-procedure)
   a. Obtain consent
   b. NPO 4 hours before procedure
   c. Horizontal for 12–24 hours after if oil based dye; head of bed raised 15–30 degrees if water-based dye
   d. Check vital signs
   e. Check voiding
   f. Encourage fluid intake
   g. Monitor for fever, stiff neck, back pain

F. Electroencephalogram (EEG)

1. **NURSING INTERVENTIONS** (pre-procedure)
   a. Obtain consent
   b. Check about giving medications before EEG
   c. No caffeine or sedatives before EEG
   d. No hair spray before EEG
2. **NURSING INTERVENTION** (post procedure): cleanse hair with acetone

G. Electromyography

1. Purpose: measure electrical activity of skeletal muscles

2. **NURSING INTERVENTIONS** (pre-procedure)
   a. Obtain consent
   b. Explain there will be some discomfort due to insertion of needle into skeletal muscles

H. Magnetic Resonance Imaging (MRI)

1. **NURSING INTERVENTIONS** (pre-procedure)
   a. Obtain consent
   b. Magnets and computers produce images of body parts
   c. Remove all metal objects, credit cards
   d. Noninvasive

"Neuro-checks"

A. **Level of Consciousness and Sensory Function**

B. **Client's Response**

C. **Pupil Size**

D. **Motor Type**

E. **Motor Strength**

F. **Reflexes**

G. **Vital Signs**

H. **Glasgow Coma Scale (normal 8–15; 7 or less indicates coma)**
1. Best eye opening response
   a. Spontaneously   =4
   b. To speech   =3
   c. To pain   =2
   d. No response   =1
2. Best motor response
   a. Obeys verbal command   =6
   b. Localizes pain   =5
   c. Flexion: withdrawal to pain   =4
   d. Flexion: abnormal (decorticate)   =3
   e. Extension: abnormal (decerebrate) =2
   f. No response to pain on any limb   =1
3. Best verbal response
   a. Oriented x 3   =5
   b. Conversation   =4
   c. Speech: inappropriate =3
   d. Sounds: incomprehensible =2
   e. No response   =1

Increased Intracranial Pressure

A. **Definition:** increase in the amount of CNS tissue, size of cerebral blood vessels, or amount of cerebrospinal fluid; intracranial pressure greater than 15 mm Hg.

B. **Causes**
1. Head injury
2. CVA
3. Brain tumor

C. Manifestations
1. Lethargic, drowsy, stupor
2. Headache
3. Nausea and vomiting, often projectile
4. Pupil changes: dilating, unequal, nonreactive
5. Changes in vital signs
   a. Widening pulse pressure
   b. Irregular respiration (Cheyne-Stokes respiration)
   c. Pulse slows, respirations decrease

D. NURSING INTERVENTIONS
1. Monitor vital signs and "neuro-checks"
2. Keep head of bed elevated
3. Avoid coughing, sneezing, suctioning
4. Maintain good respiratory exchange
5. Monitor fluid intake and output
6. Avoid opiates and sedative (contraindicated); acetaminophen *(Tylenol)* may be ordered for pain
7. Administer osmotic diuretics (e.g., mannitol *[Osmitrol]* and steroids) (e.g., dexamethasone *[Decadron]*)
8. Restrict fluids

Hyperthermia

A. Definition: body temperature above 105°F; can be caused by infection, cerebral edema, or heat

B. Hypothermia Blanket
1. Protect skin
2. Manual temperature q 4 hours

C. NURSING INTERVENTIONS
1. Monitor vital signs
2. Monitor intake and output
3. Observe skin changes
4. Prevent shivering

Epilepsy/Seizures

A. Definition: abnormal, sudden, excessive discharge of electrical activity within the brain

B. Classifications
1. Generalized (four types)
   a. Tonic-clonic (formerly grand-mal)
   b. Absence (formerly petit-mal seizures)
   c. Myoclonic
   d. Atonic ("drop-attacks")
2. Partial seizures (two types)
   a. Complex (loss of consciousness)
   b. Simple (no loss of consciousness)
3. Unclassified
   a. 50% of all seizure activity
   b. Unknown etiology

C. NURSING INTERVENTIONS
1. During seizure
   a. Maintain patent airway
   b. Protect from injury
   c. Do not restrain
   d. Turn client's head to side, prevent aspiration
2. Charting (time, aura, loss of consciousness, precipitating factors)
3. Client teaching: take medications, adequate rest, diet
4. Drug therapy
   a. Diazepam *(Valium)* is drug of choice for status epilepticus
   b. Phenytoin *(Dilantin)* side effects: gum hypertrophy, ataxia, nystagmus, hairy tongue
   c. Carbemazepine *(Tegretal)* and sodium valproates *(Depakene)* side effects: CBC rush, drowsiness, ataxia, increases GABA (an inhibitory neurotransmitter in the CNS); monitor pulmonary and cardiac status
   d. Phenobarbital *(Luminal)* side effects: drowsiness
5. Seizure precautions: bed rest with padded side rails; suction machine, diazapam *(Valium)* 10 mg and oxygen at bedside; head of bed elevated

Cerebrovascular Accident (CVA)

A. Definition: sudden loss of brain function resulting from a disruption of blood supply to part of the brain causing temporary or permanent dysfunction

B. Risk Factors
1. Hypertension
2. Smoking
3. Obesity
4. Hypercholesterolemia
5. Diabetes mellitus
6. Peripheral vascular disease

C. Manifestations

Unlimited variety of neurological deficits depending on site and size of brain involvement
1. Middle cerebral artery
   a. Hemiparesis, hemiplegia
   b. Hemianopsia
   c. Aphasia (expressive, receptive, global)
2. Internal carotid
   a. Hemiplegia
   b. Aphasia
3. Right hemispheric lesion
   a. Sensory: perception
   b. Visual: spatial
   c. Awareness of body space
   d. Great loss of functional skills
4. Left hemispheric lesion
   a. Language
   b. Speech

D. NURSING INTERVENTIONS (Same as management of unconscious client)
1. Maintain adequate airway
2. Monitor "neuro-checks" and vital signs
3. Maintain fluid and electrolyte balance
4. Establish means of communication
5. Rehabilitation phase
   a. Range of motion
   b. Bowel and bladder control
   c. Education
   d. Self-care

Transient Ischemic Attacks (TIA)

A. Definition: temporary episode of neurological dysfunction lasting only a few minutes or seconds due to decreased blood flow to the brain; warning sign of stroke, especially in first 4 weeks after TIA

B. Causes
1. Atherosclerosis
2. Microemboli from atherosclerotic plaque
3. Spasm

C. Manifestations
1. Sudden change in visual function
2. Sudden loss of sensory function
3. Sudden loss of motor function

D. Management: Surgical Carotid Endarterectomy
1. Postoperative focus: assessing for neurologic deficits; avoid flexing neck
   a. Unable to swallow (vagus)
   b. Unable to move tongue (hypoglossal)
   c. Unable to raise arm, shoulder (spinal accessory)
   d. Unable to smile (facial)
   e. Respiratory distress
2. Anticoagulant therapy: dipyridamole *(Persantine)*, aspirin

Spinal Cord Injury

A. Definition: partial or complete disruption of nerve tracts and neurons resulting in paralysis, sensory loss, altered activity, and autonomic nervous system dysfunction

B. Causes
1. Trauma
2. Infection
3. Tumors

C. Level of Injury
1. Cervical: causes quadriplegia
   a. Respiratory problems
   b. Paralysis of all four extremities
   c. Loss of bladder and bowel control
2. Thoracic injury: causes paraplegia
   a. Loss of bladder and bowel control
   b. Paralysis of lower extremities and major control of body trunk
3. Lumbar
   a. Paralysis of lower extremities (remain flaccid)
   b. Loss of bladder and bowel control

D. NURSING INTERVENTIONS

1. Immobilization
   a. Spinal board
   b. Halo traction
   c. Foster or Stryker frame
   d. Gardner-Wells traction tongs (see illustration below)
2. Providing care resulting from spinal shock (flaccid paralysis below level of injury followed by spastic reflexes)
3. Maintain respiratory function
4. Care in autonomic hyperreflexia
5. Bladder management
6. Bowel management
7. Provide decadron to reduce edema
8. Rehabilitation issues

Head Injury

A. Epidural Hematoma

1. Bleeding into space between skull and dura
2. Middle meningeal artery
3. Loss of consciousness, lucid interval, deterioration
4. Burr holes

B. Subdural Hematoma

1. Bleeding below dura
2. Usually venous
3. Acute, subacute, or chronic
4. Craniotomy

GARDNER-WELLS TRACTION TONGS

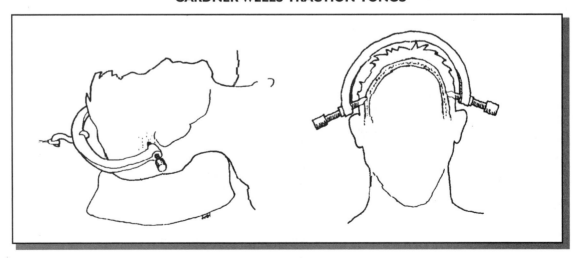

C. Basilar Skull Fracture
1. Bleeding from nose, ears
2. Otorrhea, rhinorrhea
3. Racoon's sign
4. Battle's sign
5. Watch for increased urine output

Laminectomy

A. Definition: excision of a vertebral posterior arch

B. NURSING INTERVENTIONS
1. Observe for circulatory impairment
2. Observe for loss of sensation in lower extremities
3. Observe dressing for spinal fluid leakage and bleeding
4. Log roll

Multiple Sclerosis

A. Definition: chronic, progressive disease of the CNS, characterized by small patches of demyelination in the brain and spinal cord

B. Manifestations
1. Occurs in young adults 20–40 years of age
2. Nystagmus, blurred vision, diplopia
3. Slurred hesitant speech
4. Spastic weakness of extremities
5. Emotionally labile
6. Fatigue
7. Difficulty with balance
8. Intention tremor
9. MRI-plaques on brain in 90% of patients

C. Management
1. No cure or specific treatment; long periods of remissions and exacerbation
2. During exacerbation: ACTH given
3. Stress management
4. Immunosuppressants
5. Baclofen *(Lioresal)*
6. Interferon *(Betaseron):* synthetic drug

D. NURSING INTERVENTIONS
1. Encourage active and normal life as long as possible
2. Self-catheterization
3. Daily exercise
4. Prevent injury

Parkinson's Disease

A. Definition: progressive neurologic disorder affecting the brain centers responsible for control and regulation of movement: extrapyramidal tract; loss of pigmented cells of substantia nigra and depletion of dopamine

B. Manifestations
1. Bradykinesia
2. Rigidity
3. Resting tremor
4. Expressionless, fixed gaze
5. Drooling
6. Constipation
7. Depression
8. Retropulsion, propulsion
9. Slurred speech

C. Stages
1. Unilateral flexion of upper extremity
2. Shuffling gait
3. Progressive difficulty ambulating
4. Progressive weakness
5. Disability

D. Management
1. Drug Therapy
    a. Antiparkinsonian agent (levodopa *[Dopar])*; side effects: hypotension, GI upset; administer on an empty stomach 1/2 to 1 hour before meals
    b. Antiparkinsonian agent (carbidopa *[Lodosyn]*; levodopa *[Dopar]*): side effects: hypokinesia, hyperkinesia, psychiatric manifestations
    c. Dopamine agonist: bromocriptine mesylate *(Parlodel)*
    d. Anticholinergic: (benztropine *[Cogentin]*; trihexylphenidyl *[Artane]*); side effects: dry mouth, mydriases, constipation, confusion
    e. Antiviral, antiparkinsonian: amantadine HCl *(Symmetrel)*; side effects: tremor, rigidity, bradykinesia

E. NURSING INTERVENTIONS
1. Exercise program
2. Speech therapy
3. Maintain nutrition (low protein during day, high protein during evening, semisolid foods)
4. Prevent constipation (add bran and psyllium to diet)
5. Skin and oral care
6. Safety precautions (rubber-soled shoes, low heels, grab bars)
7. Encourage self-care
8. Client teaching: avoid falls; diet, medications
9. Stereotaxic thalamotomy to decrease tremors

Myasthenia Gravis

A. Definition: disorder affecting the neuromuscular transmission of the voluntary muscle of the body; loss of acetylcholine receptors on the postsynaptic membrane of the neuromuscular junction

B. Manifestations
1. Extreme muscular weakness: increased with fatigue and relieved by rest
2. Early manifestations: diplopia, ptosis, dysphagia
3. "Mask-like" facial expression

C. Management
1. Drug therapy (anticholinesterase drugs) that increase the amount of acetylcholine in the neuromuscular function
    a. Pryidostigmine *(Mestinon)*
    b. Ambenonium *(Mytelase)*
    c. Neostigmine *(Prostigmin)*
    d. Atropine is antidote
    e. Steroids (e.g., prednisone *[Datasone]*)
2. Thymectomy (excision of the thymus)
3. Crisis
    a. Cholinergic
    b. Myasthenic
    c. Differentiate between the two with the Tensilon test: edrophonium *(Tensilon)* injected with a response expected in 30 seconds.

D. NURSING INTERVENTIONS
1. Maintain patent airway
2. Plan activities to avoid fatigue
3. Client teaching: action of drugs, manifestations of crisis
4. Give medications on time
5. Avoid quinine and morphine, antibiotics including polymyxins, aminoglycosides, tetracyclines

Meniere's Disease

A. Definition: dilation of the endolymphatic system causing degeneration of the vestibular and cochlear hair cells

B. Manifestations
1. Vertigo
2. Tinnitus
3. Sensorineural loss
4. Pressure in the ear

C. Management

1. Bed rest in position of comfort
2. Salt-free diet
3. Vasodilator
   a. Nicotinic acid
   b. Tolazone HCl *(Priscoline)*
4. Diuretics, antihistamine
5. Sedatives: IV diazepam *(Valium)*
6. Surgical division of vestibular portion of nerve or destruction of labyrinth
7. Meclizine HCl *(Antevert)*
8. Dimenhydrinate *(Dramamine)*

D. NURSING INTERVENTIONS

1. Assist in slowing down movement to avoid attacks
2. Prevent injury during attack
3. Keep room dark when photophobia present
4. Encourage client to stop smoking

Trigeminal Neuralgia (Tic Douloureux)

A. Definition: neurologic disorder specifically affecting the fifth cranial nerve

B. Manifestations

1. Excruciating recurrent paroxysms of sharp, stabbing facial pain along the trigeminal nerve
2. Affects clients in their fifties
3. Shorter intervals between attacks over time

C. Management

1. Administration of antiepileptic drugs carbamazepine *(Tegretol)* and phenytoin *(Dilantin)*
2. Alcohol injection into nerve branches
3. Surgical interventions
   a. Percutaneous radiofrequency trigeminal gangliolysis
   b. Microvascular decompression of trigeminal nerve

D. NURSING INTERVENTIONS

1. Observe and record characteristics of attack
2. Record method client uses to protect face
3. Avoid extremes of heat and cold
   a. Protective eye care
   b. Avoid hot liquids/food
4. Provide oral hygiene

Bell's Palsy (Facial Paralysis)

A. Definition: lower motor neuron lesion of the seventh cranial nerve, resulting in paralysis of one side of the face

B. Manifestations
1. Facial paralysis involving the eye
2. Tearing
3. Painful sensation in the face
4. Spontaneous recovery in 3–5 weeks

C. NURSING INTERVENTIONS
1. Administration of steroids and analgesics
2. Protection of involved eye
3. Promote active facial exercises
4. Oral hygiene
5. Teach to chew on unaffected side

Guillian-Barre Syndrome

A. Definition: an acquired acute inflammatory disease of peripheral nerves resulting in demyelination characterized by ascending, reversible paralysis

B. Manifestations
1. Disease usually preceded by an infection: respiratory or GI
2. Initial manifestations: tingling of the legs that may progress to upper extremities, trunk and facial muscles
3. Progresses to paralysis, respiratory failure
4. Recovery after several months to one year

C. NURSING INTERVENTIONS
1. No specific treatment: directed toward symptoms
2. Monitor respiratory, cardiovascular status
3. Physical therapy, occupational therapy
4. Plasmaphoresis, steroids

Detached Retina

A. Definition: occurs when the sensory retina separates from the pigment epithelium of the retina; vitreous humor fluid flows between the layers when a tear occurs in the retina

B. Manifestations
1. Gaps in vision preceded by sudden flashes of light
2. Feels like a curtain over field of vision

C. **Management**
   1. Immediate bed rest
   2. Avoid coughing, sneezing, straining
   3. Surgical intervention: scleral buckling, photocoagulation, cryosurgery

D. NURSING INTERVENTIONS: (postoperative)
   1. Bed rest with both eyes bandaged for 24 hours
   2. Avoid jarring or bumping head
   3. Client teaching

Cataract

A. **Definition: lens of the eye becomes opaque**

B. **Manifestations**
   1. Visual loss is gradual
   2. Distorted, blurred or hazy vision

C. **Management:** Surgical removal of the lens under local anesthesia, with intraocular lens implant

D. NURSING INTERVENTIONS
   1. Preoperative
      a. Mydriatics
      b. Cycloplegics
   2. Postoperative
      a. Operative eye kept covered
      b. Head of bed elevated 30–45°, do not turn client onto operative side
      c. Client teaching: avoid bending at waist, lifting, sneezing, coughing; keep fingers away from eyes
      d. Prevent vomiting
      e. Report severe pain immediately

Glaucoma

A. **Definition:** increased intraocular pressure; if uncorrected, may lead to atrophy of the optic nerve and eventual blindness

B. **Manifestations**
   1. Acute (closed angle)
      a. Results from an obstruction to the outflow of aqueous humor
      b. Severe pain in and around eye
      c. Lights have a rainbow of colors around them
      d. Cloudy and blurred vision
      e. Pupils dilate

     f.   Nausea and vomiting

     g.   Within hours may develop GI, sinus, neuro, and dental manifestations

  2. Chronic (open angle)

     a.   Insidious onset

     b.   Tired feeling in eye

     c.   Slowly decreasing peripheral vision

     d.   Halos around lights

     e.   Progressive loss of visual field

C. Management

  1. Administer drugs

     a.   Drug action

       1) Pupil contracts, iris is drawn away from cornea

       2) Aqueous humor may drain through lymph spaces (meshwork) into canal of Schlemm

     b.   Types

       1) Pilocarpine hydrochloride *(Pilocar)*; lasts 6–8 hours; drug of choice in glaucoma

       2) Acetazolamide *(Diamox)*; decreases production of aqueous humor; side effect: gastric distress

       3) Mannitol *(Osmitol)*, intravenous (systemic); reduces intraocular pressure by increasing blood osmolality; indications: useful in treatment of acute attacks of pressure and preoperatively

       4) Isosorbid *(Ismoltic)*, oral; cautions: safer than intravenous medication for cardiac clients; may cause diuresis, which is troublesome in men with prostatitis

  2. Surgical care

     a.   Procedures

       1) Iridencleisis

       2) Thermosclerectomy

       3) Trabeculectomy

     b.   Local anesthetic usually used

  3. **NURSING INTERVENTIONS**

     a.   Safety when ambulating

     b.   Liquid or low-residue diet to prevent straining on defecation

     c.   Client teaching

       1) Glaucoma is controllable, not curable

       2) Avoid emotional upsets, constrictive clothing, extreme exertion and lifting, colds

       3) Encourage moderate exercise, regular bowel habits, daily use of medicines, medical check-ups and MedicAlert bracelet

SECTION XI
REVIEW OF ONCOLOGY NURSING

Neoplastic Diseases

A. **Characteristics**
1. Etiology
   a. Healthy cells transformed into malignant cells upon exposure to certain etiological agents: viruses, chemical and physical agents
   b. Failure of immune response
2. Pathophysiology
   a. Rapid cell division
   b. Malignant cells metastasize
      1) Extending directly into adjacent tissue
      2) Permeating along lymphatic vessels
      3) Traveling through lymph system to nodes
      4) Entering blood circulation
      5) Diffusing into body cavity
3. Classification of tumors
   a. Classified according to type of tissue from which they evolve
      1) Carcinomas begin in epithelial tissue (e.g., skin, GI tract lining, lung, breast, uterus)
      2) Sarcomas begin in nonepithelial tissue (e.g., bone, muscle, fat, lymph system)
   b. Type of cell in which they arise; cell type affects appearance, rate of growth, and degree of malignancy (e.g., epithelial basal cells are basal cell carcinoma; bone cells are osteogenic carcinoma; gland epithelium are adenocarcinoma)
4. Staging
   a. Describes extent of tumor
      T = primary tumor
      N = regional nodes
      M = metastasis
   b. Describes extent to which malignancy has increased in size
      T_O = no evidence of primary tumor
      T_{IS} = carcinoma in situ
      T_1, T_2, T_3, T_4 = progressive increase in tumor, size and involvement
      T_X = tumor cannot be assessed
   c. Involvement of regional nodes
      N_O = regional lymph nodes not abnormal
      N_1, N_2, N_3, N_4 = increasing degree of abnormal regional lymph nodes

d. Metastatic development

M_O = no evidence of distant metastasis

M_1, M_2, M_3 = increasing degree of distant metastasis

B. Manifestations Suggesting Malignant Disease (ACS 7 Warning Signs)

1. Change in bowel or bladder habits
2. A sore that does not heal
3. Unusual bleeding or discharge
4. Thickening or lumps in breast or elsewhere
5. Indigestion or difficulty swallowing
6. Obvious change in wart or mole
7. Nagging cough or hoarseness

C. Cancer Therapy

1. Objective: to cure the client and to ensure that minimal functional and structural impairment results from the disease; if cure is not possible:
   a. Prevent further metastasis
   b. Relieve manifestations
   c. Maintain high quality life as long as possible
2. Surgery
   a. Radical
   b. Prophylactic
   c. Palliative
3. Chemotherapy
   a. Drugs interfere with cell division; combination of drugs usually given
   b. Common side effects
      1) Bone marrow depression
      2) Alopecia
      3) GI tract problems
      4) Elevated uric acid, crystal and urate stone formation
   c. Classification of drugs
      1) Alkylating agents: uracil mustard *(Nitrogen mustard)*, cyclophosphamide *(Cytoxan)*
      2) Antimetabolite: 5-FU *(Adrucil)*, methotrexa *(Folex)*
      3) Antibiotics: doxorubian *(Adriamycin)*, bleomycin *(Blenoxane)*, dactinomycin *(Actinomycin D)*
      4) Plant alkaloids: vincristine *(Oncovin)*, vinblastine *(Velban)*
      5) Hormones: estrogen, progesterone
      6) Miscellaneous: procarbazine *(Matulane)*

d. **NURSING INTERVENTIONS**
1) Check often for signs of bleeding or infection
2) Provide emotional support for alteration in body image and grieving
3) Give IV dose slowly to minimize toxicity; discontinue if infiltration
4) Monitor intake and output
5) Force fluids and give allopurinol *(Zyloprim)* to increase uric acid excretion
6) Provide small, frequent meals with high-calorie supplements
7) Practice good oral hygiene
8) Prevent infection

4. Radiation
   a. Purposes
      1) Curative (Hodgkin's disease)
      2) Palliative
      3) Adjunctive
   b. Types
      1) External: gamma rays

      a) **NURSING INTERVENTIONS**
        (1) Client teaching
        (2) Give antiemetic before treatment if nausea a problem; prochlorperazine edisylate *(Compazine)*
        (3) Give pain medication before treatment if needed
        (4) Psychological support
        (5) Skin care: dermatitis 3–6 weeks after start of treatment; teach client to wash with water, avoid lotions, powders, sunlight
        (6) "Wet" reaction: cleanse with warm water; keep open; may use antibiotic cream

    2) Internal: cesium needles

      a) **NURSING INTERVENTIONS**
        (1) Observe time, distance, shielding
        (2) Client teaching
        (3) Bed rest with range of motion exercise
        (4) Foley catheter
        (5) Vital signs every 4 hours
        (6) Clear-liquid or low-residue diet
        (7) If radiation source falls out, do NOT touch it with bare hands—use long forceps and put in lead container
        (8) Observe for GI or GU manifestations or skin problems

TABLE II-16.
NURSING INTERVENTIONS FOR CLIENT ON CHEMOTHERAPY

DRUGS	USES	SIDE EFFECTS	NURSING INTERVENTIONS
fluorouracil (5-FU)	Cancers of GI tract, breast, lung, uterus, ovary	Anorexia, nausea, bone marrow depression	Monitor CBC and platelets
mercaptopurine (6-MP)	Acute leukemia	Bone marrow depression	Monitor CBC and platelets
methotrexatete (Folex) (Amethopterin, MTX)	Acute leukemia	Bone marrow depression	Methotrexatete is excreted through the kidneys, so if renal function is impaired, the drug should not be given
chlorambucil (Leukeran)	Chronic lymphocytic leukemia	Bone marrow depression	Monitor CBC and platelets
cyclophosphamide (Cytoxan)	Acute lymphocytic leukemia	Bone marrow depression	Monitor CBC and platelets
mitomycin (Mutamycin)	Pancreas, stomach, breast cancer	Nausea, vomiting, bone marrow depression, severe skin reaction	Vitamin B_6 may reverse skin reaction
melphalan (Alkeran)	Cancers of the breast, ovary, testicles; multiple melanoma	Unpredictable bone marrow depression, nausea, vomiting, stomatitis	Monitor CBC and platelets; mouth care
vincristine sulfate (Oncovin)	Cancers of the breast and lung; acute leukemia	Alopecia, bone marrow depression	Monitor CBC and platelets; liquid diet for nausea

SECTION XII

REVIEW OF IMMUNOLOGIC DISORDERS

Acquired Immune Deficiency Syndrome (AIDS)

A. **Definition:** infectious disease characterized by severe deficits in cellular immune function; manifested clinically by opportunistic infection and/or unusual neoplasms

1. Etiology: human immunodeficiency virus (HIV)
2. Risk factors
   a. Unprotected intercourse with an infected or high-risk partner
   b. Intravenous drug abusers sharing needles
   c. Blood transfusions (hemophiliacs, surgical clients; blood supply testing for HIV began in 1985)
   d. Babies born to infected mothers

> **KEY INFORMATION**
> The disease has a long incubation period, sometimes up to ten years or more; therefore, manifestations may not appear until late in the infection.

3. Manifestations
   a. Malaise, weight loss
   b. Lymphadenopathy of at least 3 months
   c. Leukopenia (especially T_4 helper cells)
   d. Diarrhea
   e. Fatigue
   f. Night sweats
   g. Presence of opportunistic infections
      1) *Pneumocystis carinii* (major source of mortality)
         a) Cough
         b) Progressive SOB
         c) Low-grade fever
      2) Kaposi's sarcoma
         a) Purple-red raised lesions of internal organs and skin
         b) Poor prognosis
      3) Candidiasis
         a) Fungal infection
         b) Lesions usually in mouth

4) Herpes viruses
   a) Genital and perirectal
   b) Cytomegalovirus (CMV)
5) Cryptococcosis
6) TB
7) Diagnostic tests
   a) ELISA (enzyme linked immunosorbent assay)
   b) Western blot

8) **NURSING INTERVENTIONS**
   a) Respiratory support
      (1) Pulmonary toilet
      (2) Oxygen therapy
   b) Maintain fluid and electrolyte balance
   c) Prevent spread of infection
      (1) Blood and body fluid precautions
      (2) Do not recap needles
      (3) Wear latex gloves to handle body excreta
   d) Emotional support
   e) Skin care
   f) High-nutrition, low-residue meals
   g) Health teaching: abstinence, safer sex practices, monogamy, hand washing, use of condoms
9) Drug therapy
   a) Azidothymidine (AZT)/ zidovudine *(Retrovir)*; side effects: bone marrow depression, anemia
   b) Interferon *(Roferon)*
   c) Pentamidine *(Pentam 300)*
   d) Metronidazole *(Flagyl)* and amphotericin B *(Fungizone)* antifungal agent
   e) Anti-TB drugs as needed
   f) Acyclovir *(Zovirax)* herpes treatment

SECTION XIII

REVIEW OF BURNS

Assessment

A. **Extent of Body Surface**
1. Rule of nines
   a. Head and neck   9%
   b. Anterior trunk   18%
   c. Posterior trunk   18%
   d. Arms (9%)   18%
   e. Legs (18%)   36%
   f. Perineum   1%
2. Pediatric modifications

B. **Depth of Burn**
1. First degree
2. Second degree (partial-thickness)
3. Third degree (full-thickness)

C. **Type of Burn**
1. Thermal
2. Chemical
3. Electrical
4. Radiation

D. **Pre-Existing Physical and Psychological Status of Client**

E. **Concomitant Injuries**

F. **Pulmonary Damage**

Treatment

A. Immediate

1. Stop burning process: stop, drop and roll
2. Airway
3. Cool water for 10 minutes
4. Cover large areas with clean cloth to decrease pain
5. Chemical burns: irrigate copiously
6. Electrical burns: interrupt power source
7. Transport to emergency facility

B. Emergency Room

1. Establish client airway
2. Assessment
   a. Time of injury
   b. How injury occurred
   c. Cause of burn
   d. Treatment
   e. Medical history
   f. Age
   g. Pre-burn weight
3. 100% oxygen if burn occurred in enclosed area
4. Maintain fluid balance
5. Insert Foley catheter
6. Insert NG tube
7. Tetanus toxoid
8. Escharotomy or fasciotomy if needed

C. Hospital Care

1. Maintain airway
2. Maintain aseptic area
3. Provide fluid replacement therapy
   a. Shock phase: 24–48 hours
      1) Fluid shifts from plasma to interstitial space
      2) Hematocrit rises
      3) Metabolic acidosis
      4) Serum K^+ rises
      5) Fluid loss is plasma
      6) Protein loss
      7) Monitor vital signs
      8) Monitor urine output (50–100cc/hr)
      9) Give half of total fluids in first 8 hours

  b. Post-shock phase (diuretic phase)
    1) Capillary permeability stabilizes and fluid shifts from interstitial spaces to plasma
    2) Observe for pulmonary edema
    3) Check vital signs, central venous pressure
    4) Monitor output
    5) Check lab values

D. NURSING INTERVENTIONS
 1. Pain control
  a. Medication
  b. Positioning
 2. Meet nutritional needs
  a. NPO until bowel sounds heard
  b. Caloric needs high: 6,000–8,000 calories
  c. High-protein diet
  d. Prevent stress ulcers: Maalox q 2 hours
 3. Prevent complications
  a. Infection
    1) Asepsis: reverse isolation
    2) Wound care (debridement, hydrotherapy)
    3) Antimicrobial therapy
  b. Contractures and deformities
    1) Range of motion: first post-burn day
    2) Positioning
  c. Respiratory difficulty
    1) Airway
    2) C, T, DB (cough, turn, deep breathe)
    3) Assess for inhalation injury
      a) CO (Carbon monoxide)
      b) SO_2 (Sulfur dioxide)
      c) N_2O_2 (Nitrous oxide)
      d) Toxic fumes
    4) Give oxygen

Methods of Treating Burns

A. **Open Air or Exposure Method**
1. Allows for drainage of burn exudate
2. Eschar forms protective covering
3. Use of topical therapy
4. Skin easily inspected
5. Range of motion easier
6. Asepsis essential
7. Disadvantages
   a. Painful
   b. Heat loss
   c. Difficult to manage burns of hands and feet

B. **Occlusive (Pressure) Dressings**
1. Less pain in first 48 hours, later more painful
2. High incidence of wound sepsis
3. Contractures may occur

C. **Topical Antimicrobial**
1. Silver nitrate *(Keratolytic)*
   a. 0.5 % solution on dressing b.i.d.
   b. Dressings must be moist at all times
   c. Hypokalemia, hyponatremia, hypochloremia
   d. Discolors everything it touches
   e. Poor penetration
   f. Time consuming
2. Mafenide acetate *(Sulfamylon)*
   a. Broad spectrum
   b. Penetrates tissue wall
   c. Never use a dressing
   d. Breakdown of drug provides heavy acid load
   e. Painful
3. Silver sulfadiazine *(Silvadene)*
   a. Broad spectrum includes yeast
   b. Can be washed with water
4. Gentamicin sulfate *(Garamycin):* point 0.1 %
   a. Cream penetrates wall
   b. Nephrotoxic: monitor creatinine levels and BUN

D. Biologic Dressings

1. Allograft: same species, usually cadaver
2. Xenograft, heterograft: animal (pig or dog)
3. Amnion
4. Autograft (self)
   a. Care of donor site
   b. Care of graft site

E. Pressure Dressings

1. Decreases scarring
2. Wear 12–18 months
3. Remove only to bathe

NOTES

UNIT THREE
PSYCHIATRIC NURSING

UNIT CONTENT

SYMBOLS

 Key Points

 Nursing Interventions

 Points to Remember

SECTION I
OVERVIEW

A. **Psychiatric Nursing:** core, heart, basis, art of nursing
1. Interpersonal process
   a. Communication
   b. Caring
2. Goal
   a. Dealing with emotional responses to stress and crisis
   b. Satisfying basic needs
   c. Learning more effective ways of behaving
   d. Developing a healthful life-style
   e. Achieving a realistic and positive self-concept
3. Responsibilities
   a. Therapeutic relationship
   b. Therapeutic environment
4. Uses nursing process
   a. Assessment
   b. Diagnosis
   c. Planning
   d. Implementation
   e. Evaluation
5. Roles
   a. Counselor
   b. Teacher
   c. Advocate
   d. Leader, coordinator, manager

B. **Theoretical Models of Treatment**
1. Medical-biologic theory
   a. Oriented to diagnosing disturbances as diseases with classifiable manifestations
      1) Diagnosis
         a) History
         b) Physical
         c) DSM classification of disorders
      2) Causes
         a) Biochemical
         b) Psychological conditions
         c) Psychophysiological conditions
         d) Structural problems

b. Treatment
      1) Physical or somatic
      2) Interpersonal

   c. **NURSING INTERVENTIONS**
      1) Assist with somatic treatments
      2) Adjunct to doctor in interpersonal treatment and rehabilitation

2. Psychoanalytical model
   a. Oriented to uncovering childhood trauma and repressed feelings that cause conflicts in later life

   KEY INFORMATION
   1) Structure of the mind
      a) Id: contains instinctual primitive drives
      b) Ego: mediates demands of primitive id and self-critical superego
      c) Superego: values and mores that guide behavior
      d) Conscious: ability to recall or remember events without difficulty
      e) Unconscious: memories and thoughts that do not enter awareness

   2) Freud's psychosexual stages
      a) Oral   0–1 years
      b) Anal   1–3 years
      c) Phallic (oedipal)   3–6 years
      d) Latency   6–12 years
      e) Genital   12–young adult

   b. Treatment: clarify meaning of unconscious and conscious events, feelings, and behavior to gain insight
      1) Transference: unconscious projection of feelings onto others
      2) Free association
      3) Dream analysis
      4) Catharsis
   c. Nursing care is supportive rather than therapeutic
      1) Physical needs
      2) Safety needs
      3) Interpersonal and emotional needs

3. Psychosocial developmental model: psychosocial tasks that are accomplished throughout the life cycle
   a. Uses a interdisciplinary approach to treatment; wellness is on a continuum
   b. Types
      1) Developmental model (Erikson)
         a) Stages (see Table III-1.)
         b) Treatment
            (1) Multidisciplinary
            (2) Aim: bring client through stages

TABLE III-1.
ERIKSON'S STAGES OF DEVELOPMENT

STAGES	TASK	BEHAVIOR
Infancy (0–18 mos)	Trust vs Mistrust	Hopefulness, trusting vs Withdrawn, alienated
Early childhood (18 mos–3 yrs)	Autonomy vs Shame, doubt	Self-control vs Compliance and compulsiveness, uncertainty
Late childhood (3–5 yrs)	Initiative vs Guilt	Realistic goals: explores, tests reality vs Strict limits on self-worry
School age (5–12 yrs)	Industry vs Inferiority	Explores, persistent, competes vs Incompetent, low self-esteem
Adolescence (12–20 yrs)	Identity vs Role diffusion	Sense of self vs Confusion, indecision
Young adulthood (20–25 yrs)	Intimacy vs Isolation	Commitment in love/work/play vs Superficial, impersonal
Adulthood (25–65 yrs)	Generativity vs Stagnation	Productivity, caring about others vs Self-centered and indulgent
Old age (65 yrs–death)	Integrity vs Despair	Sense of accomplishment vs Hopelessness, depression

KEY INFORMATION

4. **Basic human needs model (Maslow):** a hierarchy of needs; a belief that needs are fulfilled in a progressive order
    a. Levels
        1) Physical
            a) Air
            b) Food
            c) Sleep
            d) Sexual expression
        2) Safety
            a) Avoiding harm
            b) Feeling secure
        3) Love and belonging
            a) Group identity
            b) Being cared about
            c) Caring for others
            d) Play
        4) Self-esteem
            a) Self-confidence
            b) Self-acceptance
        5) Self-actualization
            a) Self-knowledge
            b) Satisfying, interpersonal relationships
            c) Environmental mastery
            d) Stress management
    b. Treatment
        1) Interdisciplinary: shared roles
        2) Developmental: interpersonal view of the self
        3) Goal: fill needs in progressive manner

    c. **NURSING INTERVENTIONS**
        1) Use needs and psychosocial development for assessment
        2) Help client fulfill needs to relieve stress
        3) Help client advance through stages to become more able to fulfill own needs
        4) Help client develop new behaviors to reduce stress and prevent recurrences of mental illness and dysfunction

5. Behaviorist model (behavior modification)
    a. Changes behavior by using learning theory: replaces nonadaptive behavior with more adaptive behavior
    b. Treatment
        1) Reconditioning: unlearning learned or maladaptive behavior
        2) Reinforcement: increases the probability of behavior recurring
            a) Positive reinforcement: per contract, use rewards to increase or reinforce desired behavior (e.g., adding something such as food, attention, privileges)
            b) Negative reinforcement: per contract, extinguish undesirable behavior by removing aversive consequences (e.g., removal of imposed restrictions)

3) Positive punishment: decrease behavior by adding aversive consequences (e.g., quiet time)

4) Negative punishment: decrease behavior by withdrawing a reward (e.g., privilege such as an outing or calls)

c. Main uses

1) Children

2) Severely regressed individuals

3) Personality disorders

4) Anxiety disorders such as phobias

5) Eating disorders

d. **NURSING INTERVENTIONS**

1) Assess behavior

2) Implement reinforcement/punishment

3) Evaluate progress

6. Community mental health model (psychosocial rehabilitation)

a. Uses interdisciplinary team approach; nurse works as case manager and supervises the team

b. Orientation to countering stress in the community that precipitates psychiatric problems; emphasis is on providing treatment services in the least restrictive setting

c. Treatment

1) Primary prevention: maintenance and promotion of health by teaching (know the risk factors)

2) Secondary prevention: early diagnosis and treatment, here-and-now crisis, partial hospitalization to shorten the duration of the illness

3) Tertiary prevention: rehabilitation, follow-up to avoid permanent disability

c. **NURSING INTERVENTIONS**

1) Holistic care

2) Problem oriented using the nursing process

3) Primary, secondary, tertiary prevention

C. Treatment Modes

1. Crisis intervention

a. Definitions

1) Crisis intervention: brief treatment used to help clients cope with or adapt to stressors

2) Crisis: an acute, disequilibrating event in one's life when previous methods of problem solving are ineffective

b. Type of crisis

1) Situational (unanticipated)

2) Transitional (maturational, anticipated)

3) Cultural/social

c. Characteristics of stress

1) Physiological manifestations

2) Feelings of panic, fear, helplessness, impending doom

3) Decreased concentration and efficiency

     d. Principles of intervention
       1) Time limited (6–8 weeks)
       2) Promptness
       3) Focus on problem directly, not causes
       4) One-on-one discussion; speak openly/directly
       5) Need for support and empathy
       6) Calm, controlled atmosphere
       7) Client's responsibility to act
       8) Assess and help client use strengths and positive coping skills
       9) Collaborative effort
       10) Use all available community support
       11) Provide sense of mastery; discuss alternatives to current situation

2. Group therapy
     a. Definition: collection of individuals interacting together with a shared purpose
     b. Dynamics and concepts
       1) Process: what is said, done, or implied through actions such as nonverbal behavior allows individual feedback from other members
       2) Content: work is done to problem solve and fulfill the group functions
       3) Cohesiveness: feeling of belonging, helpfulness, problem solving, sharing
       4) Norms: standards of behavior adhered to by group
       5) Leadership: stimulate interaction so that a maximum number participate and keep the group to the goal/task
         a) Set limits
         b) Here and now; direct to current issues
         c) Provide safety
         d) Provide consistency
         e) Role model
         f) Clarifies
       6) Size and composition
         a) Seven to 10 participants is ideal
         b) Comfortable environment (physical and psychological)
         c) Homogeneous or heterogeneous
         d) 45 to 60 minute sessions

3. Types of groups
     a. Task groups
     b. Teaching groups
     c. Supportive/therapeutic
     d. Psychotherapy
     e. Peer support
     f. Self-help groups
       1) 12 Step (AA, Al-anon, Alateen, OE)
       2) Recovery, Inc.
       3) Ostomy Clubs

4. Family therapy
     a. Definition: psychotherapy in which the focus is on the family as the unit of treatment, not just one individual

    b. Concepts
       1) Systems approach: member with the manifestations/illness
       2) Scapegoating: the object of blame or displaced aggression, usually one member of the family
       3) Family involvement is necessary for treatment

    c. **NURSING INTERVENTIONS**
       1) Focus on family as a whole
       2) Empathize
       3) Help family clarify ambiguous communication patterns (e.g., double-bind)
       4) Help family change roles, rules, communication patterns
       5) Help family accept differences among members
       6) Teach family problem-solving techniques

5. Milieu therapy
    a. Definition: management of the client's environment to promote a positive living experience and facilitate recovery
    b. Concepts
       1) Individualized treatment plans
       2) Clients are involved in the therapeutic community
       3) Client government: groups and meetings between client and staff to promote shared responsibility and cooperation
       4) The environment in the facility is as close to the "real world" as possible and has potential for therapeutic value

    c. **NURSING INTERVENTIONS**
       1) Guidance in developing new ways of relating and learning to cope more effectively
       2) Helping client maintain strengths
       3) Manipulation of the environment for optimal benefit
       4) Management of day-to-day activities
       5) Management of staff through conferences, staffing, and supervision

6. Expressive therapy
    a. Definition: adjunctive therapies used to aid assessment, increase social skills, encourage expression of feelings and provide opportunities to raise self-esteem, relieve tension and be creative
    b. Types
       1) Dance: movement
       2) Recreational: picnic, volleyball
       3) Occupational: painting, hand work
       4) Art: clay, painting, drawing

    c. **NURSING INTERVENTIONS**
       1) Support and encourage client participation
       2) Communicate with staff regarding needs, interests, and any behavioral changes
       3) Support expressive therapy staff

D. Mental Health/Mental Illness Continuum (see Table III-2.)

1. Mental health
   a. Positive attitude toward self
   b. Growth, development, self-actualization
   c. Integration
   d. Autonomy
   e. Reality perception
   f. Environment mastery

2. Mental illness
   a. Problems due to stress
   b. Maladaptive behavior
   c. Disruption in ability to relate successfully with others
   d. Inability to meet basic needs in a socially acceptable way

TABLE III-2.
MENTAL HEALTH/ILLNESS CONTINUUM

ADAPTIVE		MALADAPTIVE
Healthy	◄— Neurosis —►	Psychosis
Adaptive coping (confrontation)	◄————————————►	Maladaptive coping: withdrawal or aggressiveness
Reality oriented (x3)	◄————————————►	Psychotic: denies reality, creates new environment
Interacts with real environment	◄————————————►	Hallucination/delusion
Socially acceptable behavior; insight	◄————————————►	Bizarre behavior (gesturing, posturing); little insight

3. Defense mechanisms
   a. Definition: unconscious operations used to defend against anxiety/stress and relieve emotional conflict
   b. In contrast, coping mechanisms are conscious efforts to deal with daily frustrations and conflicts

KEY INFORMATION

   c. Types
      1) Sublimation: directing energy from unacceptable drives into socially acceptable behavior (e.g., aggressive person becomes a star football player)
      2) Isolation: splitting-off response in which person blocks feeling associated with unpleasant experience (e.g., planning out funeral details of a loved one)
      3) Reaction formation: involves displaying overt behavior or attitudes in precisely the opposite direction of unacceptable conscious or unconscious impulses (e.g., feeling compassion for a person you dislike)

4) Undoing: a compulsive response that negates or reverses a previous unacceptable act (e.g., washing hands [of guilt] after touching germs)

5) Compensation: putting forth extra effort to achieve in areas real or imagined deficiency (e.g., an unpopular student excels as a scholar)

6) Projection: attributing own thoughts or impulses to another person (e.g., "You made me take a wrong turn.")

7) Introjection: incorporating the traits of others (e.g., a depressed client causes the nurse to become depressed)

8) Suppression: the conscious, deliberate forgetting of unacceptable or painful thoughts, impulses, acts

9) Repression: unconscious, involuntary forgetting of unacceptable or painful thoughts, impulses, feelings, or actions (e.g., forgetting what was on a difficult exam)

10) Denial: avoidance of disagreeable reality by ignoring or refusing to recognize it

11) Rationalization: offering a socially acceptable or logical explanation for otherwise unacceptable impulses, feelings, and behaviors (e.g., "I failed the NCLEX-RN because it is a poor test.")

12) Regression: going back to an early level of emotional development (e.g., becoming dependent on someone else for all decisions)

13) Displacement: transferring painful feelings to a neutral object (e.g., you're angry at your brother so you kick the dog)

14) Identification: the unconscious adoption of characteristics of another, generally someone who possesses attributes that are admired or envied

15) Splitting: viewing people as all good or all bad; failure to integrate positive and negative qualities

E. **Nurse/Client Relationship:** an interpersonal, collaborative helping process and organized sequence of events leading towards an identified goal
　1. Characteristics
　　a. Interpersonal; mutual growth
　　b. Helping
　　c. Organized sequence of events
　　d. Goal directed
　　e. Collaborative: contract that outlines and clarifies role expectations
　　f. Professional vs social: goal directed vs reciprocal
　　g. Designated setting and time
　　h. Confidential
　2. Phases of the nurse/client relationship
　　a. Preinteraction phase
　　　1) Gather data from secondary sources
　　　2) No prejudgement
　　　3) Assess nurse's feelings
　　　4) Assess client's feelings

b. Orientation phase: assessment
1) Introduction: purpose, roles, responsibilities
2) Establish trust
   a) Honest
   b) Nonjudgmental
   c) Empathetic
   d) Offer self
3) Assess client
   a) Orientation
   b) Activities of daily living (degree of ability to perform)
   c) Physical status
   d) Memory (recent and remote)
   e) Emotional state
   f) Intellectual capacity
   g) Family history
   h) Spiritual history
   i) Alcohol and drug history (OTC and prescription)
   j) Presenting problem
4) Formulate contract
   a) Time of meeting
   b) Confidentiality
   c) Focus: goals that are behaviorally stated
c. Working phase: planning/intervention
1) Establish specific collaborative goals
2) Explore thoughts, feelings, actions
3) Establish nursing diagnosis
4) Problem solve

KEY INFORMATION
5) Communication tools
   a) Listening: nonverbal, use eye contact
   b) Offering self: "I'll stay with you."
   c) Focusing: on "here and now" and on the client
   d) Broad openings: "How are things going today?"
   e) Clarifying: "What does that mean to you?"
   f) Sharing, perceptions: "You seem angry."
   g) Reflecting: directing back ideas, feelings, and content, "You feel tense when you fight."
   h) Restate: repeat the main thought, "You are sad."
   i) Validating: "Are you saying . . ."
   j) Empathy: stating a feeling implied by the client
   k) Giving information
   l) Silence: sitting, conveying nonverbal interest, and involvement
   m) Summarizing

6) Blocks to communication
   a) False reassurance: "Don't worry."
   b) Agreeing and disagreeing: "I think you did the right thing."
   c) Advice: "You should . . ."
   d) Judging: "That was good."
   e) Belittling: "Everyone feels like that."
   f) Defending: "All the doctors here are great."
   g) Approval: good or bad
   h) Focus on nurse: "I feel that way, too."
   i) Changing the subject
   j) Ignoring a client
   k) Changing client's words or assuming feelings

d. Termination phase: evaluation
   1) Evaluation of behavioral goals
   2) Transfer to other support systems
   3) Assess for separation reactions such as regression, acting out, anger, withdrawal
   4) Help express and work through feelings
   5) Be alert to nurse's response to separation
   6) Do not promise to continue the relationship or schedule future appointments
   7) Termination begins on admission; prepare the client from the first contact

SECTION II
ANXIETY

A. **Definition:** tension in response to a perceived physical or psychological threat (internal or external)

B. **Responses**
   1. Psychological
      a. Fear
      b. Impending doom
      c. Helplessness
      d. Insecurity
      e. Low self-confidence
      f. Anger
      g. Guilt
   2. Defense mechanisms
      a. Displacement
      b. Regression
      c. Repression
      d. Sublimation
   3. Physiological: nervous system
      a. Dry mouth
      b. Elevated vital signs
      c. Diarrhea
      d. Increased urination
      e. Palpitations
      f. Diaphoresis
      g. Hyperventilation
      h. Fatigue
      i. Insomnia
      j. Sexual dysfunction
      k. Irritability
      l. Fidgeting, pacing
   4. Behaviors
      a. Fight or flight response
      b. Talkative, giggly, angry, withdrawn

C. Levels of Anxiety (see Table III-3.)

TABLE III-3.
LEVELS OF ANXIETY

LEVEL	PHYSIOLOGIC RESPONSE	COGNITIVE STATE	BEHAVIORAL CHANGES	NURSING INTERVENTIONS
Mild (+)	Slight discomfort, restlessness; tension relief; fidgeting, tapping	Perceptual field can be heightened; learning can occur	*Restlessness (ability work toward goal) * Examine alternatives	* Listen * Promote insight, problem solving
Moderate (++)	Increased pulse, respirations, shakiness, voice tremors, difficulty concentrating	Perceptual field narrows; selective in attention	* Focus on immediate events * Benefits from guidance of others	* Calm, rational discussion * Relaxation exercises
Severe (+++)	Elevated BP, tachycardia, somatic complaints, hyperventilation, confusion	Perceptual field greatly reduced; attention scattered; cannot attend to events even when pointed out	Feelings of increasing threat; purposeless activity * Impending doom	* Listen * Encourage expression of feelings * Concrete activity (channel energy into simple tasks)
Panic (++++)	Immobility or severe hyper-activity; cool, clammy skin; pallor; dilated pupils; severe shakiness * Prolonged anxiety can lead to exhaustion	Perceptual field closed * Hallucinations or delusions may occur * Effective decision making is impossible	Mute or psychomotor agitation * May strike out physically or withdraw	* Isolate from stimuli * Stay with client * Very calm * Decrease demands * Protect client safety
* Important				

D. Maladaptive Responses to Anxiety

1. Anxiety disorders: characterized by fear that is out of proportion to external events; attacks lasting minutes to hours

    a. Panic disorders

        1) Definition: sudden onset of intense apprehension, fear or terror (panic attacks)

        2) Physical manifestations

            a) Dyspnea

            b) Palpitations

            c) Chest pain

            d) Faintness, dizziness

            e) Fear of dying or going crazy (out of control)

            f) Choking

            g) Depersonalization or derealization

            h) Hyperventilation

3) **NURSING INTERVENTIONS**
   a) Stay with client and remain calm
   b) Reassurance and support
   c) Remove stimuli
   d) Deep breaths
   e) Distraction
   f) Paper bag

b. Phobic disorders
   1) Definition: persistent or irrational fear of a specific object, activity, or situation that leads to avoidance
   2) Types
      a) Agoraphobia: fear of being away from a safe place or person in which there is no escape
      b) Simple: irrational fear of object or situation
      c) Social: fear of situations that expose
   3) Defense mechanisms
      a) Repression
      b) Displacement
      c) Avoidance

4) **NURSING INTERVENTIONS**
   a) Verbalizing thoughts/feelings
   b) Relaxation
   c) Avoid major decision making
   d) No competitive situations
   e) Behavior modifications
   f) Gradual desensitization

c. Obsessive compulsive disorders
   1) Definition: recurring obsessions or compulsions
      a) Obsessions: recurring thoughts of violence, contamination, doubt, and worry that cannot be voluntarily removed from consciousness.
      b) Compulsions: recurring, irresistible impulse to perform acts (e.g., touching, rearranging, checking, opening and closing, washing)
   2) Defense mechanisms
      a) Displacement
      b) Undoing
      c) Isolation
      d) Reaction formation
   3) Characteristics
      a) Irrational coping to handle guilt
      b) Feelings of inferiority
      c) Compulsion to repeat act
      d) Repeating act prevents severe anxiety

4) **NURSING INTERVENTIONS**
   a) Distract: substitute
   b) Do not interrupt compulsive act
   c) Allow time to complete ritual; gradually decrease the time and number of times ritual performed
   d) Provide safety
   e) Maintain structure, schedules, activities
   f) Demonstrate acceptance of individual
   g) Encourage expression of feelings
   h) Antianxiety medications may be used to relieve manifestations

2. Somatoform disorders: physical manifestations and complaints without organic impairment
   a. Conversion disorders (hysteria)
      1) Definition: alteration in physical function that is an expression of a psychological need
      2) Characteristics of manifestations
         a) Sensory: blindness, deafness, loss of sensation in extremities
         b) Motor: mutism, paralysis of extremities, ataxia, dizziness
         c) Visceral: headaches, difficulty breathing
         d) Convulsive disorder with atypical seizure response
         e) Little concern about manifestations: la belle indifference
         f) Usually one major manifestation
         g) Defense mechanism: repression of conflict and conversion of anxiety into manifestations
         h) Primary gain: suppressing conflict
         i) Secondary gain: sympathy or avoidance of unpleasant activity gained

      3) **NURSING INTERVENTIONS**
         a) Redirect away from manifestations
         b) Encourage expression of feelings
         c) Alternatives for dealing with stress
         d) Stress reduction techniques
         e) Relaxation techniques
         f) Counter secondary gain by involving client in activities of daily living

   b. Hypochondriasis
      1) Definition: exaggerated preoccupation with physical health, not based on real organic disorders
      2) Characteristics
         a) Multiple manifestations
         b) Worried/anxious about manifestations
         c) Seeks medical care frequently

      3) **NURSING INTERVENTIONS**
         a) Help client express feelings
         b) Set limits on rumination
         c) Do not feed into the manifestations

3. Psychophysiological/psychosomatic disorders
   a. Definition: stress-related medical disorders; psychosocial factors predispose client to episodes of illness and influence the progression of manifestations; can be fatal if not treated adequately
   b. Defense mechanisms
      1) Repression
      2) Introjection
   c. Types
      1) Migraine
      2) Ulcerative colitis
      3) Peptic ulcer
      4) Eczema
      5) Cancer

   d. **NURSING INTERVENTIONS**
      1) Care for physical signs
      2) Provide attention and security
      3) Help client express feelings
      4) Teach problem solving so client may gain control
      5) Relaxation techniques (e.g., biofeedback imagery, progressive relaxation)
      6) Life-style changes

4. Dissociative disorders (hysterical neuroses)
   a. Definition: splitting off an idea or emotion from one's consciousness; "psychological flight" from anxiety
   b. Types
      1) Multiple personality
      2) Psychogenic fugue
      3) Psychogenic amnesia
      4) Depersonalization

   c. **NURSING INTERVENTIONS**
      1) Assessment to rule out organic pathology
      2) Help client recognize when dissociation occurs
      3) Help client link thoughts, feelings, and behavior
      4) Individual, group, and family psychotherapy

5. Expressive therapy for maladaptive responses to anxiety
   a. Client with poor concentration: group work, simple tasks
   b. Client with hyperactivity: decrease external stimuli, one-to-one interaction, walks, uncompetitive activities

6. Somatic treatment for maladaptive responses to anxiety, insomnia, and stress-related conditions
   a. Antianxiety agents: anxiolytic, minor tranquilizers (see Table III-4.)

TABLE III-4.
ANTIANXIETY AGENTS AND SIDE EFFECTS

CHEMICAL CLASS	GENERIC NAME	TRADE NAME	DAILY DOSE
Benzodiazepine compounds	chlordiazepoxide	*Librium*	15 –100 mg
	diazepam	*Valium*	5 – 40 mg
	oxazepam	*Serax*	15 –120 mg
	clorazepate	*Tranxene*	7.5– 60 mg
	lorazepam	*Ativan*	1 – 6 mg
	alprazolam	*Xanax*	.5– 4 mg
	clonazepam	*Klonopin*	.5– 2 mg
Mephenesin-like compounds	meprobamate	*Miltown* *Equanil*	800–1,600 mg
Sedating antihistamines	hydroxyzine	*Vistaril* *Atarax*	75–400 mg
Beta-blockers	propranolol	*Inderal*	
Anxiolytics	buspirone	*BuSpar*	30–60 mg

SIDE EFFECTS	NURSING INTERVENTION
1. Dry mouth	1. Provide candies, fluids
2. Blurred vision	2. Will disappear within a week
3. Urinary retention	3. Monitor intake and output; for distention, run water
4. Drowsiness/sedation	4. Instruct client not to operate machines; do not give with other CNS depressants
5. Ataxia	5. Use side rails if needed; stay with client if out of bed
6. Tremors	6. Observe severity
7. Hypotension	7. Take frequent BP
8. Tolerance	8. Observe for proper usage and effect; withdraw gradually

DRUG INTERACTIONS
- CNS depressants—action potentiated; avoid alcohol
- Tolerance does develop; discontinue slowly to minimize symptoms & rebound symptoms of insomnia or anxiety
- Elderly more vulnerable to side effects/safety risk
- Possible paradoxical reactions in children/elderly

SECTION III
SCHIZOPHRENIA

A. **Definition:** group of psychotic disorders characterized by regression, thought disturbances (including delusions and hallucinations), bizarre dress and behavior, poverty of speech, abnormal motor behavior, and withdrawal

B. **Overview**
   1. Bleuler's four A's
      a. Autism: preoccupation with self and inner experience
      b. Affect: feeling tone is flat, blunted or inappropriate
      c. Ambivalence: conflicting strong feelings that may confuse, frighten or immobilize
      d. Loose association: disrupted/disorganized thinking
   2. Appearance: disheveled
   3. Other major manifestations
      a. Delusions: fixed false beliefs; can be paranoid, grandiose, or somatic delusions
      b. Hallucinations: sensory perceptions without any environmental stimuli (e.g., hearing voices, seeing spiders, smelling foul)
      c. Illusions: misidentification of actual environmental stimuli; client may see an electrical cord as a snake
      d. Ideas of reference: personalizing environmental stimuli (e.g., client believes static on telephone is wiretapping)
      e. Neologisms: made up words
      f. Circumstantiality: can't come to point, includes nonessential details
      g. Blocking: interrupt flow of speech due to distracting thoughts, words, ideas, subjects
      h. Regressive behavior: behavior appropriate at earlier stage of development
      i. Poor interpersonal relationships
      j. Declining ability to work, socialize and care for self
   4. Characteristics and defense mechanisms
      a. Depersonalization: feel alienated from self, no ego boundaries
      b. Projection
      c. Regression
      d. Denial
      e. Fantasy world

C. **Schizophrenic Disorders**
   1. Types
      a. Disorganized: incoherent, severe thought disturbance, shallow, inappropriate, often silly behavior and mannerisms

    b. Catatonic
        1) Stupor: lessening of response
        2) Excitement: increase in activity
        3) Waxy flexibility: bizarre posturing
        4) Negativism: doing the opposite of what is being asked
        5) Mutism: continuous refusal to speak
    c. Paranoid
        1) Hallucination: grandiose or persecutory
        2) Delusions: persecution and grandeur
        3) Emotions: angry, suspicious, argumentative, mistrust, excessive religiosity
    d. Undifferentiated
        1) Mixed characteristics
        2) Meets criteria of more than one type
    e. Residual
        1) Has had acute episode of illness in past
        2) Not overtly psychotic or displaying positive manifestations
        3) May demonstrate negative manifestations

2. **NURSING INTERVENTIONS**
    a. Physical care
    b. Safety
    c. Increase trust
    d. Increase self-esteem
    e. Orient to reality
    f. Provide structure to the day
    g. Involve family
    h. Interactions should be simple and concrete; often nonverbal and short
    i. Help work through regressive behavior
    j. Decrease bizarre behavior, anxiety, agitation, aggression
    k. Deal with hallucinations
        1) Distraction
        2) Do not confront
        3) Point out that you do not share the same perception
        4) Get to feeling level
        5) Avoid being alone (client will hallucinate more)
        6) Engage in activities (e.g., current events discussion groups)

D. Paranoid Personality Disorder

1. Definition: insidious development of a permanent and unshakable delusional system accompanied by preservation of clear and orderly thinking

2. Characteristics

   a. Projection: unacceptable feelings are attributed to others
   b. Delusions of grandeur and/or persecution
   c. Ideas of reference (e.g., personalizing environmental stimuli)
   d. Resistance to treatment
   e. Loneliness and distrust
   f. Refusal to eat
   g. Suspiciousness and fear
   h. Emotional expressions are appropriate to content of delusional system
   i. Argumentative and hostile

3. **NURSING INTERVENTIONS**

   a. Persecutory delusions
      1) Do not argue or confront
      2) Interject reality when appropriate
      3) Get to feeling level
      4) Discuss topics other than delusions
   b. Aggression and hostility
      1) Monitor
      2) Help client express self verbally
      3) Set limits and offer alternatives
      4) Provide outlets for aggression
      5) Remind client of consequences of inappropriate behavior
      6) Keep a distance
      7) Have back up
      8) Don't respond with aggression; use calm, controlled tone
      9) Use speed
      10) Use direct, simple statements
      11) Decrease stimulation with time out or seclusion
      12) Medication
      13) Keep other clients away
      14) Seclude if necessary
   c. Fear of being poisoned
      1) Serve food in containers
      2) Medications should be wrapped or in containers
      3) Do not covertly put meds in juice
      4) Open meds in presence of client
   d. Attitude of superiority
      1) Small groups, ratio of one nurse to one client
      2) Activities that ensure success
      3) Limits without judging
      4) Increase self esteem
      5) Descale, talk about feelings

E. Pervasive Developmental Disorders

1. Autistic disorders
   a. Characteristics
      1) Lack of interest in human contact
      2) Obsessional attachments to inanimate objects
      3) Compulsive need for following routines
      4) No or abnormal social play
      5) Impaired in ability to form peer relationships
      6) Autoerotic behavior (rocking, excessive masturbation)
      7) Abnormal nonverbal communication
      8) Abnormal production of speech and content
      9) Impaired ability to sustain a conversation
      10) Self-mutilation (e.g., head banging)
      11) Distressed by slight environmental changes
      12) Restricted range of interest

   b. **NURSING INTERVENTIONS**
      1) Assess social and physical aspects of client
      2) Assess family understanding and coping
      3) Facilitate communication (verbal and/or nonverbal)
      4) Goal: maintain optimum level of functioning and prevent regression
      5) Techniques to use
         a) Story telling
         b) Painting
         c) Poetry
         d) Imitation
      6) Prioritize care
         a) Safety
         b) Communication
         c) Re-education
      7) Involve and educate family

2. Attention-deficit/hyperactivity disorder
   a. Characteristics
      1) Fails to complete task
      2) Easily distracted
      3) Difficulty concentrating
      4) Acts before thinking, impulsive
      5) Has difficulty sitting still
      6) Does not seem to listen
      7) May talk incessantly

   b. **NURSING INTERVENTIONS**
      1) Assist to communicate effectively
      2) Set stage for improving ego function
      3) Help learn more adaptive coping behaviors
      4) Techniques to use
         a) Play therapy
         b) Cognitive-behavioral
         c) Family therapy
         d) Psychopharmacology (methylphenidate *[Ritalin]*)

F. **Medications:** Antipsychotics (For Schizophrenic and Paranoid Behavior Patterns)
   1. Block dopamine receptors
      a. Target positive manifestations
         1) Negativism
         2) Combativeness
         3) Disorganization
         4) Hallucinations, delusions
         5) Hostility
         6) Suspiciousness
         7) Seclusiveness
         8) Self-care deficits
      b. Negative manifestations not affected
         1) Apathy
         2) Withdrawal
         3) Insight
         4) Lack of interest
         5) Blunted affect
         6) Judgement
   2. Antipsychotic agents (major tranquilizers or neuroleptic agents) (see Table III-5.)

TABLE III-5.
ANTIPSYCHOTIC AGENTS AND SIDE EFFECTS

CHEMICAL CLASS	GENERIC NAME	TRADE NAME	DOSAGE
Phenothiazine, aliphatic	chlorpromazine	*Thorazine*	30–1,200 mg
Phenothiazine, piperidine	thioridazine, mesoridazine	*Mellaril* *Serentil*	30–600 mg 100–400 mg
Phenothiazine, piperazine	fluphenazine perphenazine trifluoperazine	*Prolixin* *Trilafon* *Stelazine*	5–20 mg 6–24 mg 2–20 mg
Thioxanthene, piperazine	thiothixene	*Navane*	6–60 mg
Butyrophenone	haloperidol	*Haldol*	6–20 mg
Dihydroindolone	molindone	*Moban*	150–225 mg
Dibenzoxazepine	loxapine clozapine	*Loxitane* *Clozaril*	60–100 mg 300–600 mg
Benzisoxazole	risperidone	*Risperdal*	1–4 mg
Thienobenzo diazepine	olanzopine	*Zyprexia*	5–15 mg

SIDE EFFECTS	NURSING INTERVENTIONS
Sedation	Most common in low-potency antipsychotics; ask physician if entire dose can be given at bedtime
Extrapyramidal effects: parkinsonian symptoms (e.g., fine hand tremors, pill rolling, drooling, muscle stiffness)	Report to the physician; specific medication may be changed; antiparkinsonian medication is given to control manifestations
Dystonias: muscle spasm of the face and neck; eyes rolling back in head	Report to physician; usually an antiparkinsonian medication is given (P.O., IM, or IV) and the antipsychotic medication changed
Akathesia: restlessness, inability to sit still	Call physician; if treated with antiparkinsonian medications, may need to change antipsychotic medication
Tardive dyskinesia: lip smacking, sucking, tongue protrusion, jerking of the head and neck, extension and flexion of the fingers, back and forth movement of spine, movement of the arms	Careful observation in early steps of treatment; discontinue medication at first sign to prevent permanent disability
Anticholinergic • Dry mouth	Provide candies, fluids
• Constipation	Laxatives, diet
• Urinary retention	Monitor intake and output
• Blurred vision	Client teaching: will disappear within a week
• Nasal congestion	Increase humidity (showers help)
Hypotension	Monitor BP frequently, sitting and standing; caution client to stand up slowly

TABLE III-5.
ANTIPSYCHOTIC AGENTS AND SIDE EFFECTS (CONTINUED)

SIDE EFFECTS	NURSING INTERVENTIONS
Photosensitivity	Sunscreen; cover up with clothing
Agranulocytosis	Observe for sign of infection and report immediately if present; discontinue medication
Retinopathy	Sunglasses
Neuroleptic malignant syndrome	Discontinue medication and report immediately if manifestations occur (altered consciousness, unstable BP&P, fever, muscle rigidity, diaphoresis and tremors)
Endocrine Breast enlargement	Yearly breast exams
Decreased libido; ejaculatory imcompetence	Decrease dose or change to high-potency drugs
Appetite increase, weight gain	Exercise/diet regimen

DRUG INTERACTIONS
MAO inhibitors Anticonvulsives CNS depressants Lithium

1. Drugs to control extrapyramidal reaction (CNS)
    a. Commonly used
        1) Trihexyphenidyl *(Artane)*
        2) Benztropine Mesylate *(Cogentin)*
        3) Procyclidine *(Kemadrin)*
        4) Biperiden *(Akineton)*
    b. Side effects: anticholinergic
        1) Blurred vision
        2) Dry mouth
        3) Constipation
        4) Urinary retention
        5) Drowsiness
        6) Nervousness
    c. General information
        1) Geriatric information
        2) Abuse potential

SECTION IV
MOOD DISORDERS AND ASSOCIATED BEHAVIORS

A. Depression and Elation

1. Definition
   a. Depression: mood state of gloom, despondency, and dejection with accompanying physical, cognitive and behavioral responses
   b. Mania: predominant mood is elevated; great amount of activity
2. Continuum of emotional responses (see Table III-6.)

TABLE III-6.
CONTINUUM OF EMOTIONAL RESPONSES

ADAPTIVE RESPONSES		MALADAPTIVE RESPONSES
Sadness Grief	Dysthymic Cyclothymic Reactive Exogenous	Major depression Bipolar disorder Endogenous
No treatment ——————— Psychotherapy ——————— Medications		
Duration of illness increases ————————————————⟶		

3. Range and severity of moods
   a. Grief: takes 2 years for full recovery; a normal process
      1) Precipitating factors
         a) Death in family
         b) Separation
         c) Divorce
         d) Physical illness
         e) Work failure
         f) Disappointment
      2) Stages (Kubler-Ross)
         a) Denial
         b) Anger
         c) Bargaining
         d) Depression
         e) Acceptance

3) **NURSING INTERVENTIONS**
   a) Acceptance
   b) Encourage expression of feelings
   c) Help through

4) Unresolved grief produces psychotic and neurotic manifestations such as chronic depression, psychosomatic disorders, acting out behavior

b. Moderate mood disorders
   1) Types
      a) Dysthymia: chronically depressed mood
      b) Cyclothymic: cycles of depression and hypomania (not as severe as mania)
   2) Characteristics: depression (dysthymia)
      a) Pessimism
      b) Insomnia or hypersomnia
      c) Social withdrawal
      d) Feelings of worthlessness, not caring, little pleasure, irritability
      e) Low energy level

c. Severe mood disorders
   1) Major depression
      a) Weight gain or loss of over 10 pounds
      b) Sleep disturbances
      c) Loss of pleasure or interest in usual activities, including sex
      d) Low energy, fatigue
      e) Feelings of helplessness and hopelessness
      f) Decreased concentration
      g) Psychomotor retardation or agitation
      h) Anger turned inward
      i) Cannot make decisions
      j) Suicidal ideation
      k) Delusional about guilt, unworthiness, sin
      l) Social withdrawal
      m) Persistent physical manifestation such as headaches, digestive disorders, chronic pain
      n) Pack of self care
   2) Mania's characteristics: client may be or display
      a) Extroverted
      b) Flight of ideas
      c) Accelerated speech
      d) Accelerated motor activity
      e) Anger turned outward
      f) Impulsive
      g) Arrogant, demanding, controlling behavior with underlying feelings of vulnerability and inadequacy
      h) Delusions of grandeur

d. **NURSING INTERVENTIONS**
1) Depression
a) Structure environment and time; promote client's physical well being
b) Safety: suicide precautions
c) Communication to decrease loneliness
d) Reestablish sleep patterns
e) Set limits on behavior
f) Build trust, short frequent visits
g) Discourage decision making; increase skill slowly
h) Schedule nonintellectual activities such as leather work, sanding
i) Encourage goal setting to provide success
2) Mania
a) Provide for physical welfare
b) Frequent small feedings, finger foods
c) Safety: protect from impulsive activity
d) Reduce external stimuli (client responds to environment)
e) Communicate calmly
f) Milieu activities such as walks, ball tossing, creative writing, and drawing; avoid competitive games

e. Suicide
1) Definition: self-imposed death steming from depression, especially hopelessness and negative feelings about the future
2) High risk groups: depressed, hallucinating, delusional, organic mental disorders, substance abusers, adolescents, chronic or painful illness, elderly, sexual identity conflicts
3) Danger signs
a) Specific plan
b) Giving away personal items, completing wills, finalizing personal/business matters
c) Making amends
d) Change in behavior in a depressed client
e) Gesture or history of attempt
f) Verbal statement

4) **NURSING INTERVENTIONS**
a) Crisis intervention
b) Take all gestures seriously
c) Suicide precautions
(1) Stay with client
(2) Safety contract
(3) Remove sharp and harmful objects
d) Personal contact providing care, concern, neutral tone, hope, goals
e) Provide diversional activities with increasing numbers of people

B. Treatments

1. Antidepressant agents
   a. Thymoleptic agents (see Table III-7.)
   b. MAO inhibitors (see Table III-8.)
2. Antimania agents/mood stabilizers (see Table III-9.)

TABLE III-7.
ANTIDEPRESSANT AGENTS: THYMOLEPTIC AGENTS

CHEMICAL CLASS	GENERIC NAME	TRADE NAME	DOSAGE
Tricyclic antidepressants	imipramine	*Tofranil*	50–300 mg
	desipramine	*Norpramin*	75–300 mg
	amitriptyline	*Elavil*	50–300 mg
	nortriptyline	*Aventyl*	20–150 mg
	protriptyline	*Vivactil*	15– 60 mg
	doxepin	*Sinequan*	75–300 mg
	amoxapine	*Asendin*	150–300 mg
Tetracyclic antidepressant	maprotiline	*Ludiomil*	75–300 mg
Newer antidepressants	trazodone	*Desyrel*	50–600 mg
	bupropion HCl	*Wellbutrin*	300–450 mg
	fluoextine	*Prozac*	20– 80 mg
	sertraline	*Zoloft*	50–200 mg
	paroxetine	*Paxil*	20– 50 mg
	venlafaxine HCL	*Effexor*	75–225 mg

TABLE III-7.
ANTIDEPRESSANT AGENTS: THYMOLEPTIC AGENTS (CONTINUED)

SIDE EFFECTS	NURSING INTERVENTIONS
Anticholinergic effects	
Dry mouth	Increase fluids, good oral hygiene
Constipation	Bulk, diet, exercise, stool softeners
Urinary retention	Urecholine, monitor intake and outflow
Blurred vision	Corrective lenses or pilocarpine drops, large print
Aggravated glaucoma	Ophthalmologist consult
Cardiovascular effects	
Postural hypotension	Take BP regularly, sitting and standing
Direct effects on the heart: tachycardia, arrhythmia, conduction defects	Use smaller divided doses in clients with known heart disease; avoid in those with cardiac conduction defects or recent MI
Fluid retention: can lead to CHF	Check vital signs regularly; weigh client daily; check for fluid retention
Allergic reactions	
Rashes	Observe and report to physician
Photosensitivity	Provide sunscreen, protect skin with clothing, observe carefully, report, provide comfort measures
Insomnia	Single morning dose
Tremors and seizures	Observe carefully; advise client to avoid caffeine
Excessive perspiration	Observe, report, provide comfort measures
Erection/orgasm difficulty	Lower dose or switch to less anticholinergic preparation
Anxiety, restlessness	Observe, report, may have to discontinue
DRUG	**NURSING INTERVENTIONS**
MAO inhibitors	14-day waiting period before changing from MAOI to antidepressant or vice versa
Antihypertensives and heart medications	Causes hypotension or hypertension
Antacids	Inhibits absorption
Antipsychotics	Potentiates anticholinergic effects
CNS depressants/alcohol	Effects are potentiated

TABLE III-8.
ANTIDEPRESSANT AGENTS: MAOI'S

CHEMICAL CLASS	GENERIC NAME	TRADE NAME	DOSAGE
MAO	isocarboxazid phenelzine tranylcypromine	*Marplan* *Nardil* *Parnate*	10–30 mg 45–90 mg 20–30 mg

SIDE EFFECTS	NURSING INTERVENTION
Hypertensive crisis: elevated BP, palpitations, diaphoresis, chest pain, and headache that can lead to intracranial hemorrhage and death	Teach clients to avoid foods with high tyramine content such as aged cheeses, fermented foods, chocolate, liver, bean pods, yeast, sausage and bologna, beer, chianti, and vermouth wines: limit amounts of ETOH, sour cream, yogurt, raisins, soy sauce; teach clients to avoid OTC and prescription medications such as antidepressants, sedatives, cough and cold preparations, which interact to produce hypertensive crises
Anticholinergic disturbances: dry mouth, constipation	Increase fluids, bulk in diet, and exercise
CNS effects: drowsiness, fatigue, headache, restlessness	Some can be expected to last for a short period; increase activity, short afternoon nap
Orthostatic hypotension (drop in BP due to change in position)	Monitor BP frequently, lying, sitting, standing; teach to rise slowly.
Delay in ejaculation/orgasm	Take dose in morning if sexual activity is in evening
Insomnia	Give single morning dose; relax several hours before bedtime

DRUG INTERACTIONS	SIDE EFFECTS
Tricyclic antidepressants	Hypertensive crisis
CNS depressants	Decrease liver function
Dibenzoxapines	Hypertensive crisis
Amphetamines	Potentiate action
Antihypertensives (diuretics)	Decrease action

TABLE III-9.
ANTIMANIA AGENTS/MOOD STABILIZERS

CHEMICAL CLASS	GENERIC NAME	TRADE NAME	DOSAGE

Lithium*
 	
* Blood levels
.5–1.5 meq/liter:
   therapeutic
Above 1.5 meq/liter:
   toxic
2.0 mEq/liter:
   lethal
	Lithium	*Eskalith*
		Lithonate
		Lithotabs
		Lithobid
			600–2,100 mg

Anticonvulsant	Carbamazepine Valproic acid	*Tegretol* *Depakote*	200–1,600 mg 500–1,000 mg

SIDE EFFECTS	NURSING INTERVENTIONS

	Interventions for all side effects
	  Instruct client of short duration
	  Observe client carefully for changes in manifestations
	  Lithium work-up: renal, thyroid, EKG
	  Regular physicals
	  Check blood levels
	  Lower doses in geriatric clients

Initial therapy Fine tremor	Eliminate caffeine; adjust dose.
Transient nausea	Use of side rails; assist when up
Drowsiness, lethargy	Avoid using machinery
Loose stools, abdominal discomfort	Take with meals; change to slower release form

Polyuria
  Thirst
  Weight gain, fatigue	

Toxic levels
  Vomiting
  Diarrhea
  Lethargy
  Muscle twitching
  Ataxia
  Slurred speech
  Coma, seizure, cardiac arrest
	Careful observation for and of blood levels as sodium decreases and lithium levels increase; hold doses and obtain blood level; liver function/hematology levels need to be monitored with valproic acid

DRUG INTERACTIONS	EFFECTS
Diuretics Antipsychotics Sodium bicarbonate ECT /surgery Pregnancy	Increase risk of lithium toxicity Neurotoxicity, especially in elderly Promote excretion, lowering serum level May cause neurotoxicity Crosses placental barrier

3. ECT (electroconvulsive therapy)
   a. Characteristics
      1) Used mainly with depressed clients
      2) Used after other methods have been tried and failed
      3) Grand-mal seizure induced by passing an electric current through the temporal lobes and hypothalamus for .1–1 second
      4) Slight grimace and/or plantar flexion and toe movement may be observable
      5) Dose: 6–10 treatments 3 times a week

   b. **NURSING INTERVENTIONS**
      1) Obtain informed consent
      2) NPO after midnight
      3) Take baseline vital signs
      4) Remove prosthesis and jewelry
      5) Bladder emptied
      6) Medications
         a) General anesthesia
         b) Muscle relaxant: succinylcholine chloride *(Anectine)*
         c) Barbiturate to induce anesthesia: methohexital *(Brevital Sodium)*
         d) Atropine sulfate *(Donnatal):* diminishes secretions and blocks vagal reflexes
      7) Recovery
         a) Take vital signs q 15 minutes
         b) Maintain a patent airway
         c) Position on side to prevent aspiration
         d) Provide orientation to time, place, situation
         e) Assist to ambulate
         f) Resume normal eating and activity as soon as possible
         g) Reassure that memory loss is temporary up to 2 months
         h) Symptomatic treatment of headache, nausea

SECTION V
PERSONALITY DISORDERS

A. Definition: individual personality traits reflecting chronic, inflexible and maladaptive patterns of behavior that impair social and occupational functions

B. Causes
1. Genetic abnormalities
2. Learned responses
3. Deficiencies in ego and superego development
4. Unresponsive, inappropriate parent-child relationship
5. Early separation

C. Manifestations
1. Antisocial: sociopathic/psychopathic
   a. Superficial charm, wit, intelligence; manipulative, often seductive behavior
   b. Inability or refusal to accept responsibility for self-serving, destructive behavior
   c. Failure at school and work; delinquency, rule violations, inability to keep a job
   d. Promiscuity, desertion, two or more divorces or separations
   e. Repeated substance abuse
   f. Thefts, vandalism, multiple arrests
   g. Inability to function as a responsible person; no give or take
   h. Fights, assaults, abuse of others
   i. Impulsiveness, recklessness, inability to plan ahead
   j. Inappropriate affect: not sorry for violating others, no guilt
   k. Does not change with punishment
   l. Does not seek treatment
2. Borderline
   a. Impulsive and unpredictable behavior in self-damaging areas: spending, sex, gambling
   b. Unstable and intense interpersonal relationships, rapid attitude shifts, idealization, devaluation
   c. Inappropriate, intense anger
   d. Manipulative, splitting behaviors
   e. Identity disturbance with uncertain self-image and imitative behavior
   f. Unstable affect with rapid mood swings
   g. Intolerance of being alone, chronic feelings of emptiness or boredom
   h. Self-destructive behavior: suicidal gestures, self-mutilation, frequent accidents and fights

3. Dependent: does not accept responsibility
    a. Passive and self-conscious
    b. Overly compliant, clinging behavior, avoiding independence, leaving major decisions to others, subordinating own needs to those of others
4. Passive aggressive: resistance expressed indirectly
    a. Intentional inefficiency, chronic lateness, procrastination; reluctance to accept responsibility to make decisions
    b. Complaining and blaming behavior; feelings of confusion and mistreatment
    c. Fear of authority

D. NURSING INTERVENTIONS
1. Be aware of own feelings
2. Patience, persistence, consistency, flexibility; develop client trust
3. Direct approach: confrontation
4. Teach social skills
5. Reinforce appropriate behavior
6. Set limits
7. Encourage verbal expression of feelings
8. Encourage responsibility and accountability
9. Help delay gratification
10. Protect other clients from verbal and physical abuse
11. Clear rules; regulations, and consequences for rule violation
12. Contract for behavioral changes
13. Group treatment; identify manipulation

SECTION VI

CHEMICAL DEPENDENCE/ABUSE

A. **Substance-Related Disorders**
1. Definition
   a. Abuse: drug use leading to legal, social, and medical problems
   b. Addiction: refers to physical dependence
   c. Dependence: need resulting from continued use; results in mental/physical discomfort upon withdrawal of the substance
2. Contributing factors
   a. Genetic predisposition
   b. Peer pressure and social approval
   c. Low self-esteem
   d. Low frustration tolerance
   e. Availability
3. Defense mechanisms
   a. Denial
   b. Rationalization
   c. Intellectualization
   d. Projection
   e. Blaming
4. Behavioral effects
   a. Reduces anxiety
   b. Sense of well-being
   c. Inhibits self-control
   d. Dependence: physical and psychological addiction
   e. Tolerance: need for increasing amounts to achieve the same effect
5. Alcohol dependence/abuse
   a. General characteristics
      1) Abuse vs dependence
      2) Central nervous system depressant with progression from relaxation to slurred speech and impaired motor activities to stupor and anesthesia
      3) Blood alcohol concentration (BAC)
         a) Number of mg of alcohol diluted in each 100 ml of blood
         b) 0.10% BAC is the legal level for driving
         c) Liver detoxifies alcohol at 3/4 oz/hour
         d) 3/4 oz = 12 oz beer or 4 oz wine or 1 shot of whiskey

4) Stages of alcohol dependence
   a) Relaxation: freedom from anxiety
   b) Tolerance: increasingly higher amount needed to reach the same effect
   c) Loss of control
   d) Blackouts: fugue-like state where client acts normally but remembers nothing for that period of time
   e) Progression: tolerance reverses
5) Physical effects occur in all systems
   a) Nervous system: psychosis, dementia, seizure disorders
      (1) Wernicke-Korsakoff's syndrome (thiamine & niacin deficiency)
      (2) Alcoholic dementia: memory and intellectual loss
   b) Cardiac: arrhythmias, myopathy, hypertension
   c) GI: gastritis, cirrhosis, pancreatitis, hypoglycemia, ulcers, esophageal varices
   d) Respiratory: COPD, pneumonia, cancer
   e) Genitourinary system: fetal alcohol syndrome, decreased libido
   f) Skin and skeletal: ulcers, spider angiomas, fractures
6) Psychological and social effects
   a) Erratic, impulsive, abusive behavior
   b) Poor judgment, loss of memory
   c) Family problems
   d) Depression, low self-esteem
   e) Suicide
   f) Job loss

b. Withdrawal
   1) Definition: physical manifestations developing 6–8 hours after abstinence from alcohol
   2) Manifestations (autonomic nervous system)
      a) Shakiness
      b) Anxiety
      c) Mood swings
      d) Insomnia
      e) Impaired appetite
      f) Some confusion
      g) Elevated vital signs

c. Delirium tremens (DTs)
   1) Definition: acute medical condition occurring usually 2–4 days after abstinence, potentially fatal
   2) Manifestations
      a) Confusion
      b) Disorientation
      c) Visual and auditory hallucinations
      d) Convulsions
      e) All manifestations of withdrawal

d. Medical treatment
  1) Inpatient detoxification: 3–7 days; purpose is to medically manage withdrawal and prevent DTs
     a) Antianxiety medications
     b) Fluids and vitamins
     c) Antidiarrheal medications
     d) Seizure precautions: anti-seizure medications and magnesium sulfate
     e) Provide symptomatic relief: fluids, analgesics, sleeping medications
     f) Diet: high-protein, high-carbohydrate, low-fat
  2) DTs
     a) Quiet, moderately lit area
     b) Decreased stimuli
     c) Reality orientation
     d) Avoid restraints
     e) Seizure precautions

e. **NURSING INTERVENTIONS**
  1) Administer medications and treatments as ordered
  2) Observe for physical complications
  3) Rest and nutrition
  4) Observe for manifestations of depression and suicide
  5) Provide firm limits
  6) Provide support
  7) Be nonjudgmental
  8) Avoid being manipulated
  9) Monitor visitors
  10) Assist in identifying use of defense mechanisms (denial)
  11) Encourage rehabilitation programs and aftercare (e.g., Alcoholics Anonymous [AA])
  12) Educate and support family; discuss support groups such as Al-Anon and Alateen

f. Rehabilitation: 30-day programs essential to recovery; use education, family therapy, and psychotherapy

g. Aftercare
  1) AA: 12-step program of sobriety
  2) Antabuse: medication used to prevent use of alcohol; aversion therapy
     a) Sensitizes the client to alcohol
     b) If alcohol is used, client suffers headache, vomiting, nausea, flushing, hypotension, tachycardia, dyspnea, chest pain, palpitations, confusion, respiratory and circulatory collapse, convulsions, death
     c) Avoid drinking for 2 weeks after last dose
     d) Warn client that alcohol is present in cough medicines, rubbing compounds, vinegars, aftershave lotions, and some mouthwashes

h. Special groups
  1) Teenagers: 40–65%
  2) Elderly: increasing

6. Drug abuse/dependence
   a. General characteristics
      1) Abuse vs dependence
      2) Effect on CNS depends on the type of substance
      3) Psychological and social effects
         a) Isolation and withdrawal
         b) Family and work problems
         c) Loss of property
         d) Incarceration
      4) Physical effects
         a) Endocarditis/AIDS
         b) Hepatitis B
         c) Pulmonary emboli
         d) Gangrene
         e) Malnutrition
         f) Trauma
         g) Psychosis
   b. Common drugs abused (see Table III-10.)
   c. Medical treatment (see Table III-10.)

   d. NURSING INTERVENTIONS
      1) Carry out medical regime
      2) Observe for manifestations of withdrawal
      3) Provide quiet, safe environment
      4) Monitor visitors
      5) Be nonjudgmental, accepting, firm attitude
      6) Set limits
      7) Monitor nutrition
      8) Promote sleep
      9) Refer for detoxification, rehabilitation, and aftercare
      10) Support family in seeking help (Al-Anon)

   e. Rehabilitation: 30 days to 2 years; change life-style
   f. Aftercare: lifelong AA, NA (Narcotics Anonymous), CA (Cocaine Anonymous), etc.

Substance Abuse

Substance abuse is the term used to designate the use of psychoactive drugs, including alcohol, to the extent of significant interference with the user's physical, social, and or emotional well-being. It is characterized by preoccupation with the drug and loss of control over its use. If the quantity and duration of abuse is sufficient, physical dependence may develop with tolerance and risk of a withdrawal syndrome when drug use is terminated. (see Table III-10.)

TABLE III-10.
SUBSTANCE ABUSE

DRUG	MANIFESTATIONS OF INTOXICATION	WITHDRAWAL SYNDROME	METHOD OF DETOXIFICATION
Hallucinogens: psychedelics, LSD, mescaline peyote, marijuana	Flushing of skin, dilated pupils, transient increase in pulse rate and blood pressure, hallucinations, psychosis, marked anxiety, depression, suicidal thoughts, confusion, paranoia	None	None required; "bad trips" can be treated with diazepam (Valium) or, more simply, by "talking down" through verbal reassurance and emotional support; flashbacks may occur for several months
Phencyclidine (PCP, angel dust)	Vertical or horizontal nystagmus, increased BP and heart rate, ataxia, marked anxiety, emotional liability, dysarthria, euphoria, agitation, delusions, grandiosity, irrationality, violence, synthesis (seeing colors when loud sound is heard); sensation of slowed time; can lead to dangerous behavior	None	Minimize social stimulation and control environment; administer ascorbic acid (Vit. C tabs or cranberry juice); do not "talk down"; treat with Valium if excited; if psychotic, admit to psychiatric unit and treat with antipsychotic medication
Stimulants: amphetamine, amyl nitrate, cocaine (see separate category)	Restlessness, irritability, anxiety, tachycardia, cardiac arrhythmia, paranoia, psychosis with clear sensorium, elation, grandiosity, psychotic behavior, perspiration or chills, nausea and vomiting; weight loss with prolonged use	Use of high doses associated with a rapidly developing syndrome on withdrawal: - persecutory delusions - ideas of reference - aggressiveness and hostility - anxiety - psychomotor agitation - suicidal; Prolonged, heavy use yields withdrawal syndrome after after 2–4 days of depression and fatigue	None usually required; psychiatric hospitalization for severe
Cocaine	Same as amphetamines; overdose: syncope, chest pain, seizures, death may result from cardiac and respiratory failure: high dose use: visual and tactile hallucinations and "cocaine bugs;" a "rush" of increased self-confidence and well-being, confusion, anxiety, paranoia; headache, palpitations followed by "crashing"	Sleepiness, depression, lack of energy or motivation, poor concentration, irritability, "cocaine craving," psychosis	Hospitalization for high-dose "crack" or freebase use or the polyaddicted; others treated in out-patient programs

TABLE III-10.
SUBSTANCE ABUSE (CONTINUED)

DRUG	MANIFESTATIONS OF INTOXICATION	WITHDRAWAL SYNDROME	METHOD OF DETOXIFICATION
Opiates: heroin, morphine, *Dilaudid, Demerol, Percodan,* codeine, Opium, methadone	Mitosis, euphoria, drowsiness, dysphoria, apathy, psychomotor retardation, slurred speech, impaired attention or memory, impaired social judgment; chronic use can lead to malnourishment, criminal behavior, sexually transmitted disease, HIV/AIDS with IV drug use	Withdrawal begins after 8–12 hours and lasts 3–5 days; severity varies with extent of abuse; lacrimation, rhinorrhea, sweating, piloerection, diarrhea, yawning, mild hypertension, tachycardia, fever, insomnia, dilated pupils, restlessness, abdominal cramps, anxiety	Can be accomplished "cold turkey" or medically managed with anti-anxiety agents, methadone or clonidine *(Catapres)*
Sedative-Hypnotics: barbiturates, *Equanil, Miltown,* benzodiazepines, *Ativan, Librium, Valium, Klonopin, Xanax*	Mental impairment, confusion, nystagmus, motor incoordination, ataxia, depression, dysarthria; frequently used by alternating with alcohol: which can lead to overdose	Weakness, insomnia, nausea and postural hypotension develop within first 48 hours and last 5–7 days; seizures may occur at any time, especially within first few days; delirium may develop between the 3rd-7th days and last 3–5 days	Can be medical emergency; hospitalization required and pentobarbital or phenobarbital used to prevent precipitous withdrawal
Sleep Agents: *Dalmane, Restoril, Halcion, Ativan*	Can have paradoxical response, hyperactivity in elderly, children		

SECTION VII
ORGANIC MENTAL DISORDERS

A. **Normal Aging**
1. Life cycle changes
   a. Physical health
   b. Emotional: integrity, despair
   c. Intellectual changes
   d. Social changes such as retirement, widowhood
2. Special characteristics
   a. Life review
   b. Legacy
   c. Dealing with loss

B. **Organic Mental Disorders (OMD):** psychological and behavioral problems resulting from organic conditions; may be reversible or irreversible
1. Delirium: acute brain syndrome; decreased attention and level of awareness; usually temporary and reversible; rapid onset; identifiable stressor
   a. Disturbance
      1) Disturbances in sleep and wakefulness
      2) Attention: easily distracted, illusions
      3) Restless and disoriented
      4) Difficulty concentrating
      5) Disorganized speech
   b. Causes
      1) Medical
      2) Surgical
      3) Pharmacological
      4) Neurological
   c. Stages
      1) Restless and talkative
      2) Slurred and incoherent speech
      3) Purposeless hyperactivity
      4) Excitation or stupor

2. Dementias
   a. Definition: sustained and often progressive intellectual impairment
   b. General manifestations
      1) Lingering
      2) Gradual, progressive
      3) Language disorders (e.g., confabulation, blocking)
      4) Motor impairment
      5) Disintegrating personality
      6) Disintegrating behavior
      7) Memory impairment (short term)
      8) Judgment impairment
      9) Thinking impairment (abstract)
      10) Degeneration (1–10 years post-onset)
   c. Types
      1) Wernicke-Korsakoff's syndrome (dementia associated with alcoholism): not reversible
         a) Memory (long or short term); impairment is predominant
         b) Confabulation
         c) Polyneuritis
         d) Flat affect
         e) Ataxia
         f) Confusion
         g) Learning impaired
      2) Alzheimer's disease (primary degenerative dementia)
         a) Onset: 45 years or older
         b) Progressive and chronic
         c) Cognitive function with behavior changes
         d) Prognosis: live up to 15 years from onset
         e) Three phases
            (1) Forgetfulness
               (a) Anxiety
               (b) Recent memory impaired
               (c) Shortened retention
            (2) Confusion
               (a) Orientation disturbance
               (b) Concentration decreases
               (c) Forget words
               (d) Denial
            (3) Dementia
               (a) Disorientation
               (b) Anxiety, denial
               (c) Delusions, hallucinations, paranoia
               (d) Agitation
               (e) Physical deterioration
      3) Multi-infarct dementia: difference from Alzheimer's is mainly its step-wise progression, rather than gradual decline; trauma induced (stroke, neurosurgery)

3. **NURSING INTERVENTIONS:** allow as much independence as possible
    a. Physical
        1) Medical care: physical problems
        2) Adequate nutrition: provide finger foods, tolerate poor manners
        3) Exercise and rest: range of motion exercises, walks, naps, keep awake during the day
        4) Elimination: monitor intake and output, diet, limit fluids at bedtime, use stool softeners, toilet at regular intervals
    b. Activities of daily living
        1) Break down tasks into short simple steps
        2) Provide clear expectations
        3) Allow ample time
        4) Remain with client
        5) Assist with grooming and hygiene
        6) Matter-of-fact manner (avoid embarrassment)
    c. Safety
        1) Rugs
        2) Driving
        3) Light at night (sundown)
        4) Medications (side effects: grogginess and confusion)
        5) Wandering (do not confine)
        6) Clutter
    d. Cognitive
        1) Eliminate multiple stimuli
        2) Short, simple conversation (slow, distinct, soft voice)
        3) Only small decisions
        4) Break down tasks (e.g., dressing)
        5) Accompany verbal with nonverbal cues
        6) Consistency: establish routine, familiar caregivers
        7) Orient x 3
        8) Use visual cues such as pictures, labels, calendar, clock
        9) Remove harmful objects
    e. Social
        1) Provide human contact
        2) Groups
        3) Children
        4) Activities such as gardening, music
    f. Families
        1) Explain disorder
        2) Explain regression and provide activities such as photo albums, music, games
        3) Resources: Alzheimer's Disease and Related Disorders, Inc.
        4) Discuss need for family to obtain support/relief
        5) Counseling is necessary at times

SECTION VIII
EATING DISORDERS

A. Anorexia/Bulimia
1. Definitions
   a. Anorexia: refusal to eat and relentless self-induced pursuit of thinness; up to 21% die
   b. Bulimia: binge-purge cycle of eating
2. Causes
   a. Adolescent struggle for independence and control
   b. Feelings of control are related to body
   c. Family problems: denial, conflict avoidance, enmeshment
   d. Society promotes thinness, dieting
3. Comparison (anorexia and bulimia)
   a. Obedient, bright, ambitious
   b. Perfectionist, type A personalities
   c. Low self-esteem
   d. Preoccupied with food
   e. Depression
   f. Manipulation
4. Contrast:

ANOREXIA	BULIMIA
Younger (18–20 yrs)	Older
Unable to maintain body weight at 85% of expected body weight	Weight fluctuates considerably
Amenorrhea	Amenorrhea
Starvation	Binge eating
Don't admit abnormal eating patterns	See patterns and fears loss of control
Intense fear of becoming obese	Hide food, hoard
Prefers health foods	Prefers high-calorie food
Preoccupation with buying, planning and preparing foods	Repeated crash dieting, use of laxatives, diuretics, amphetamines
Rigorous exercise	Abuse of alcohol and/or drugs, petty crime
Still views self as overweight	Aware that behavior is abnormal

5. Effects
    a. Anorexia: holding in
        1) Skeletal muscle atrophy; emaciated
        2) Loss of fatty tissue
        3) Hypotension
        4) Constipation
        5) Susceptible to infections
        6) Blotchy, sallow skin
        7) Lanugo
        8) Dryness and loss of hair
        9) Amenorrhea
        10) Electrolyte imbalance
        11) Cause of death: cardiac dysrhythmia; arrest
    b. Bulimia: letting go
        1) Electrolyte imbalance
        2) Dental caries
        3) Erosion of tooth enamel
        4) Gingival infections
        5) Susceptible to infections
        6) Bingeing
        7) Vomiting
        8) Use and abuse of laxatives and diuretics

6. **NURSING INTERVENTIONS**
    a. May need hospitalization
    b. Provide nutrition
        1) Monitor intake and output
        2) Vigilance 30–60 minutes after eating
        3) Help with relaxation prior to eating
        4) Enforce a behavior modification plan
        5) Positive reinforcement for weight gain
        6) Parenteral feedings as needed
    c. Teach coping skills
        1) Encourage recognition and verbalization of feelings
        2) Reinforce realistic perception of weight and appearance
        3) Assertiveness training
        4) Allow control
        5) Acceptance of self responsibility
        6) Limit setting and consistency
    d. Family
        1) Therapy
        2) Education
    e. Refer to self-help groups
        1) American Anorexia/Bulimia Association, Inc.
        2) Anorexia Nervosa and Associated Disorders (ANAD)

SECTION IX
DEVELOPMENTAL DISABILITIES

A. **Definition:** adaptive ability compromised by an alteration in the pattern or rate in stages of development during childhood: functional limitations in self care, learning, mobility, self-direction, self-sufficiency in independent living; diagnosis based on IQ and socially adaptive behavior

B. **Causes**
  1. Genetic
     a. Chromosomal
        1) Down's syndrome (formerly called mongoloidism): congenital mental retardation with motor involvement
        2) Klinefelter: gonadal defect with subnormal intelligence and social adaptation
     b. Errors of metabolism
        1) PKU: accumulation of phenylalanine, which is toxic to the brain; retardation may be avoided by strict dietary avoidance of phenylalanine
        2) Tay-Sachs: inherited disorder of lipid metabolism causing mental retardation, blindness and muscle weakness
  2. Acquired
     a. Prenatal: viruses, toxins
     b. Perinatal: anoxia, injury, prematurity
     c. Post-natal: infections, poisons, trauma, deprivation

C. **Levels of Mental Retardation:** based on IQ level (normal range is 80–110)
  1. Mild
     a. Social and communication skills
     b. Social and vocational skills, minimal self-support
     c. May be self-sufficient and independent as adult
     d. IQ range: 50–70
  2. Moderate
     a. Can care for self
     b. Poor awareness of social conventions
     c. May learn to count
     d. May contribute to own support under close supervision
     e. IQ range: 35–49
  3. Severe
     a. Poor motor and speech
     b. May learn simple work tasks

           b. IQ range: 20–34
    4. Profound
           a. Very limited self-care
           b. IQ range: below 20

D. Client with a developmental disability has a full range of emotions and may be subjected to the full range of emotional illnesses

E. NURSING INTERVENTIONS
    1. Know growth and development
    2. Observe child and parents together
    3. Assess physical status
    4. Denver development test
           a. Gross motor
           b. Language
           c. Fine motor
           d. Personal, social
    5. Help parents with grieving; suggest parent support groups
    6. Counsel and teach parents care; train parents as case managers
    7. Encourage parents to get help and rest through respite care; make sure parents know all available resources (e.g., medical, social, educational, legal, community, etc.)
    8. Prevention
           a. Health teaching, such as nutrition, obstetrical care
           b. Immunizations
           c. Prenatal counseling/family planning
           d. Psychological needs

SECTION X

FAMILY VIOLENCE

(see also: Unit IV, Section VIII)

A. **Definition:** abuse of a violent physical or verbal nature within a family, which crosses socioeconomic, religious, racial, and cultural lines

B. **Types of abuse**
   1. Physical: pushing, hitting, throwing
   2. Psychological: verbal degradation
   3. Sexual: wife, child, friend
   4. Neglect: medical, physical, psychological
   5. Social: isolation
   6. Material: theft

C. **Abused Persons**
   1. Wives
   2. Husbands
   3. Children
   4. Elderly

D. **Characteristics of Abuser**
   1. Low self-esteem
   2. Uses alcohol and/or drugs
   3. Projects anger
   4. Anxious
   5. Depressed
   6. Has come from an abusive household (victimization)
   7. Socially isolated
   8. Impulsive, immature
   9. Guilt ridden

E. **Characteristics of Abused Persons**
   1. Victims of child abuse
   2. Accepts responsibility for others (co-dependency issues)
   3. Helpless
   4. Suicidal at times
   5. Submissive
   6. Frightened (may be harmed/killed)
   7. Emotionally dependent
   8. Elderly often emotionally, materially abused

F. General Manifestations of Abused Persons

1. Psychological manifestations
   a. Sleep disorders: as nightmares
   b. Headaches
   c. Anxiety
   d. Depression
   e. Suicidal ideation
   f. Substance abuse
   g. Disruptive behavior at home, school, work
   h. Teen runaway behavior
   i. Frequent emergency room visits

G. Signs of Abuse in Children (see Table III-11.)

TABLE III-11.
SIGNS OF ABUSE IN CHILDREN

TYPE	PHYSICAL	BEHAVIORAL
Physical abuse	- Multiple injuries and/or in various stages of healing - Unexplained bruises, burns, fractures or lacerations - Incongruence between explanation and injury - X-rays show numerous injuries	- Wary of strangers - Labile behavior - Depressed, frightened, stiff, rigid, distant, does not seek out parents
Physical neglect	- Appearance: poor hygiene and dress - Medical and physical problems unattended	- Fatigue - Withdrawal - Substance abuse
Sexual abuse	- Venerial disease - Pregnancy - Pain or itching in vaginal area; difficulty walking or sitting	- Unusual sexual behavior or knowledge - Poor peer relations - Reports of sexual assault
Emotional abuse		- Decreased self-esteem - Lack of emotional response (no tears) - Hypochondriasis (vague complaints) - Slowed growth and development - Sleep disorders or neglect - Behavioral extremes - Deliquent (runs away)

H. NURSING INTERVENTIONS

1. Ask in detail about manifestations
2. Build trust
3. Be nonjudgemental
4. Do not give advice
5. Determine seriousness of battering: if child, call proper authorities
6. Assist to identify support system
7. Identify resources for housing, money, legal aid, vocational counseling, crisis center for therapy
8. Call proper authorities

SECTION XI

RAPE

(see also: Unit IV, Section VIII)

A. Characteristics
1. Crime of violence: force, penetration, lack of consent
2. Motives: power, anger, intimidation
3. Myths
   a. Provoked by victim's actions
   b. Victim promiscuous
   c. Women can avoid rape; cannot be raped against their will
   d. Rape is an impulsive act
   e. Rapists are abnormal
   f. Elderly are not raped
   g. Women frequently get revenge by accusing men of rape

B. Post-Traumatic Stress Disorder
1. Disorganization
2. Reorganization
3. Physical, emotional, and behavioral stress

C. NURSING INTERVENTIONS
1. Crisis intervention
   a. Empathetic, understanding approach
   b. Provide safe and secure environment
   c. Encourage verbalization about feelings
   d. Clarify what happened
   e. Offer support and reassurance
   f. Referrals for ongoing counseling
2. Emergency action
   a. Allow choices (loss of control)
   b. Provide evidence collection
   c. Provide documentation
   d. Offer comfort and privacy
   e. Schedule follow-up
3. Encourage use of groups to provide support
4. Help with psychological trauma
   a. Disrupted relationships
   b. Phobias
   c. Nightmares
   d. Flashbacks
   e. Family and sexual relations
5. Talking and working through feelings

SECTION XII
LEGAL ASPECTS OF PSYCHIATRIC NURSING

A. Types of Admissions
1. Voluntary
   a. Persons admit themselves
   b. Client consents to all treatment
   c. Client can refuse treatment, including drugs, unless danger to self or others
2. Involuntary judicial process
   a   Initiated when someone files a petition
   b. Certification of the likelihood of serious harm to self or others, or unable to care for self
   c. Under 18: parents can confine with confirmation by a neutral fact finder
   d. Must be released at end of statutory time or put on voluntary status or have a hearing

B. Judicial Precedents
1. Rights: unless incompetent, client maintains all previous rights
2. Right to treatment: efforts by staff consistent with medical knowledge
   a. Humane psychological and physical environment
   b. Qualified personnel and adequate nursing
   c. Individual treatment plan
3. Competency hearings
4. Least restrictive alternative

C. Informed Consent Required
1. ECT
2. Medications
3. Seclusion
4. Restraint

D. Insanity as a Defense
1. Insanity: determined in court; legal terminology
2. McNaughten rule: at the time of the crime, the individual didn't know the nature and quality of the act or didn't know right from wrong
3. Present
   a. Does client know right from wrong?
   b. Was client mentally ill at time of the crime?
   c. Is client able to conform to the requirements of the law?

E. Clients' Rights
1. Right to treatment
2. Access to stationery and postage
3. Access to unopened mail
4. Visits by physician, attorney, clergy
5. Visits by other people
6. Keep personal possessions
7. Keep and spend money
8. Storage space for personal items
9. Telephone access
10. Hold property, vote, marry
11. Make wills, contracts
12. Educational resources
13. Sue, be sued
14. Challenge hospitalization

NOTES

UNIT FOUR
WOMEN'S HEALTH NURSING

Unit Content

 Key Points　　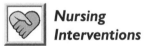 **Nursing Interventions**　　 **Points to Remember**

SECTION I
REVIEW OF FEMALE REPRODUCTIVE NURSING

Pregnancy

A. **Anatomy and Physiology of the Female Reproductive Tract**
1. External genitalia
   a. Mons pubis
   b. Labia majora
   c. Labia minora
   d. Clitoris
   e. Vestibule
      1) Urethral orifice
      2) Skene's glands
      3) Hymen and vaginal introitus
      4) Bartholin's glands
   f. Perineum
2. Internal genitalia
   a. Fallopian tubes
   b. Uterus
      1) Fundus
      2) Cervix
   c. Vagina
   d. Ovaries

B. **Fertilization and Fetal Development**
1. Conception (fertilization)
   a. Definition: union of sperm and ovum
   b. Conditions necessary for fertilization
      1) Maturity of egg and sperm
      2) Timing of deposit of sperm
         a) Lifetime of ovum is 24 hours
         b) Lifetime of sperm in the female genital tract is 72 hours
         c) Ideal time for fertilization is 48 hours *before* to 24 hours *after* ovulation
         d) Menstruation begins approximately 14 days *after* ovulation

3) Climate of the female genital tract
  a) Vaginal and cervical secretions are less acidic during ovulation (sperm cannot survive in a highly acidic environment)
  b) Cervical secretions are thinner during ovulation (sperm can penetrate more easily)

c. Process of fertilization (7–10 days)
  1) Ovulation occurs
  2) Ovum travels to fallopian tube
  3) Sperm travel to fallopian tube
  4) One sperm penetrates the ovum
  5) Zygote forms (fertilized egg)
  6) Zygote migrates to uterus
  7) Zygote implants (nidation) in uterine wall
  8) Progesterone and estrogen are secreted by the corpus luteum to maintain the lining of the uterus and prevent menstruation until placenta starts producing these hormones; (note: progesterone is a thermogenic hormone that raises body temperature—an objective sign that ovulation has occured)

d. Placental development
  1) Chorionic villi develop that secrete Human Chorionic Gonadotropin (HCG), which stimulates production of estrogen and progesterone from the corpus luteum
  2) Chorionic villi burrow into endometrium, forming the placenta
  3) The placenta secretes HCG, human placental lactogen (HPL), and (by week three) estrogen and progesterone

e. Fetal membranes develop and surround the embryo-fetus
  1) Amnion: inner membrane
  2) Chorion: outer membrane
  3) Umbilical cord
    a) Two arteries carrying deoxygenated blood to placenta
    b) One vein carrying oxygenated blood to fetus
    c) No pain receptors
    d) Encased in Wharton's jelly
    e) Covered by chorionic membrane

f. Amniotic fluid
  1) Production origins
    a) Maternal serum during early pregnancy
    b) Fetal urine in greater proportion during latter part of pregnancy
    c) Replaced every 3 hours
    d) 800–1,200 ml at end of pregnancy
  2) Functions
    a) Protection from trauma and heat loss
    b) Facilitates musculoskeletal development by allowing for movement of the fetus
    c) Facilitates symmetric growth and development
    d) Source of oral fluid for fetus

g. Placental transfer of material to and from the fetus
   1) Diffusion across membrane (e.g., gases, water, electrolytes)
   2) Active transport via enzyme activity (e.g., glucose, amino acids, calcium, iron)
   3) Pinocytosis: minute particles engulfed and carried across the cell (e.g., fats)
   4) Leakage: small defects in the chorionic villi cause slight mixing of material and fetal blood cells

C. Fetal Development
1. Pre-embryonic: first two weeks
2. Embryonic: three to seven weeks
3. Fetal: eight to 40 weeks
   a. Fullterm: 38 to 42 weeks
   b. Preterm: less than 38 weeks
   c. Post-term: more than 42 weeks

D. Terminology
1. Gravida
   a. Definition: number of times pregnant, including present pregnancy
   b. Variations: primigravida, multigravida
2. Para
   a. Definition: number of pregnancies delivered after the age of viability, whether born alive or dead
   b. Variations: nullipara, primipara, multipara

3. Five-digit system
   a. G: gravida
   b. T: term infants
   c. P: preterm
   d. A: abortions
   e. L: living

Teratogenic Effects on Fetal Development

A. Teratogen
1. Definition: nongenetic factor producing malformations of the fetus; greatest effect on those cells undergoing rapid growth, thus time is important (e.g., ears and kidneys)
2. Types
   a. Chemical agents (e.g., insecticides)
   b. Radiation
   c. Drugs (e.g., alcohol, tetracycline, chemotherapeutic agents, phenytoin *(Dilantin)*, narcotics, nicotine, mega-vitamins)
   d. Bacteria and viruses
      1) Syphilis
         a) Spirochete does not cross placenta until after 18th week; treat as soon as possible; can treat later since penicillin does cross placenta
         b) Can cause late abortions, stillbirths, and congenitally infected infants

2) Gonorrhea: causes injury to eyes at birth
3) T.O.R.C.H.: severe effects on the fetus
   a) Toxoplasmosis: protozoan contracted by ingesting raw meat or feces of infected animal (e.g., cats)
   b) Rubella: first trimester most serious; causes congenital heart problems, cataracts, hearing loss
   c) Cytomegalovirus (CMV): member of the herpes family; causes congenital and acquired infection; principal organs affected: liver, brain, and blood
   d) Herpes simplex virus, Type 2 (HSV-2)
      (1) Transmitted to infant vaginally in intrauterine cavity or during delivery; do not deliver vaginally if active lesions are present
      (2) Affects blood, brain, liver, lungs, CNS, eyes, skin
      (3) Perinatal mortality: 96%; 50% of survivors have neurological or visual abnormalities
4) Chlamydia: causes conjunctivitis and pneumonia in the newborn
5) AIDS
   a) Transmitted via breast milk
   b) 30% chance of transmission in utero or during delivery
   c) Treatment of client while pregnant can reduce chance of transmission to fetus to approximately 8%

Signs of Pregnancy

A. Presumptive (subjective)
1. Amenorrhea: missed periods
2. Nausea/vomiting: morning sickness, probably due to HCG; usually lasts about 3 months
3. Fatigue: first trimester
4. Urinary frequency: caused by enlarging uterus pressing on bladder
5. Breast changes: tenderness and tingling, nipples pronounced, full feeling, increased size, areola darker
6. Quickening: mother's perception of fetal movement around 16–18 weeks; fluttering sensation

B. Probable (objective)
1. Chadwick's sign: bluish coloration of the mucous membranes of the cervix, vagina, and vulva
2. Goodell's sign: softening of cervix; occurs beginning of the third month
3. Hegar's sign: softening of the isthmus of the uterus, between the body of the uterus and cervix; occurs about the sixth week
4. Enlargement of abdomen: uterus just above symphysis at 8–10 weeks; at umbilicus at 20–22 weeks
5. Braxton-Hicks contractions: painless contractions occurring at irregular periods throughout pregnancy; felt most commonly after 28 weeks
6. Uterine souffle: soft blowing sound; blood flow to placenta same rate as maternal pulse

7. Pregnancy test positive: HCG in serum/urine
8. Ballottement: can push fetus and feel it rebound
9. Pigmentation changes: increased pigmentation, chloasma, linea nigra, and striae gravidarum

C. Positive
1. Fetal heartbeat: by Doppler at 8–10 weeks
2. Fetal movements: felt by examiner
3. Fetal outline: on sonogram

Assessment of Date of Delivery

A. Nagele's rule: first day of last menstrual period (LMP) minus three months plus seven days; in most cases, add one year

B. Other parameters: fundal heights, quickening, sonograms

Physical Adaptations and Discomforts of Pregnancy

Table IV-1.

ADAPTATIONS TO PREGNANCY

Adaptations to Pregnancy	Trimester	Interventions
G.I.: Nausea/vomiting	1	Small frequent meals; eat crackers or dry toast before getting up in the morning; eat dry meals; drink liquids between meals
Constipation, flatulence and heartburn	2, 3	Exercise; increase fluid and fiber in diet; stool softeners if recommended by physician
Bleeding gums; epulis	2, 3	Use soft toothbrush for dental care
Gallstones	2, 3	Avoid fatty foods
Heartburn	2, 3	Small frequent meals; avoid spicy, fatty foods; no sodium bicarbonate as antacid; antacids as recommended by physician
Urinary Tract: Frequency during first and third trimester due to pressure on bladder.	1, 3	Void when first urge felt; wear a pad if leaking
Glomerular filtration rate (GFR) increases (glycosuria)		
Increase in urinary infections	2,3	Increase fluid intake
Breasts: Increase in size and nodularity, striae	1	
Tenderness and tingling	1	Wear good supportive bra
Hypertrophy of Montgomery tubercles	2	
Darkening of areola	2	
Colostrum secreted	2, 3	
Vagina: Epithelium undergoes hypertrophy and hyperplasia		
Increased vascularity		
Increased pH: good for growth of Candida (thrush)	1, 2, 3	Report itching and burning to physician
Increase in discharge; leukorrhea is common	1	Promote cleanliness by bathing daily; avoid douching; avoid nylon undergarments

Table IV-1.
ADAPTATIONS TO PREGNANCY (CONTINUED)

Adaptations to Pregnancy	Trimester	Interventions
Respiratory System: Increase in volume of up to 40–50% between 16–34th week		
Diaphragm is pushed upward; ribcage flares out; breathing changes from abdominal to chest		
Increase in oxygen consumption by 15%		
Stuffiness, epistaxis, and changes in voice occur as a result of increased estrogen levels	1	Cool moist air may help; avoid over-the-counter decongestants and sprays
Dyspnea	3	Proper posture; sleep with head propped up
Skin: Areola darkens Abdominal striae, linea nigra		
Diaphoresis	2, 3	Daily bathing; powder
Chloasma: mask of pregnancy		
Vascular spider nervi; chest, neck, arms, and legs		
Metabolism/nutrition: Basal metabolic rate increased by 20%		
Water retention: edema	2, 3	Elevate legs and feet when sitting; avoid prolonged standing; do not wear garters or clothing with restrictive bands around the legs; avoid crossing legs at knees

Weight gain: 20–25 lbs. recommended
  - Adequate protein intake, especially for teens
  - Increase iron during last eight weeks		

Pica: craving for nonnutritive substances	2, 3	Eat well-balanced diet
Perineum: Increased vascularity		
Venous congestion of the perineum	2, 3	Kegal exercises

Table IV-1.
ADAPTATIONS TO PREGNANCY (CONTINUED)

Adaptations to Pregnancy	Trimester	Interventions
Cardiovascular: Cardiac output increases by 30% Blood volume progressively increases and peaks around 30–40 weeks at 47% above pre-pregnant state Plasma volume increases greater than RBC and hemoglobin, resulting in "pseudo anemia" Pulse rate increases by 10–15 beats/minute; BP drops slightly in second trimester due to peripheral dilatation effects of progesterone; returns to normal by third trimester Varicose veins may develop	2, 3	Elevate legs; avoid standing for long periods of time; avoid constrictive clothing
Uterus: Growth is influenced by estrogen 500–1,000-fold increase in capacity Cervical secretions form mucus plug		
Endocrine: Increase in size and activity of thyroid Increase in size and activity of anterior lobe of pituitary Increase in size and activity of adrenal cortex Increase in production of relaxin causes joint and back pain.	2, 3	Pelvic rock; good body mechanics; supportive shoes

Emotional and Psychological Adaptations to Pregnancy

A. **Stressors**
   1. Circumstances of pregnancy
   2. Meaning of pregnancy to the couple
   3. Responsibilities associated with parenthood
   4. Resources available to family

B. **Development Tasks of Pregnancy**
   1. First trimester: accept the biological fact of pregnancy; it is common to feel ambivalent early in pregnancy
   2. Second trimester: accept growing fetus as a baby to be nurtured
   3. Third trimester: prepare for the birth and parenting of the child

C. **Emotional Responses**
   1. Self concept related to body image
   2. Mood swings related to biophysical and social changes
   3. Ambivalence related to fear and anxiety
   4. Sexual concerns related to biophysical changes

Prenatal Care

A. **Assessment**
   1. Complete history
   2. Lab work: complete blood count (CBC), blood type and Rh, irregular antibody, Rubella, VDRL/FTA-ABS/RPR, hepatitis B surface antigen, HIV antibody (with client's consent)
   3. Vital signs, weight, urine test for protein and glucose
   4. Physical exam: fundal height, fetal heart rate (FHR), fetal activity
   5. Internal exam
      a. Adequate pelvic outlet, signs of pregnancy (First visit)
      b. Cervical changes (e.g., "ripe cervix") (last weeks)
      c. Vaginal smear for Neisseria gonorrhoeae, chlamydia, group B strep, HPV cultures, and pap test
   6. Psychosocial assessment

B. Health Teaching

1. Nutrition
2. Discomforts

3. Danger signs
   a. Bleeding
   b. Rupture of membranes (ROM)
   c. Contractions (Braxton-Hicks contractions usually go away when position is changed)
   d. Signs of pregnancy induced hypertension (PIH)/toxemia
      1) Edema of hands and face, sudden weight gain
      2) Headache, blurred of vision, spots before eyes, dizziness
      3) Decrease in urinary output
   e. Burning on urination
   f. Fever
   g. Significant decrease in fetal activity
4. Childbirth education and alternative methods of birth
   a. Read method (Grantly Dick-Read)
      1) Natural childbirth
      2) Abdominal breathing
      3) Fear-tension-pain cycle
   b. Lamaze method
      1) Prepared childbirth
      2) Labor coach
      3) Chest breathing
   c. LeBoyer
      1) Birth without violence
      2) Concerned with possible negative effect a traumatic birth can have upon an infant
   d. Birthing chairs
   e. Alternate positions
   f. Birthing rooms
   g. Birthing centers
   h. Delivery by midwife
5. Rest and exercise

SECTION II

REVIEW OF
LABOR AND DELIVERY

Components of Labor

A. Power (Uterine Contractions)

1. Frequency: from the beginning of one contraction to the beginning of the next contraction
2. Duration: from the beginning of one contraction to the end of that same contraction
3. Intensity: strength of contraction, measured with fingertips lightly on the fundus (mild, moderate, and strong); accurate measurement can only be made with an internal monitor
4. Regularity: establish a pattern that increases in frequency and duration
5. Effacement: thinning of cervix, 0–100%
6. Dilatation: opening of cervix, 0–10 cms

B. Passenger (Fetus)

1. Lie: relationship of the cephalocaudal axis of the infant to the cephalocaudal axis of the mother
   a. Transverse lie
   b. Longitudinal lie
2. Presentation: body part of the passenger that enters the pelvic passageway first is called the "presenting part"
   a. Cephalic
      1) Vertex: occiput
      2) Brow: sinciput
      3) Face: mentum
   b. Breech
      1) Complete: sacrum
      2) Frank
      3) Footling
   c. Shoulder
3. Position: relationship of the landmark on the presenting fetal part to the front, sides, and back of the maternal pelvis
   a. Pelvis is divided into six areas: anterior, transverse, or posterior; left or right side
   b. Fetal landmarks are: occiput (O), mentum (M), sacrum (S), and scapula (Sc)
   c. Most common is left occiput anterior (LOA)

4. Attitude/habitus: to the relationship of the fetal parts to one another, usual is "fetal position"
5. Station: the relationship between the presenting part and the ischial spines; 0-station is engagement
6. Cardinal movements of descent
   a. Descent
   b. Flexion
   c. Internal rotation
   d. Extension
   e. External rotation or restitution

C. **Passageway (Maternal Pelvis)**
1. False pelvis helps support pregnant uterus
2. True pelvis forms bony canal; inlet, pelvic cavity, outlet
3. Types
   a. Gynecoid: normal female (50%), best for delivery
   b. Android: normal male (20%), not favorable
   c. Platypelloid: flat female pelvis (5%), not favorable
   d. Anthropoid: apelike (25%), favorable
4. Cephalo-pelvic disproportion (CPD)

D. **Psyche**
1. Physical preparation for childbirth
2. Cultural heritage
3. Previous experience
4. Support systems
5. Self-esteem

Signs of Impending Labor

A. **Lightening**

B. **Braxton-Hicks Contractions**

C. **Weight Loss (one to three pounds)**

D. **Cervical Changes**

E. **Increase in Back Discomfort**

F. **Bloody Show**

G. Rupture of Membranes

1. Client should contact physician

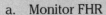

2. **NURSING INTERVENTIONS**

   a. Monitor FHR

   b. Check for prolapsed cord

   c. Test vaginal secretions for alkalinity with nitrozine paper

   d. Watch for signs of infection/meconium

H. Sudden Burst of Energy

Stages of Labor

Table IV-2.
STAGES OF LABOR

Stages	Characteristics	Interventions
First Stage: "stage of dilatation") begins true labor; ends with complete cervical dilatation; composed of of three phases	Duration: primigravida 3.3–19.7 hours; multigravida 0.1–14.3hours	Admission; assessment: medical and OB history, vital signs, FHRs signs of labor, weight, vaginal exam (if no active vaginal bleeding)
Latent phase	0–4cm dilatation; mild to moderate contractions q 15–20 min, lasting 10–30 seconds; backache, cramping, bloody show; mother talkative, cheerful, anxious	Diversional activities; time contractions; assess maternal-fetal status; pelvic rock; promote hydration; use breathing patterns; evaluate labor progress
Active phase	5–7cm dilatation; strong contractions q 3–5 minutes, lasting 30–60 seconds	Assess maternal-fetal status; backrubs; comfort measures; mother may feel apprehensive; provide encouragement; provide analgesia or anesthesia if requested and is appropriate; promote hydration and elimination; keep perineum clean; promote rest between contractions; evaluate labor progress
Transitional phase	8–10cm dilatation; strong contractions of 2–3 min, lasting 50–90 seconds; legs may cramp; nausea/vomiting, perspiration on forehead and upper lip; dark, profuse bloody show; mother may have amnesia between contractions, is irritable, anxious, and self-oriented	Assess maternal-fetal status; provide much reassurance; provide comfort measures; pant/blow with pushing urges; be supportive and help mother maintain control with breathing, etc; evaluate labor progress

Table IV-2.
STAGES OF LABOR (CONTINUED)

Stages	Characteristics	Interventions
Second stage ("stage of delivery"): begins with complete dilatation of the cervix and ends with delivery	Duration: primigravida .3–1.9 hrs; multigravida .9–.69 hours; contractions 2–3 minutes, lasting 50–90 seconds; client has urge to push and is exhausted	Assess maternal-fetal status; coach pushing; promote comfort; record time of delivery, episiotomy/lacerations, medications, or anesthetics; evaluate labor progress
Third stage ("placental stage"): begins with delivery of infant; ends with delivery of placenta	Mild contractions continue until placenta expelled, normally within 30 minutes; client may have to push to help expel placenta	Assess maternal status, blood loss; note time of placenta delivery; administer an oxytocic after placenta separation, if ordered; promote bonding
Fourth stage ("stage of recovery"): the first hour after delivery or until stable	Cramping uterine discomfort; rubra vaginal discharge with small clots; discomfort if episiotomy done; client feels happy, relieved, excited	Assess vital signs (BP, P and R) fundus, lochia, bladder and perineum q 15 min. for 1st hr., q 30 min. second hr.; temp. x1; encourage hydration and elimination; promote comfort; ice to perineum if painful; promote bonding

A. Initial Care of Newborn
1. Maintain patent airway by suction, position
2. Maintain temperature: dry, place baby on mother or under radiant heat source
3. APGAR score: performed at one and five minutes after birth
   a. Five areas scored: heart rate, respiratory effort, muscle tone, reflex irritability, color
      1) 7–10: good
      2) 3–6: moderately depressed
      3) 0–2: severely depressed
4. Eye prophylaxis: silver nitrate ($AgNO_3$), erythromycin or tetracycline (protects against infections caused by chlamydia & gonorrhea)
5. Identification
6. Vitamin K *(AquaMEPHYTON)*

TABLE IV-3.
MEDICATIONS USED IN LABOR AND DELIVERY

NAME: GENERIC (TRADE)	USE
1. Oxytocin *(Pitocin)*	Induces labor, stimulates labor, or contracts uterus after delivery
2. Methylergonovine maleate *(Methergine)*	Contracts uterus after delivery
3. Ritodrine hydrochloride *(Yutopar)*	Treats premature labor
4. Terbutaline sulfate *(Brethine)*	Treats premature labor
5. Hydralazine hydrochloride *(Apresoline)*	Treats high blood pressure
6. Magnesium sulfate *(Epsom Salt)*	Controls convulsions when used with PIH; treats premature labor
7. Calcium gluconate *(generic only)*	Antidote for magnesium sulfate toxicity
8. Rh(D)immune globulin *(RhoGAM)*	Prevents sensitization of Rh^- mother carrying Rh^+ fetus
9. Naloxone HCl *(Narcan)*	Treats respiratory depression
10. Betamethasone *(Celestone)*	Stimulates lung development in premature infant
11. Prostaglandin E_2 gel *(Prepidil)*	Softens and thins cervix

Table IV-4.
ANALGESIA/ANESTHESIA FOR LABOR AND DELIVERY

A. **Analgesics**: butorphanol tartrate *(Stadol)*, nalbuphine hydrochloride *(Nubain)*, merperidine hydrochloride *(Demerol)*; often mixed with hydroxyzine HCl *(Vistaril)* or promethazine HCl *(Phenergan)* to potentiate; do not give if within 2 hours of delivery (infant may be depressed and require naloxone HCl *[Narcan]*)

B. **Local anesthetic**: given locally into perineal tissue during second stage just prior to delivery

C. **Paracervical**: numbs cervix; good for 1st stage of labor; should not be given after dilation of 8 cms (danger of injecting fetal head); can cause fetal bradycardia

D. **Pudendal**: numbs vagina and perineum; good for 2nd stage, large episiotomy, or if anterior-posterior repair is to follow delivery

E. **Epidural**: numbs from the waist down
   1. Nursing interventions: take BP q 5 minutes until stable; assess bladder; assist in turning and pushing; hydrate client; assess fetal heart rate
   2. Complications: hypotension and fetal distress; turn client on side, increase IV rate, give oxygen

F. **Saddle (spinal)**: numbs from waist down
   1. Complications: headaches, may need blood patch
   2. Nursing interventions: use good body mechanics when moving client

G. **General**: used primarily for emergency cesarean section or vaginal birth

Operative Obstetrics

A. **Episiotomy**
   1. Definition: incision made into the perineum during delivery
   2. Purpose
      a. To spare muscles from overstretching/lacerations; to avoid difficulty holding urine in later life
      b. Limit pressure on infant's head

   3. **NURSING INTERVENTIONS**
      a. Assess for healing, infection, laceration of the anal sphincter, hemorrhage
      b. Teach Kegel exercises

B. **Forceps**
   1. Definition: obstetric instrument used to aid in delivery
   2. Indications
      a. Poor progress
      b. Fetal distress
      c. Persistent occiput posterior position
      d. Exhaustion (maternal)

3. **NURSING INTERVENTIONS**
   a. Assess infant for intracranial hemorrhage, facial bruising, facial palsy
   b. Assist with delivery as needed
4. Complications
   a. Lacerations to cervix or vagina
   b. Rupture of the uterus

C. **Vacuum Extraction**
   1. Definition: an OB procedure using a suction cup to aid in delivery
   2. Indications
      a. Poor progress
      b. Fetal distress
      c. Occiput posterior/occiput transverse position
      d. Exhaustion (maternal)

3. **NURSING INTERVENTIONS**
   a. FHR q 5 minutes
   b. Assess for cerebral trauma
   c. Inform parents that caput will disappear in a few hours

D. **Cesarean Section** (c-section)
   1. Definition: incision into abdominal wall and uterus to deliver fetus
   2. Types
      a. Low transverse: decrease chance of uterine rupture with future pregnancies; less bleeding after delivery
      b. Classical: good for emergency delivery; provides more room
   3. Indications
      a. Fetal distress
      b. CPD
      c. Placenta previa/abruptio
      d. Uterine dysfunction
      e. Prolapsed cord
      f. Diabetes/toxemia
      g. Malpresentation

3. **NURSING INTERVENTIONS**
   a. Postoperative assessment
   b. Postpartum assessment
4. VBAC (vaginal birth after c-section)

E. **Induction of Labor**
   1. Definition: process of initiating labor
   2. Indications
      a. Maternal disease: cardiac, PIH
      b. Placental malfunctions (e.g., partial previa)
      c. Fetal conditions (e.g., anomaly, death)

3. Methods used to soften cervix
   a. Prostaglandin E_2 gel
   b. Laminaria: be alert for contraindications such as asthma, nonreassuring FHR, pelvic infection, ROM, vaginal bleeding
4. Methods used to initiate induction
   a. Oxytocin *(Pitocin)*
   b. ROM (amniotomy)

5. **NURSING INTERVENTIONS**
   a. Assessment of FHR
   b. Assess for prolapsed cord, ruptured uterus
   c. STOP Pitocin if contraction longer than 90 seconds or at signs of fetal distress

SECTION III
REVIEW OF
POSTPARTAL ADAPTATION

Review of Physical Changes

A. Puerperium
1. Definition: period of time during which the body adjusts and returns to a near pre-pregnancy state; usually lasts six weeks
2. Uterus (involution)
   a. Fundus is at umbilicus after delivery; 1 fingerbreadth above umbilicus 12 hours after delivery; decreases 1 fingerbreadth a day; by 10th day, is at symphysis pubis
   b. Fundus involutes faster if client breast feeds infant
3. Lochia
   a. Definition: vaginal discharge following delivery
   b. Color
      1) Rubra (1–3 days)
      2) Serosa (3–10 days)
      3) Alba (3–6 weeks)
   c. Odor: if foul smelling, may indicate infection
   d. Amount: moderate at first, will increase with activity

e. Afterpains: due to involution of uterus; more severe with multiple births (e.g., twins), polyhydramnios; administration of oxytocin, breastfeeding

f. Menstruation: resumes in about 6–8 weeks in non-nursing mothers; and can vary with nursing mothers

4. Perineum
   a. Episiotomy or laceration
      1) Edema
      2) Pain

5. Gastrointestinal
   a. Sluggish bowels
   b. Increased appetite

6. Urinary tract
   a. Lessened sensation of bladder fullness
   b. Urinary retention
   c. Difficulty urinating

7. Temperature
   a. First 24 hours, there can be an increase up to 100.4°F due to dehydration; exhaustion
   b. WBC normally elevated

8. Skin diaphoresis
   a. Diuresis
   b. Night sweats
   c. Increased output

9. Postpartal chill
   a. Neurologic or vasomotor response to impending delivery
   b. Normal immediately following delivery

Psychological Adaptation

A. Self Concept
   1. Body image
   2. Fatigue
   3. Discomfort

B. Maternal Role/Reva Rubin's stages
   1. Taking-in phase: lasts about 2 days; mother focused on self; passive, dependent, fingertip touching
   2. Taking-hold phase: increasing independence, ready to learn
   3. Letting-go phase

C. Postpartum Depression
   1. Mood swings, depression
   2. Usually peaks on 5th day, if lasts longer than 10 days, notify physician
   3. Related to hormonal changes and fatigue; if continues, must seek professional help

SECTION IV
REVIEW OF
POSTPARTAL NURSING ASSESSMENT

A. Physical Assessment
1. Breasts
2. Fundus
3. Lochia
4. Episiotomy
5. Bladder
6. Bowels/hemorrhoids
7. Homans' sign
8. Signs of infection

B. NURSING INTERVENTIONS
1. Pain relief medications
2. Episiotomy: sitz bath, sprays, ointments, Kegel exercises
3. Hemorrhoids: sitz bath, Tucks wipes, witch hazel, ointments
4. Engorgement
   a. Non breast feeding
      1) Don't stimulate breasts
      2) Support bra 24 hrs/day
      3) Pain medication
      4) Ice
   b. Breast feeding
      1) Frequent nursing
      2) Hot shower
      3) Massage

C. Client Education
1. Perineal care
2. Restrictions
3. Rest/activity
4. Infant care
   a. Bath
   b. Cord care
   c. Circumcision care

    d. Feeding
        1) Breast feeding
            a) Advantages/disadvantages
            b) Getting started: frequent feedings, positions
            c) Nipple care: airing nipples after feeding
            d) Milk let down reflex: caused by release of oxytocin/prolactin
            e) Growth spurts
            f) Introducing solids/weaning
            g) Freezing milk
        2) Bottle: teach formula preparation
5. Sexual relations/contraception
6. Exercises

SECTION V

REVIEW OF
REPRODUCTIVE RISK

Pregnancy

A. High-Risk Pregnancy
1. Younger than 16 and older than 35 years of age
2. Above gravida 4
3. Over- or underweight
4. Drug and alcohol abuse; smoking
5. Previous blood transfusions
6. Poverty income level
7. Less than high school education
8. Unmarried
9. Unwanted pregnancy
10. Little prenatal care
11. Difficulty conceiving
12. Medical problem or pregnancy induced disease

B. Medical Problems
1. Cardiac problems
   a. Pathophysiology
      1) Pregnancy expands plasma volume, which increases cardiac output and causes an increased work load on the heart
      2) Can result in congestive heart failure or death
   b. Prognosis
      1) Occurs in 1% of all pregnant women
      2) Danger of maternal death
         a) When blood volume peaks at end of 2nd trimester (30–50% increase in volume)
         b) During labor: increase of up to 20% from "milking" effect of contractions
         c) During delivery: due to sudden increase in volume at birth when uterus contracts fully
   c. Prenatal care
      1) Prevent infection
      2) High-protein diet, restrict weight gain, do not limit salt unless ordered
      3) Monitor for anemia
      4) Anticoagulant therapy: use heparin *(Hep Lock)*, NOT warfarin sodium *(Coumadin)*
      5) Decrease activity, encourage rest, reduce stress
   d. Labor and delivery
      1) Avoid frequent changes of position
      2) Avoid pain by use of medication, epidural
      3) Avoid c-section; deliver vaginally with epidural and forceps
      4) ECG, FHM and oxygen
      5) Monitor IV carefully
      6) Use oxytocin *(Pitocin)* with caution
   e. Postpartum
      1) Critical time: first 48 hours after delivery (congestive heart failure)
      2) Watch for hemorrhage if oxytocin *(Pitocin)* not used
      3) Monitor intake and output (cardiac failure)
      4) No stockings
      5) Assess for infection: prophylactic antibiotics may be given
      6) Plan for discharge: client will need help; ability to breast feed
2. Diabetes mellitus
   a. Pathophysiology affecting pregnancy
      1) Maternal insulin: does not cross placenta; by 12 weeks fetus makes insulin, but this does not lower blood sugar level (maternal control)
      2) First trimester: fetus draws large amounts of glucose for growth; so maternal need goes way down, may not need any insulin
      3) Second trimester: HPL and other hormones secreted by the placenta after the 18th week of pregnancy have anti-insulin effect; need for insulin will increase
   b. Prenatal care
      1) Blood sugar control imperative for good outcome
      2) High incidence of congenital anomalies and still births if client not in good glucose control

c. Labor and delivery
   1) Assess infant for maturity and well-being by amniocentesis, stress and nonstress testing, estriol levels
   2) c-section after 37 weeks may be necessary if placenta deteriorates
d. Postpartum
   1) Insulin: need drops rapidly after delivery of placenta
   2) Assess infant for hypoglycemia
   3) Assess client for infection
e. Complications
   1) PIH
   2) Polyhydramnios
   3) Hypo/hyperglycemia
   4) Fetal death
   5) Macrosomia (dystocia)
   6) Spontaneous abortion
f. Gestational diabetes (2nd to 3rd trimester)
   1) May be controlled by diet alone
   2) 10–15% of clients need insulin
   3) Normal after delivery; increased risk of being diabetic later in life

C. Hyperemesis Gravidarum
1. Definition: excessive vomiting
2. Etiology: may be hormonal or psychological

3. **NURSING INTERVENTIONS**
   a. IV therapy; monitor intake and output; introduce foods slowly
   b. Decrease stress; psychiatric care
   c. Assess for metabolic acidosis (check for breath odor)

D. Polyhydramnios
1. Definition: excessive amniotic fluid
2. Etiology
   a. Maternal diseases (toxemia, diabetes)
   b. Fetal malformation (esophagus not complete)
   c. Erythroblastosis
   d. Multiple pregnancies
3. Treatment
   a. Relieve pressure by amniocentesis
   b. Delivery

E. Abortion
1. Definition: expulsion of the fetus, usually before 20 weeks gestation (spontaneous or induced)
2. Etiology
   a. Abnormal fetus
   b. Infection
   c. Anomaly of reproductive tract
   d. Injury
   e. Unwanted pregnancy

3. Terminology
   a. Spontaneous: miscarriage
   b. Therapeutic: termination of a pregnancy by medical intervention
   c. Criminal: abortion done outside medical facilities; against the law

4. **NURSING INTERVENTIONS**
   a. Save all pads and any tissues passed
   b. Assess for shock, infection, DIC, thrombophlebitis
   c. Administer RhoGAM if Rh negative
   d. Provide emotional support: do not give false encouragement

F. Ectopic Pregnancy
   1. Definition: pregnancy that occurs outside the uterus; usually in the fallopian tube, but can be on the ovary, abdomen or interligaments
   2. Etiology
      a. Malformations of tubes
      b. Pelvic inflammatory disease (PID)
      c. Tumors
      d. Adhesions
   3. Manifestations
      a. Sharp abdominal pain (rupture of tube)
      b. Shock
      c. Mild manifestations initially (e.g., spotting)
   4. Diagnosis/treatment
      a. Culdocentesis (blood doesn't clot)
      b. Removal of tube; may need blood transfusion

5. **NURSING INTERVENTIONS**
   a. Watch for shock
   b. Provide usual postop care
   c. Provide emotional support; fear of happening again

G. Hydatidiform Mole/Molar Pregnancy
   1. Definition: abnormal degeneration of the products of conception
   2. Etiology
      a. Abnormal ova
      b. Protein deficiency
   3. Manifestations
      a. Bleeding: spotting to profuse; pass tan-colored, grape-like clusters
      b. Severe nausea and vomiting
      c. Increased levels of HCG
      d. Signs of pregnancy induced hypertension (PIH) before 24th week
      e. Uterus enlarges at a rapid rate
   4. Diagnosis/treatment
      a. Lab values for increased HCG
      b. Sonogram
      c. Remove products by D&C
      d. Follow client closely for possible cancer; discourage client from becoming pregnant until cancer is ruled out

5. NURSING INTERVENTIONS
   a. Provide usual postop care: watch for hemorrhage
   b. Must have close follow-up for cancer

H. Incompetent Cervix
   1. Definition: defect in the cervix that prevents carrying a pregnancy to term
   2. Manifestation: client has repeated 2nd trimester spontaneous abortions
   3. Treatment: surgical procedures to close cervix (Shirodkar or Cerclage)
   4. Prior to delivery: suture removed

I. Pregnancy Induced Hypertension (PIH)
   1. Definition: hypertensive disorder of pregnancy occurring after the 20th week or early post partum
   2. Pathophysiology: Increased sensitivity to angiotension II causes cyclic vasospasms leading to vasoconstriction; this is responsible for most or all symptoms of PIH
   3. Terminology
      a. Pre-eclampsia: mild or severe depending upon degree of manifestations
      b. Eclampsia: convulsions occurs
   4. Manifestations
      a. Edema: mild to severe swelling of hands, face; pitting of legs
      b. Proteinuria: from 1 gm/24 hours to 5 gm or more/24 hours
      c. Hypertension: from 140/90 (or increase of 30/15 above base) to 160/110 or increase in systolic of 50 above base
      d. Decrease in urinary output (must have at least 30ml/hour)
      e. Weight gain from edema
      f. Headaches, visual disturbances, vasospasm
      g. Hemoconcentration
      h. Epigastric pain
   5. Occurrence
      a. Primigravida with age extremes
      b. Any chronic medical condition that affects the vascular system (e.g., diabetes mellitus, chronic hypertension, kidney disease)
      c. Family history
      d. Multiple pregnancies (e.g., twins, triplets)
      e. Dietary deficiencies, especially protein

6. **NURSING INTERVENTIONS** (depends upon degree of illness; status can change very quickly):
   a. Assess vital signs, weight, edema, protein in urine
   b. Provide diet high in protein, adequate fluid intake, do not restrict salt unless ordered
   c. Promote bedrest, controlled environment, lying on left side
   d. Monitor intake and output
   e. Institute seizure precautions have suction and oxygen ready
   f. May have to stabilize client and deliver baby
      1) Check reflexes, then give magnesium sulfate ($MgSO_4$); have calcium gluconate at beside (must be given slowly)
      2) Assess for precipitous delivery and abruptio placenta
7. HELLP syndrome: hemolysis, elevated liver enzymes, and low platelet count

J. Abruptio Placenta
   1. Definition: premature separation of the placenta from the uterus
   2. Etiology
      a. Trauma
      b. PIH
      c. Multiparity
      d. Cocaine use
   3. Manifestations
      a. Bleeding: either internal or external
      b. Boardlike abdomen, severe pain, tenderness, lack of contractions
      c. Bradycardia or no fetal heart rate (uteroplacental insufficiency)
   4. Treatment
      a. Usually immediate c-section
      b. Treat for blood loss

5. **NURSING INTERVENTIONS**
   a. Observe for shock
   b. Monitor vital signs, FHR
   c. Assess for diffuse intravascular coagulation (DIC), infection, anemia

K. Placenta Previa
   1. Definition: placenta attaches low in the uterus, either near or covering the cervical os
   2. Etiology
      a. Older mothers
      b. Multiparity
   3. Types
      a. Total: completely covers cervix
      b. Partial: partial covering of cervical os
      c. Low lying: near to cervical os
   4. Manifestations: painless, bright red bleeding after the 7th month (bleeding may be intermittent)

5. **NURSING INTERVENTIONS** (depends on type, severity, and gestational age):
   a. Can vary from bed rest to immediate c-section, may need blood
   b. Observe for hemorrhage; count pads; monitor vital signs and FHR; be prepared for emergency c-section; provide emotional support
   c. Do not perform vaginal exams

Labor and Delivery

A. Fetal Distress
1. Etiology
   a. Uteroplacental insufficiency
      1) Acute uteroplacental insufficiency
         a) Excessive uterine activity associated with oxytocin *(Pitocin)*
         b) Maternal hypotension: epidural, venacaval compression, supine position, internal hemorrhage
         c) Placental separation: abruptio, previa
      2) Chronic uteroplacental insufficiency
         a) PIH
         b) Diabetes
         c) Postmaturity

   b. **NURSING INTERVENTIONS**
      1) Position client on side
      2) Start IV
      3) Administer oxygen
      4) Notify physician
      5) Monitor FHR continuously

B. Umbilical Cord Compression
1. Etiology
   a. Prolapsed cord
      1) Causes: abnormal presentation, inadequate pelvis, presenting part at high station, multiple gestation, prematurity, PROM, polyhydramnios
      2) Complications: fetal asphyxia

      3) **NURSING INTERVENTIONS**
         a) Keep hand in vagina; push presenting part away from cord
         b) Continuously assess fetal welfare by pulsation of the cord
         c) Place client in Trendelenburg or knee-chest position
         d) Prepare for c-section; type and cross match blood; start IV; obtain consent
   b. Nuchal cord

C. PROM (Premature Rupture of Membrane)
   1. Etiology
      a. Infection
      b. Trauma

   2. **NURSING INTERVENTIONS**
      a. Assess FHR
      b. Assess for infection

D. Premature Labor
   1. Etiology
      a. Chronic pyelonephritis
      b. Incompetent cervix
      c. Multiple pregnancy
      d. History of premature births
      e. Sepsis
      f. Placental disorders

   2. **NURSING INTERVENTIONS**
      a. Place client on bed rest
      b. Assess for signs of infection; monitor vital signs, FHR
      c. Administer ritodrine HCl *(Yutopar),* terbutaline *(Brethine)* or magnesium sulfate as ordered to stop premature labor
      d. Provide emotional support
      e. Administer betamethasone *(Celestone)* to promote fetal lung development
      f. Delivery if near term

E. Emergency Childbirth
   1. Have mother pant, unless breech
   2. Support perineum
   3. If membranes not ruptured, do so
   4. Feel for cord around infant's neck; gently slip over head
   5. Clear out mucous; keep infant dry and warm
   6. Do not cut cord
   7. Deliver placenta: expect gush of blood and lengthening of cord; save placenta
   8. Massage client's uterus to shrink it; place infant on client's breast

F. Amniotic Fluid Emboli
   1. Definition: amniotic fluid in blood stream
   2. Often happens at delivery
   3. Emergency situation, often fatal

G. Dystocia

1. Definition: prolonged, difficult labor
2. Etiology
   a. Dysfunction of uterine contractions
   b. Abnormal position
   c. Cephalopelvic disproportion (CPD)
   d. Maternal exhaustion

3. **NURSING INTERVENTIONS**
   a. Depends upon cause
   b. Can vary from rest to c-section

Postpartum

A. Hemorrhage

1. Definition: loss of more than 500 ml of blood, or blood loss of more than 1% of body weight after delivery
2. Etiology
   a. Early: atony
   b. Late: retained placenta
   c. Lacerations, hematomas

3. **NURSING INTERVENTIONS**
   a. Atony: massage fundus first, assess bladder, administer oxytocic medications; (prostaglandin F2a) (carboprost tromethamine) may be ordered if these measures don't stop the bleeding; do not give to clients with asthma; PID; cardiac, pulmonary, renal or hepatic conditions
   b. Retained placenta, lacerations and hematoma: surgery may be necessary

B. Thromboembolic Disease

1. Etiology
   a. Normal changes in blood during pregnancy
   b. Stasis

2. **NURSING INTERVENTIONS**
   a. Assess temperature, Homans' sign
   b. Ambulate to prevent stasis
   c. Elevate client's leg; provide heat, blood thinner, antibiotics
   d. Do NOT rub

C. Infection

1. **NURSING INTERVENTIONS**
   a. Assess for signs of infection; check vital signs, pain, chills, lochia
   b. Antibiotic therapy
2. Complications
   a. Pulmonary embolism
   b. Peritonitis
   c. Pelvic cellulitis

Fetal Assessment

A. **Sonogram**
1. Purpose
   a. Locate placenta
   b. Diagnose multiple pregnancy
   c. Identify some congenital anomalies
   d. Determine gestational age

2. **NURSING INTERVENTIONS**
   a. Client must have full bladder
   b. Provide client education

B. **Fetal Monitoring**
1. Purpose
   a. Determine FHR: normal is 110–160 bpm
   b. Recognize periodic changes in FHR
   c. Determine frequency and duration of contractions
2. Types
   a. Auscultation with fetoscope; palpation
   b. External electronic monitoring
   c. Internal electronic monitoring
      1) Provides actual intrauterine pressures
      2) Provides beat-to-beat variability of the FHR, which is an indication of the sympathetic and parasympathetic nervous system status
3. Periodic changes
   a. Early decelerations: head compression
   b. Variable decelerations: cord compression
   c. Late decelerations: uteroplacental insufficiency
   d. Accelerations: usually a sign of fetal well-being
4. Variability
   a. Long-term
   b. Short-term

C. **Non-Stress Test (NST)**
1. Purpose
   a. Assess fetal well-being
   b. Look for increase in FHR (accelerations) with fetal activity (reactive NST)

A non-reactive, non-stress test is NOT reassuring

D. **Contraction Stress Test**
1. Types
   a. Oxytocin challenge test (OCT)
   b. Nipple stimulation test

2. Purpose
   a. Look for three contractions in 10 minutes
   b. No late decelerations determines fetal well-being

This is a negative CST and IS reassuring

E. Biophysical Profile
   1. Purpose
      a. Determine fetal well-being after questionable NST
      b. Determine amount of amniotic fluid

   2. **NURSING INTERVENTIONS**
      a. Provide client education
      b. Provide emotional support

F. Amniocentesis
   1. Purpose
      a. Determine fetal anomalies, sex, fetal maturity
      b. Determine L/S ratio, bilirubin levels, creatine levels

   2. **NURSING INTERVENTIONS**
      a. Provide client education
      b. Assess for premature labor
      c. Provide RhoGAM for Rh negative client

G. Chorionic Villi Sampling
   1. Purpose
      a. Determine fetal anomalies, genetic defects
      b. Early test: 8–10 weeks

   2. **NURSING INTERVENTIONS**
      a. Provide client education
      b. Provide RhoGAM for Rh negative client

SECTION VI

REVIEW OF NEWBORN

Initial Assessment

A. Vital Signs
   1. Temperature range is 97–99°F; if too high: dehydration, sepsis, brain damage, overheated; if too low: infection, brain stem injury, cold
   2. Heart rate range is 120–150 beats per minute, dependent upon state; murmur is common at first from transient patent ductus arteriosus
   3. Respirations
      a. 30–50/minute
      b. Distress: nasal flaring, intercostal or xiphoid retractions, expiratory grunt, tachypnea
   4. BP is 80/40 at birth, 100/50 by the 10 day

B. Head
   1. Measure
   2. Assess fontanels
      a. Anterior: diamond shaped, closes at 18 months
      b. Posterior: triangular shaped, closes at 8–12 weeks
      c. Bulging: increased intracranial pressure, depressed, dehydration
   3. Molding
   4. Caput succedaneum
   5. Cephalohematoma

C. Eyes
   1. Blue-gray color
   2. Strabismus is common
   3. Small hemorrhage (clears in a few weeks)
   4. Cataracts

D. Ears
   1. Low-set ears are associated with anomalies
   2. Infants hear acutely as mucous is absorbed

E. Nose
   1. Patency: infants are nose breathers; can smell
   2. Symmetry

F. Mouth

  1. Sucking reflex

  2. Epstein pearls

  3. Thrush

  4. Palate intact

G. Breast

  1. Engorgement

  2. Amount of breast tissue

H. Abdomen

  1. Measure

  2. Palpate for masses

  3. Umbilical cord

    a. Three vessels (one vein, two arteries)

    b. Will fall off in 10 days; assess for infection

I. Skin

  1. Normal variations

    a. Acrocyanosis: immature circulation

    b. Milia

    c. Toxic erythema

    d. Vernix

    e. Mongolian spots: birth marks

    f. Stork bites

  2. Color

J. Skeletal

  1. Clavicles

  2. Hips

K. Genitals

  1. Female

    a. Swollen

    b. Pseudo menstruation

    c. Vaginal tag

  2. Male

    a. Swollen

    b. Hypospadias

    c. Phimosis

    d. Testicles

L. Elimination

  1. Void in first 24 hours: pink stains from urates

  2. Patent rectum: meconium during first 24 hours

Assessment for Gestational Age

A. Physical Assessment (first 24 hours)
1. Resting posture
2. Vernix distribution
3. Skin
4. Nails
5. Lanugo
6. Sole creases
7. Skull firmness
8. Breast tissue
9. Ear formation and cartilage
10. Genitalia
11. Recoil

B. Neurological Exam (after 24 hours)
1. Ankle dorsiflexion
2. Square window sign
3. Popliteal angle
4. Heel-to-ear maneuver
5. Scarf sign
6. Neck extensors
7. Neck flexors
8. Horizontal position
9. Major reflexes
    a. Sucking
    b. Rooting
    c. Grasping
    d. Moro
    e. Tonic neck

C. NURSING INTERVENTIONS
1. Weigh daily: initial loss of 10% is normal
2. Nutrition: record daily intake and number of wet and dry diapers
3. Regulate temperature
4. Circumcision: discuss options with parents
    a. Permit signed
    b. Assess for hemorrhage, infection
5. Tests
    a. Phenylketonuria (PKU), Guthrie test: 24 hours after first milk feeding, again in 4–6 weeks
    b. Dextrostix: assess blood sugar level
    c. Cultures: if possible infection
6. Parent education: general care such as feeding; bathing, dressing, cord, and circumcision care
7. Promote attachment
8. Assess need for parental support after discharge

SECTION VII
REVIEW OF
HIGH-RISK NEWBORN

Premature Newborn

A. Definition: gestational age of less than 37 weeks, regardless of weight

B. Physical Adaptation
1. Respiratory
   a. May lack surfactants
   b. At risk for respiratory distress syndrome (RDS)
      1) Retractions
      2) Nasal flaring
      3) Expiratory grunt
      4) Tachypnea
      5) Needs mechanical ventilation, oxygen, continuous positive airway pressure (CPAP)
2. Nutrition (fluid and electrolyte)
   a. May lack gag and sucking reflex if under 34 weeks
   b. Fed by gavage or hyperalimentation
3. Circulatory
   a. Patent ductus arteriosus is common
   b. Persistent fetal circulation
4. Complications
   a. Hypothermia
   b. Hypocalcemia
   c. Hypoglycemia
   d. Hyperbilirubinemia
   e. Birth trauma
   f. Sepsis
   g. Intracranial hemorrhage
   h. Necrotizing enterocolitis
   i. Apnea

5. **NURSING INTERVENTIONS**
   a. Monitor vital signs
   b. Maintain temperature
   c. Assess hydration, nutrition
   d. Promote attachment and bonding between parents and newborn

Small for Gestational Age (SGA)

A. Definition: any newborn who falls below the tenth percentile on the growth chart at birth

B. Etiology
1. Placental insufficiency
2. PIH
3. Multiple pregnancy
4. Poor nutrition
5. Smoking, drugs, alcohol
6. Adolescent pregnancy

C. Complications
1. Perinatal asphyxia
2. Meconium aspiration syndrome
3. Hypoglycemia
4. Hypothermia
5. Infections

D. NURSING INTERVENTIONS
1. Support respirations
2. Provide neutral thermal environment
3. Provide adequate nutrition
4. Observe for complications
5. Protect from infection
6. Support parents; promote bonding

Large for Gestational Age (LGA)

A. Definition: newborn whose weight is at or above the 90th percentile

B. Etiology
1. Diabetes
2. Genetic predisposition
3. Congenital defects

C. Complications
1. Birth trauma (e.g., fractured clavicle)
2. Hypoglycemia
3. Polycythemia
4. If mother diabetic, same risk and care as premature infant

D. NURSING INTERVENTIONS
1. Assess for trauma
2. Assess for congenital abnormalities
3. Assess for hypoglycemia, especially if infant of diabetic mother (IDM)

Postmature Infant

A. Definition: gestational age of over 42 weeks

B. Complications
1. Aging of placenta
2. Difficult delivery

Jaundice (Hyperbilirubinemia)

A. Causes
1. Physiological
   a. Never seen during first 24 hours; usually appears by third day
   b. Immature liver
2. Bruising
3. ABO incompatibility
4. Rh incompatibility (erythroblastosis fetalis)
   a. Rh⁻ mother and Rh⁺ baby
   b. Kernicterus can lead to brain damage, anemia, hepatosplenomegaly
   c. Treatment
      1) Phototherapy, sunlight, exchange transfusion
      2) RhoGAM administered at 28 weeks gestation and within 72 hours of delivery
      3) Note: RhoGAM also given to all Rh negative mothers who abort after the 8th week of gestation
5. Breast feeding

Substance Abuse and the Newborn

A. Drug Dependent
1. Manifestations of withdrawal
   a. Early manifestation: irritability
   b. Sneezing, nasal stuffiness
   c. High pitched cry
   d. Tremors
   e. Perspiration
   f. Feeding problems
   g. Transient tachypnea

2. **NURSING INTERVENTIONS**
   a. Prevent overstimulation to prevent possible seizures
   b. Swaddle; hold infant firmly
   c. Medications as ordered
   d. Small, frequent feedings

B. **Fetal Alcohol Syndrome**
   1. Etiology: consumption of alcoholic beverages during pregnancy
   2. Manifestations
      a. Feeding problems
      b. Distinctive facial features
      c. CNS dysfunction
      d. Withdrawal manifestations

   3. **NURSING INTERVENTIONS**
      a. Protect infant from injury
      b. Administer medications
      c. Monitor fluid therapy
      d. Decrease stimuli
      e. Provide support for parents to care for possibly difficult infant
      f. Provide social service referral

SECTION VIII
REVIEW OF GYNECOLOGY

Vaginal Infections

A. Candidiasis (Yeast)
  1. Manifestations
     a. Cheeselike discharge
     b. Itching

  2. **NURSING INTERVENTIONS**
     a. Nystatin *(Mycostatin)*
     b. Cleanliness
     c. Treat both partners

B. Trichomoniasis (sexually transmitted)
  1. Manifestations
     a. Frothy, yellow discharge
        b. Itching
        c. Burning

  2. **NURSING INTERVENTIONS**
     a. Metronidazole *(Flagyl);* no alcohol consumption
     b. Treat both partners

C. Condyloma (sexually transmitted)
  1. Manifestations: presence of soft grayish-pink lesions on perineum

  2. **NURSING INTERVENTIONS**
     a. Application of podophyllum resin
     b. Cryosurgery or laser surgery
     c. Linked to cervical cancer
     d. Close follow-up with pap smears

Cancer

A. Cervical
1. Manifestations
   a. Bleeding between periods or after intercourse, douching
   b. Leukorrhea
   c. Pap smear
2. Treatment
   a. Hysterectomy
   b. Radiation
   c. Laser surgery

B. Endometrium
1. Manifestations
   a. Post-menopausal bleeding
   b. Abnormal bleeding
2. Treatment
   a. Radium
   b. X-ray therapy
   c. Hysterectomy

   1) **NURSING INTERVENTIONS**
      a) Assess for grieving
      b) Preop teaching
      c) Provide postop care
      d) Assess psychosexual needs

C. Ovarian
1. Manifestations (usually late in diagnosing)
   a. Back discomfort
   b. Ascites
2. Treatment: oophorectomy

D. Breast
1. Manifestations
   a. Nontender lump (often in upper outer quadrant of breast)
   b. Dimpling
   c. Asymmetry
   d. Nipple changes (bleeding or retraction)
2. Treatment
   a. Mastectomy (lumpectomy, simple or radical)
   b. Radiation
   c. Chemotherapy

3. **NURSING INTERVENTIONS**
   a. Close follow up with mammogram, breast self-examination (BSE)
   b. Provide emotional support
   c. Provide client education

Uterine Disorders

A. **Myomas**
1. Definition: benign fibroid tumors of the uterine muscle
2. Etiology: African-Americans over age 30 who have never been pregnant
3. Manifestations
    a. Pain
    b. Hypermenorrhea
4. Treatment: myomectomy

B. **Endometriosis**
1. Definition: endometrial tissue located outside of uterus
2. Manifestations
    a. Severe dysmenorrhea
    b. Lower abdominal pain, pain during intercourse, back and rectal pain
    c. Abnormal bleeding
3. Treatment
    a. Oral contraceptives (hormone therapy)
    b. Surgery
    c. Pregnancy

Tubal Disorder

A. **Pelvic Inflammatory Disease (PID)**
1. Etiology
    a. Infections
    b. Venereal disease
2. Manifestations
    a. Vaginal discharge: foul smelling, purulent
    b. Pain in abdomen, lower back
    c. Elevated temperature, nausea, vomiting

3. **NURSING INTERVENTIONS**
    a. Antibiotic therapy
    b. Client education

Menopause

A. **Definition:** cessation of menstruation for one year

B. **Manifestations**
1. Hot flashes
2. Palpitations
3. Diaphoresis
4. Osteoporosis

C. Nursing interventions
1. Assess psychosocial response
2. Discuss merits of estrogen therapy, including prevention of osteoporosis, heart disease

Battering and Rape/Assault

(see also: Unit III, Sections X-XI)

A. Battering
1. 50% of all women will be battered at some time
2. Battering may start or worsen during pregnancy
   a. Lead to miscarriage
   b. Lead to drug and alcohol abuse
   c. Spousal battering may lead to infant battering; first few days after birth, infant is at highest risk
3. Good nursing assessment and documentation is of prime importance; can lead to early intervention

B. Rape (Assault)
1. Legal (not medical) term; differs in different states (must have absence of consent); medical terms: alleged rape or alleged sexual assault
2. Rape trauma syndrome: acute phase (disorganization), then long-term process of reorganization

3. **NURSING INTERVENTIONS** (documentation is important)
   a. Obtain completed consent forms
   b. History: medical, obstetrical, sexual; describe assault and activity since
   c. Physical exam: do NOT undress client at first
      1) Examine clothes, vagina (without lubrication)
      2) Perform tests for gonorrhea and syphilis; send to venereal disease research lab (VDRL)
      3) Take x-rays and photographs
   d. Treatment: provide emotional support; prophylaxis for infection, tetanus; estradiol *(Estinyl)* for prevention of pregnancy (if indicated); medical follow-up to repeat culture for gonorrhea, VDRL, AIDS, and to assess healing
   e. Provide follow-up counseling

Infertility

A. Definition: decreased capacity to conceive

B. Etiology
1. Abnormal genitalia
2. Absence of ovulation
3. Blocked fallopian tubes
4. Altered vaginal pH
5. Sperm deficiency or decreased motility

C. Diagnosis
1. Assessment of male
2. Assessment of female

D. Management
1. Medication
   a. Clomiphene citrate *(Clomid)* or menotropins *(Pergonal);* associated with multiple births
   b. Hormone replacement
2. Artificial insemination
3. In vitro fertilization

E. NURSING INTERVENTIONS
1. Provide emotional support
2. Provide client education

Family Planning

A. Nursing Assessment
1. Determine client's knowledge about and previous experience with family planning
2. Determine client's need for genetic counseling
3. Identify infertility problems

B. Types
1. Natural (rhythm) method
   a. Use of calendar, basal body temperature and cervical mucus
   b. **NURSING INTERVENTION:** teach method

2. Oral contraceptives
   a. Side effects similar to pregnancy: initial discomforts, hypertension, clotting problems, fluid retention
   b. Do not use if family history of clotting problems or cancer; client is over 35

   c. **NURSING INTERVENTIONS**
      1) Teach method
      2) Assess for complications (increased BP)
3. Injectable contraceptive
   a. Medroxyprogesterone acetate *(Depo-Provera)*
      1) Long-acting contraceptive
      2) Administered every three months via IM injection
4. Implants
   a. Levonorgestrel *(Norplant)*
   b. Discuss ethical issues
5. Intrauterine device (IUD)
   a. High risk of PID, ectopic pregnancy, perforation of uterus; periods may be heavy (anemia)

b. **NURSING INTERVENTIONS**
   1) Need for follow-up
   2) Client should get regular pap tests
   3) Teach client to feel for strings frequently

6. Mechanical barriers
   a. Diaphragm

   1) **NURSING INTERVENTIONS**
      a) Teach client how to insert diaphragm
      b) Teach client how to use spermicidal jelly
      c) Teach client to leave in 6–8 hours after intercourse
      d) Teach client to have diaphragm refitted if client gains or loses weight, after childbirth

   b. Condom

   1) **NURSING INTERVENTIONS:** female condom (vaginal sheath)
      a) Teach client to use with spermicide
      b) Protects against STDs, including HIV
   2) **NURSING INTERVENTIONS:** male condom
      a) Teach client to leave space at end
      b) Teach how to prevent slipping or tearing during removal
      c) Protect against STDs, including HIV

   c. Cervical cap: can be left in place up to 12 hours

7. Chemical barriers

   a. **NURSING INTERVENTIONS**
      1) Teach client about possible allergic reactions
      2) Teach client how to clean equipment
      3) Warn client not to douche for 6–8 hours after intercourse

8. Sterilization
   a. Tubal ligation

   1) **NURSING INTERVENTIONS**
      a) Discuss permanency
      b) Discuss methods of obstructing tubes

   b. Vasectomy

   1) **NURSING INTERVENTIONS**
      a) Discuss permanency
      b) Warn client of need for negative sperm count three times before attempting unprotected intercourse

9. Unreliable methods
   a. Withdrawal/coitus interruptus
   b. Douching

NOTES

UNIT FIVE
PEDIATRIC NURSING

UNIT CONTENT

SYMBOLS

 Key Points

 Nursing Interventions

 Points to Remember

SECTION I
GROWTH AND DEVELOPMENT

Characteristics of Development

A. Lifelong Process

B. Critical Periods

C. Proximodistal

D. Cephalocaudal

Life Span and Development of the Infant

BIRTH–12 MONTHS

1. Physical characteristics
   a. Height: increases by 50% in first year
   b. Weight: birth weight doubles at 6 months; birth weight triples at 12 months
   c. Head: 70% of adult size at birth; 80% of adult size by end of first year
      1) Posterior fontanel: closes by 2 months of age
      2) Anterior fontanel: closes between 12 to 18 months of age
   d. Dentition
      1) Drools at four months
      2) Primary teeth (see Table V-1.)
         a) By 12 months: six primary teeth (age of child in months minus 6 = number of teeth)
         b) by 2-1/2 years: all 20 primary teeth

TABLE V-1.
SCHEDULE OF PRIMARY TOOTH ERUPTION

ERUPTION	LOWER	UPPER
Central incisor	6 months	7–1/2 months
Lateral incisor	7 months	9 months
First molar	12 months	14 months
Cuspid	16 months	18 months
Second molar	20 months	24 months

3) **NURSING INTERVENTIONS**
   a) Avoid medications that may stain teeth (e.g., tetracycline, iron)
   b) Increased drooling, finger sucking, biting on objects are all indicators of teething
   c) Cool or cold items are soothing (teething ring)
   d) Use acetaminophen *(Tylenol)* for continued irritability

  e. Reflexes
   1) Rooting (disappears by 3–4 months)
   2) Tonic neck (disappears by 3-4 months)
   3) Palmar grasp (disappears by 3–4 months)
   4) Moro (disappears by 3–4 months)
   5) Sucking (continues throughout infancy)
   6) Stepping (disappears by 3–4 months)

  f. Vital signs
   1) Pulse ranges from 100–140 beats/minute, may even be as high as 160 beats/minute depending upon activity
   2) Respirations range from 30–40/minute
   3) Immature thermoregulatory mechanisms
   4) Crying will increase all vital signs

2. Nutrition
  a. Infant feeding
   1) Allow infant to set own schedule
   2) Breast or bottle feeding depends upon mother's preference
   3) Vitamin supplements at the discretion of the physician; usually begun around 3–4 months (vitamin D and iron); flouride supplements for breast-fed infants
   4) Caloric requirements range from 110 to 120 calories/Kg/d
   5) Once dentition occurs, avoid nighttime bottle with juice or formula (it increases the incidence of dental caries ["bottle mouth" caries])

  b. Introduction of solid foods
   1) Physiologic readiness
    a) Tongue extrusion reflex (fades by about four months)
    b) Digestive enzymes
    c) Motor skills: sit with support; head and neck control
    d) Interest in solid food

   2) Nutritional guidelines
    a) Solids usually begun around 4–6 months
    b) Introduce foods one at a time, at every 4–7 days (observe for allergy)
    c) Sequence usually followed at one month intervals:
     (1) Rice cereal (good source of iron; avoid wheat)
     (2) Fruits and vegetables (yellow, then green)
     (3) Meats (begin with chicken, turkey)
     (4) Egg yolks (avoid egg whites)

d) Begin table foods around 8–12 months
   (1) Avoid nuts, foods with seeds, raisins, popcorn, grapes (risk for aspiration)
   (2) Finger foods enhance thumb-finger apposition
e) When switching from formula to cow's milk, avoid skim milk (not enough fat); infant needs whole milk
f) As amount of solids increases, reduce quantity of milk (no more than 30 oz/day)
g) Never mix food, medication with the formula
h) Avoid sweeteners such as honey or corn syrup (risk of botulism)

c. Weaning
   1) Usually begins around 4–6 months with sips from a cup; can use training cup with sipper tube and/or handles
   2) Introduce cup gradually
   3) Remove one bottle or breast feeding at a time; remove nighttime feeding last
   4) By 12–14 months, should be able to drink from a cup

d. Nutritional concerns
   1) Colic
      a) Seen in infants younger than 3 months
      b) Paroxysmal abdominal pain associated with crying and accumulation of gas
      c) Associated with overfeeding, air swallowing, maternal insecurity

      d) **NURSING INTERVENTIONS**
         (1) Slower feedings with frequent burping
         (2) Avoid excessive feedings
         (3) Increase TLC between mother and baby
         (4) Teach various feeding and holding techniques
   2) Iron deficiency anemia
      a) Result of poor diet or low-iron stores in the newborn
      b) Seldom seen in first six months due to iron stores inherited from mother
      c) Most frequently seen in children between 6 months and 1 year who ingest large quantities of milk
      d) RBCs appear microcytic and hypochromic
      e) Prevention: use of an iron-fortified formula and/or cereal
      f) Ferrous salts *(Feosol)* is the drug of choice

      g) **NURSING INTERVENTIONS**: client education
         (1) Administer between meals
         (2) Administer with citrus juice for greater iron absorption
         (3) Liquid preparations may stain teeth
         (4) May cause tarry stools

3. Activity/rest
   a. Normal infants sleep 14–16 hours a day
   b. Nocturnal pattern of sleep develops by 3–4 months

4. Motor skills
   a. 2 months
      1) Smiles socially
      2) Differentiated cry
      3) Turns head from side to side
   b. 3 months
      1) Follows object 180° horizontal and vertical (20/100 visual acuity at birth)
      2) Discovers hands
      3) Reaches for object
      4) Lifts head off bed; bears weight on forearms
   c. 4 months
      1) Recognizes familiar objects; moves extremities in response
      2) Sits with support
      3) Reaches for object
      4) Laughs aloud
      5) Begins to recognize parent
      6) Rolls back to side
      7) Almost no head lag
   d. 5–6 months
      1) Rolls over completely
      2) Bangs with object held in hand
      3) Vocalizes displeasure when object taken away
      4) Rakes object
      5) No head lag
   e. 6–8 months
      1) Holds own bottle (6 months)
      2) Transfers toy (7 months)
      3) Pincer grasp begins (8 months)
      4) Cries when scolded
      5) Sits alone (8 months)
      6) Creeps and crawls (9 months)
   f. 10–12 months
      1) Pulls self to feet (9 months)
      2) Stands alone
      3) Walks with help
      4) Uses spoon, with spilling
      5) Cruises (9 months); crawls well (10 months)
      6) Claps hands on request
      7) Imitates behavior
      8) Smiles at image in mirror
5. Language development
   a. Vocalizes (distinct from crying) by 3–4 months
   b. Recognizes "no" by 9 months; name by 10 months
   c. Two to three words in addition to "mama", "dada" by 12 months

6. Developmental stages
    a. Psychosocial development (Erikson)
        1) Trust vs. mistrust
        2) Quality of caregiver/child relationship
    b. Cognitive development (Piaget)
        1) Sensorimotor phase
            a) Reflexive
            b) Imitates and recognizes new experiences
        2) Object permanence
            a) Understands that self and object are separate (10 months)
            b) Will search for lost object (12 months)
            c) Separation anxiety (8–12 months)
7. Play
    a. Solitary
    b. Characteristics
        1) 0–3 months: verbal, visual, tactile stimuli
            a) Toys should be brightly colored, washable
            b) Enhance eye-hand coordination
                (1) Mobiles, cradle gyms
                (2) Busy box, toys with faces
            c) Stimulate auditory senses (e.g., rattles, music box)
            d) Different textures, sizes, shapes
        2) 4–6 months: initiates, recognizes new experiences
            a) Mobility increasing
            b) Hand coordination increasing
            c) Memory begins
            d) Types of toys
                (1) Mirrors to see image
                (2) Chewable, large toys
                (3) Brightly colored rattles, beads
                (4) Squeeze toys, teething rings
                (5) Remove cradle gym to avoid accidents
        3) 6–12 months
            a) Increasing self awareness
            b) Repeats pleasurable activities
            c) Object permanence
            d) Imitates behavior at 10 months; "peek-a-boo"
            e) Increased desire to explore
            f) Types of toys
                (1) Large boxes, kitchen utensils
                (2) Water play with supervision
                (3) Texture play: sand, dirt
                (4) Pouring, filling, dumping
                (5) Playing with food (beginning of self feeding)

  c. Safety measures

    1) Toys should be large; short strings

    2) Constructed of nontoxic materials

    3) Always supervise

    4) Inspect toys for problems

      a) Rough edges

      b) Parts that can be pulled off and swallowed or aspirated

8. Health maintenance

  a. Safety

    1) Avoid overstimulation, rough handling

    2) Limit setting should involve redirecting behaviors to safer activities

    3) Childproof the environment

  b. Immunizations (see Table V-10. on p. 301)

    1) Hepatitis B: birth, two months, six months

    2) DTP, OPV, HIB: two, four, and six months (timing of 3rd OPV optional)

    3) Acetaminophen *(Tylenol)* given prophylactically to lessen fever from DTP

    4) Pertussis held if temp > 105°F after previous DTP or if child has history of neurologic disorder

  c. Infant restraints

    1) Semi-reclining seat that faces rear until 20lbs/10kg

    2) Use car seat belt to anchor restraint

    3) Middle of car's back seat is the safest area

    4) Infant restraints should not be used in front seat, especially with passenger-side airbag

  d. Aspiration of foreign objects

    1) Common problems include food, buttons from clothing, baby powder, and older sibling's toys

    2) Emergency measures for choking infant

      a) Five backblows, five chest thrusts (repeat until successful)

      b) No blind finger sweep

9. Health deviations

  a. Accidents (leading cause of death over one year of age)

    1) Falls (depth perception develops by 7–9 months)

    2) Suffocation/aspiration/drowning

    3) Burns

  b. Anticipatory guidance

    1) Put gates at top and bottom of stairs

    2) Put pots on back burners of stove

    3) Place electrical cords out of reach

    4) Put safety plug covers in all electrical outlets

    5) When feeding, do not prop bottle

    6) Never leave alone on bed or table top; avoid infant walkers

    7) Avoid plastic bags

    8) Use infant restraints

    9) Supervise near any source of water (including tub, buckets, toilet)

Life Span and Development of the Toddler

12 MONTHS–36 MONTHS

1. Physical characteristics
   a. Appearance is potbellied, long legged, clumsy
   b. Slowing rate of growth for height and weight (adult height = approximately double height at 2 years)
   c. Dentition
      1) 20 teeth by end of toddler period (2-1/2 years)
      2) Visits dentist by age 2
      3) Adult should brush child's teeth (by 2 years)
      4) Nursing caries (only water should be in bottle at bedtime)
   d. Vital signs
      1) Pulse: ranges from 80–110 beats/minute
      2) Respirations: range from 25–35/minute
      3) Blood pressure: average is 100/70
2. Nutrition
   a. Growth lag (100 kcal/kg)
   b. Expresses independence through food preferences; food fads are common
   c. Wants to feed self; very ritualistic, messy
   d. Space meals with frequent nutritious snacks (cheese, PB & J)
   e. Small portions (physiologic anorexia)
   f. Child should participate in family meals
   g. Fluid requirements: 115 ml/kg/day
   h. 2–3 cups of milk/day
3. Activity/rest
   a. Sleeps 10–12 hours with naps
   b. Routines/rituals are reassuring
   c. Nightmares/night terrors are possible
4. Motor skills
   a. 13–16 months
      1) Uses spoon and cup, but will spill
      2) Will crawl when in hurry
      3) Walks without help (since about 13 months)
      4) Climbs up and down stairs with buttocks
      5) Loves containers of all kinds
      6) Mimics housework
      7) Scribbles with crayon held in fist
      8) Pulls from sitting to standing without help
      9) Stacks 2–3 blocks (15 months)
      10) Throws and drops things (15 months)

b. 18 months
1) Runs clumsily; falls often
2) Kicks small ball
3) Throws ball overhand
4) Jumps in place
5) Pulls and pushes toys
6) Uses spoon and cup without spilling
7) Removes clothes (e.g., shoes, socks)
8) Stacks 3–4 blocks (18 months)

c. 2 years
1) Walks up and down stairs
2) Runs well
3) Climbs
4) Turns knobs to open door; unscrews lids
5) Turns pages in book one at a time
6) Dresses self in simple clothing
7) Tower of five blocks

d. 2-1/2 to 3 years
1) Holds crayon with fingers
2) Strings beads
3) Confuses right and left
4) May have daytime bowel and bladder control
5) Jumps with both feet

5. Language development
a. Ten words by 18 months
b. May say "no" when agreeing (means "yes")
c. Uses two- to three-word phrases by 2 years; vocabulary of 300 words; verbalizes needs (toileting, food, drink); uses pronouns
d. Gives first and last name by 2-1/2 years

6. Developmental stages
a. Psychosocial development (Erikson)
1) Autonomy vs. shame/doubt (1–3 years)
a) Egocentric
b) Transitional objects
c) Uninhibited at showing independence
d) Negativism/temper tantrums
2) Child gains control of body, excretions

b. Cognitive development (Piaget)
1) Sensorimotor (12–24 months)
a) Objects are cause of action
b) Memory increasing
c) Separation anxiety
2) Preoperational (24 months–4 years)
a) Concrete thinking begins
b) Symbolic play increases
c) Increasing use of speech
d) Egocentric

7. Play
   a. Parallel play
      1) No sharing
      2) Ownership determined by possession of object
      3) Short attention span
   b. Purposes of play
      1) Increase motor skills
      2) Decrease anxieties
      3) Mode of exercise
      4) Learn about body
      5) Fantasy
      6) Form of socialization

   c. Types of activities
      1) Gross motor
         a) Jungle gym
         b) Push pull toys
         c) Tricycle (2-1/2–3 years)
      2) Fine motor
         a) Crayons, paints, paper
         b) Building blocks
         c) Musical toys
         d) Smearing (12–18 months)
            (1) Playdough
            (2) Water play
         e) Pounding boards
      3) Enjoys being read to
8. Health maintenance
   a. Toilet training (18 months–2 years)
      1) Physiologic readiness (sphincter control at approximately 18 months)
      2) Imitation; potty chair
      3) Respect autonomy needs (psychologic readiness)
      4) Praise and reward
      5) May not be complete until 4 to 5 years of age (nocturnal control often delayed)
   b. Discipline
      1) Toddlers are negative and ritualistic
      2) Limits must be simple and consistent
      3) Difficult due to intellectual functions
      4) Parental example; removal of privileges
   c. Safety
      1) Precautions
         a) Childproof the environment
         b) Post emergency room and poison control phone numbers
         c) Infant restraints (may switch to forward facing car seat when child weighs approximately 20lbs/10kg)
         d) Supervised play

2) Immunizations (see Table V-10. p. 301)
   a) MMR: 15 months
   b) HIB: 15 months
   c) DTP, OPV: 18 months
   d) Varicella zoster (chicken pox): after 12 months
9. Health deviations
   a. Accidents
      1) Motor vehicles: passengers, pedestrians
      2) Burns
      3) Drowning/suffocation/aspiration
      4) Falls
      5) Poisoning
         a) Lock all medications or potentially toxic substances
         b) Use child-resistant caps appropriately
         c) Never refer to medications as candy
         d) Have syrup of ipecac in the home
         e) Have phone number for poison control posted by telephone
   b. Anticipatory guidance
      1) Supervise closely near any source of water
      2) Store flammables, lighters out of reach
      3) Use child restraints in vehicles
      4) Avoid foods easily aspirated

Life Span and Development of the Preschooler

THREE–FIVE YEARS
1. Physical characteristics
   a. Average four year old is 40 inches and 40 pounds
2. Nutrition
   a. Growth lag (90 kcal/kg)
   b. Encourage finger foods (e.g., cheese, fruit)
   c. Food jags are common
   d. Allow child time to finish playing before meal time; give 5-minute warning
   e. Give small portions of food
   f. Fluid requirements drop to 100 ml/kg
3. Activity/rest
   a. May give up nap but needs quiet time
   b. Peak time for sleep disturbances
      1) Refusal to go to bed: child resists bedtime; comes out of room frequently
         a) **NURSING INTERVENTIONS**
            (1) Consistent bedtime
            (2) Ignore attention seeking behaviors
            (3) Avoid bringing child into parents' bed
            (4) Transitional object may be helpful

    2) Nighttime fears
       a) Child resists bed because of fears (e.g., dark, "monsters")

       b) **NURSING INTERVENTIONS**
         (1) Calmly reassure child
         (2) Use of night-light may be helpful
         (3) Monitor bedtime television viewing

4. Motor skills

  a. Three years
    1) Dresses with supervision; needs help with buttons
    2) Rides tricycle
    3) Tower of nine–10 blocks
    4) Climbs stairs with alternate feet
    5) Pours fluid from a pitcher
    6) Copies a circle or cross
    7) Can perform simple household tasks

  b. Four years
    1) Hops and skips on one foot
    2) Walks upstairs without use of handrail; alternates feet walking downstairs
    3) Uses scissors
    4) Throws overhand
    5) Copies square and triangle
    6) Brushes teeth
    7) Laces shoes but cannot tie

  c. 5 years
    1) Skips and hops on alternate feet
    2) Walks backwards
    3) Can master two-wheel bike
    4) Uses simple tools
    5) Roller skates
    6) May master tying shoes
    7) Prints first name
    8) Dominant hand established

5. Language development

  a. Three years
    1) Vocabulary of 900 words
    2) Talks constantly regardless of whether anyone is listening
    3) Complete sentences of 4–5 words

  b. Four years
    1) Vocabulary of 1,500 words
    2) Questions constantly
    3) Exaggerates; tells "tall tales"
    4) May stutter
    5) May pick up profanity from others

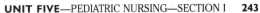

    c. 5 years
      1) Vocabulary of 2,000 words
      2) Uses all parts of speech
      3) Speech 100% intelligible to others
      4) Some sounds still imperfect
      5) Names colors, coins, days of week

5. Developmental stages
    a. Psychosocial development (Erikson)
      1) Initiative vs guilt (3–6 years)
        a) Vigorous behavior
        b) Limit testing
        c) Pursues a goal; sometimes in conflict with others
      2) Child develops a conscience
    b. Cognitive development (Piaget)
      1) Preoperational (2–7 years)
        a) Egocentric in thought and behavior
        b) Concrete, tangible thinking
        c) Vivid imagination
          (1) Magical thinking (e.g., thoughts can cause events)
          (2) Peak age for fears
        d) Animism
    c. Socialization

      1) 3 years
        a) May have an imaginary friend
        b) Increased ability to separate from parents
      2) 4 years
        a) May be bossy and impatient
        b) Privacy and independence become important
      3) 5 years
        a) Less rebellious; more responsible
        b) Cares for self and hygiene needs with minimal supervision
    d. Sexuality
      1) Knows own sex and sex of others by three years
      2) Always determine what child wants to know before answering questions
      3) Answer questions honestly and simply
      4) Masturbation is normal, healthy expression, if not excessive
      5) Sexual exploration demonstrated in playing doctor

7. Play
    a. Cooperative play beginning
      1) Enjoys loud, physical activities
      2) More socialization during play
      3) Self-criticism or boasting evident
      4) Peers increasing in importance, but relationships are loose and fluid; change constantly

b. Purposes of play
1) Increase coordination
2) Decrease tension, anxiety
3) Deal with fantasies
4) Enhance self-esteem
5) Sense of power, control
6) Increase knowledge of self
c. Materials
1) Physical: bat, ball, sand box, sled, bike, puzzles
2) Dramatic: dress-up clothes, dolls, costumes; imitate adult behavior
3) Creative: pens, paper, crayons, paint, scissors, playdough, record player, chalk
8. Health maintenance
a. Safety
1) Maintain safe environment
a) Lock up flammables, medications, and toxic substances
b) Supervise play
c) Teach water safety (swimming)
d) Teach traffic (pedestrian) safety
e) Automobile safety
(1) Use of car seat until approximately 4 years, 40lbs; may depend on local laws
(2) Small child safer with booster seat
(3) Use of seat belt
2) Immunizations (see Table V-10. p. 301)
a) Pre-kindergarten boosters given at five years (DTP, OPV, MMR)
b) May catch up on "missed" immunizations required for school attendance
b. Discipline
1) Consistent limit setting
2) "Time-out" for misbehavior
a) Effective if used consistently
b) Time-out: one minute per year of child's age

Life Span and Development of the School-Age Child

SIX YEARS–12 YEARS
1. Physical characteristics
a. Grows 1–2 inches/year
b. Gains 3–7 pounds/year
c. Pubescent changes may begin to appear
1) Girls: by approximately 10–12 years
2) Boys: by approximately 12–14 years
d. Vital signs approach adult normals
1) Pulse: ranges from 60–80 beats/min
2) Respirations: range from 18–20/min
3) Blood pressure: averages 90–110/55–60

e. Dentition
   1) Permanent teeth begin erupting about six years (see Table V-2.)
   2) Erupting permanent teeth loosen primary teeth; child wiggles out primary teeth
   3) 32 permanent teeth by 18 years of age
   4) May wear braces (orthodontia)

TABLE V-2.
SCHEDULE OF PERMANENT TOOTH ERUPTION

ERUPTION	AGE
First molar	5 1/2–6 years
Medial incisor	6–7 years
Lateral incisor	7–8 years
Cuspid	10–12 years
Bicuspid	10–11 years
Bicuspid	11–12 years
Second molar	12–13 years

2. Nutrition
   a. Influenced by peers, mass media in food selections
   b. "Junk food" (empty calories), "fast food" preferred
   c. Obesity possible if inadequate exercise
   d. Nutritious snacks are useful, should be encouraged
3. Activity/rest
   a. Sleeps 8–10 hours/day with vivid dreams
   b. Somnambulism (sleep walking) is common
4. Motor skills
   a. Gross-motor skills
      1) Roller skates
      2) Bicycles
      3) Swimming
      4) Competitive sports
      5) Skate boards
   b. Fine-motor skills
      1) Cursive writing
      2) Musical instruments
      3) Arts and crafts
5. Language development
   a. Masters all sounds by 7-1/2–8 years
   b. Uses telephone
   c. Reads and writes

6. Developmental stages
   a. Psychosocial development (Erikson)
      1) Industry vs inferiority (6–12 years)
         a) Primary tasks relate to learning skills, activities
         b) Child may display pride, diligence, cooperation, loyalty or aggression, bossiness, irritation, disrespect
         c) Family life continues to be important but child begins to branch out (e.g., peers, teachers)
         d) Afraid of failure; embarrassed by poor grades
      2) Child develops self-esteem
   b. Cognitive development (Piaget)
      1) Concrete operations (7–11 years)
         a) Conservation of matter
         b) Classifies and sorts; enjoys collecting
         c) Concrete logic and problem solving
         d) Less self-centered
      2) Inductive thinking
   c. Socialization
      1) Prefers peers of same age and sex
      2) Can share and cooperate
      3) Responds positively to rewards
      4) Enjoys scouts, clubs, team sports (e.g., recreation leagues)
      5) Cliques may become evident (9–10 years)
      6) May be left alone for short periods (10–12 years)
   d. Sexuality
      1) Answer questions openly and honestly
      2) Approach sexuality as a normal biological function
      3) Pre-adolescents need specific, age-appropriate information about puberty, physical changes (10–12 years)
      4) Develops interest in opposite sex (10–12 years)
7. Play
   a. Cooperative
   b. Characteristics
      1) Clubs (8–10 years)
      2) Gangs (10–12 years)
      3) Best friends (9–10 years)
      4) Secrets
      5) Wants to know how things are made
   c. 6–8 years
      1) Table games
      2) Collections
      3) Radio
   d. 9–12 years
      1) Community sports
      2) Group play
      3) Creative: dance, art, music

8. Health maintenance
   a. Safety
      1) Prevention
         a) Focus on teaching child to be safe
         b) Not under parental supervision at all times
      2) Immunizations
         a) MMR booster (if not given pre-kindergarten) at 11–12 years
         b) Varicella zoster (chicken pox) for susceptible children (can be given anytime after 1 year of age)
   b. Common problems
      1) Swearing
      2) Lying
      3) Cheating
      4) Stealing
      5) Nail biting
      6) Sibling rivalry
         a) Often jealous of younger/older sibling
         b) May violate "personal space" or take belongings
         c) Parent may get pulled into sibling dispute
         d) Encourage parent not to become involved except in case of physical/emotional harm
   c. Discipline
      1) Avoid punitive measures
      2) Consistency
      3) Withdrawal of privileges
      4) Use of "time-out"
   d. Stress and coping
      1) School-age children face enormous societal pressures
      2) Do not have cognitive skills to deal with these pressures
      3) Professionals need to be aware that sleep problems, enuresis, changes in appetite, or behavioral problems may be indicative of inadequate coping
      4) Use stress reduction techniques
9. Health deviations
   a. Accidents
      1) Motor vehicles (use seat belts)
      2) Fractures due to increased activity (use helmets and other protective gear)
      3) Firearms
      4) Drowning
   b. School phobia
      1) Fear or dread of school
      2) Manifestations
         a) Physical complaints voiced on weekday mornings
            (1) Nausea and vomiting
            (2) Anorexia
            (3) Abdominal pain (i.e., "stomach ache")

        b) Manifestations subside once child is at home

        c) Abrupt onset

        d) More common in females

    3) Etiology

        a) Teacher/child mismatch

        b) Fear of failure

        c) Bully

        d) Inappropriate dress

        e) Physical defect

        f) Separation anxiety

    4) Treatment

        a) Identify cause

        b) Support child in attending school daily

        c) Professional (psychiatric) help may be required in severe cases

Life Span and Development of the Adolescent

12 YEARS–18 YEARS

1. Physical characteristics
   a. Very individualized
   b. By 17 years, 100% of adult stature
   c. Vital signs reach adult norms
   d. Dentition
      1) 3rd molars (wisdom teeth) by approximately 18 years
      2) Orthodontia
   e. Sexual maturation/puberty
      1) Female
         a) Breast enlargement (approximately 11 years)
         b) Pubic hair
         c) Growth spurt
         d) Menarche (i.e., onset of menstruation)
            (1) Approximately 12-1/2 years
            (2) Ovulation approximately 6 months–1 year after menarche
      2) Male
         a) Pubic hair
         b) Growth of external genitalia
         c) Growth spurt/increased muscle mass
         d) Voice changes
         e) Ejaculation/nocturnal emission
         f) Axillary and facial hair
2. Nutrition
   a. Growth spurt
   b. Increased protein, iron, and calcium needs

3. Activity/rest
   a. Sleep needs increase due to growth demands
   b. Tire easily
4. Motor skills
   a. Characteristics
      1) Risk takers
      2) Sense of indestructibility
      3) Appear gawky and clumsy
      4) General increase in physical and psychomotor skills enhance self-esteem
5. Language development
   a. Sophisticated ability to communicate via verbal and written word
   b. Use of slang prominent
6. Developmental stages
   a. Psychosocial development (Erikson)
      1) Identify formation vs. identify diffusion (12–18 years)
         a) Stable, coherent picture of self
         b) Incorporate changes in body into identity
         c) Identify future career goals
      2) Adolescent makes identity commitments
   b. Cognitive development (Piaget)
      1) Formal operations (11+ years)
         a) Future perspective
         b) Ability to hypothesize
      2) Abstract thinking
   c. Socialization
      1) Emancipation from family
      2) Less adult supervision
      3) Peer group major influence; has strong need to belong
      4) Employment
   d. Sexuality
      1) Establishes sexual identity and orientation
      2) Experiments with intimate relationships
      3) Common issues
         a) Sexually transmitted disease
         b) HIV
         c) Adolescent pregnancy
7. Play
   a. Reflects psychosocial needs (e.g., cliques, peers, dating)
   b. Group activities (e.g., sports)
8. Health maintenance
   a. Safety
      1) Accident prevention
         a) Focus on educating adolescent to make safe choices
         b) Be alert to signs of depression, substance abuse

2) Immunizations (see Table V-10., p 301)

    a) Td (Tetanus-diptheria) needed every 10 years

    b) Hepatitis B if not previously immunized

b. Discipline

  1) Increased independence

  2) Consistency

c. Stress and coping

  1) Faced with enormous societal pressures

  2) Feels pressure to belong, conform, achieve

  3) Common reactions to stress

    a) Early adolescent: mood swings, self-centered

    b) Middle adolescent: rebellious behavior

    c) Later adolescent: conceals anger, better coping skills

  4) Common problems

    a) Runaways

    b) Eating disorders

    c) Substance abuse

      (1) Non-prescription, illicit, or street drugs

      (2) Alcohol

      (3) Tobacco

9. Health deviations

a. Accidents

  1) Motor vehicles

    a) Driver's education

    b) Drunk driving

  2) Firearms

  3) Drowning

b. Homicide

c. Suicide

SECTION II

THE HOSPITALIZED CHILD

Stress of Hospitalization

A. Regression
1. Usually healthy adaptation to hospitalization
2. Respect child's use of this defense mechanism
3. Assist child to achieve past developmental levels

B. Reaction to Hospitalization
1. Protest: strong, conscious need for parent; may be confused, frightened, crying
2. Despair: mourning period; may be withdrawn, apathetic
3. Denial: represses true feelings; feels parent has failed; interested in surroundings but not mom
4. Separation can be overwhelming for clients younger than 6 years old

C. Developmental Factors
1. Infant: trust vs mistrust; stress of hospitalization related to:
   a. 0–6 months: loss of consistent care giver
   b. 6–12 months: strong need for mother; stress of hospitalization related to separation anxiety
2. Toddler: autonomy vs shame/doubt; stress of hospitalization related to:
   a. Separation, loss of significant other
   b. Loss of mobility due to restraints, crib
   c. Inconsistent care giving; needs rituals, consistency
3. Preschooler: initiative vs guilt; stress of hospitalization related to:
   a. Separation anxiety
   b. Loss of control due to decreased mobility, increased dependence
   c. Threats to body integrity may cause increased aggression
   d. Concept of illness
      1) Magical thinking (i.e., feels thoughts can cause illness)
      2) May believe illness or hospitalization is punishment

4. School age child: industry vs inferiority; stress of hospitalization related to:
   a. Loss of control
   b. Separation from: peers, school, after school activities
   c. Type of illness: acute vs chronic
   d. Concept of illness
      1) Perceives an external cause for illness
      2) May view illness as a result of "doing something wrong"
5. Adolescent: identity vs role diffusion; stress of hospitalization related to:
   a. Threats to body image
   b. Loss of control
   c. Separation from peers, schools, activities
   d. Concept of illness
      1) Believes self to be invulnerable
      2) Understands internal cause of disease
      3) Can cooperate with treatment plan if understands immediate benefits

D. Reaction to pain
   1. Rule of thumb: assume that if a procedure would be painful for an adult, it is also painful for a child
   2. Developmental assessment of pain
      a. Infant
         1) Generalized body response of rigidity, thrashing
         2) Loud crying, facial expression
      b. Toddler
         1) Localized response; will withdraw from pain
         2) Physical resistance after painful stimulus
      c. Preschooler
         1) Verbalizes pain
         2) Attempts to avoid painful stimulus
         3) May view pain as punishment
      d. School-aged child
         1) Verbalizes pain
         2) Stalling behavior; vocal protest
         3) Recognizes physical cause of pain
      e. Adolescent
         1) Sophisticated verbal expression of pain
         2) Less resistance offered; physical, vocal
         3) Understands physical and psychological pain

3. **NURSING INTERVENTIONS** (strategies for pain management)
   a. Age-appropriate assessment
     1) Ask child with age-appropriate language
     2) Use pain rating tool (e.g., Baker-Wong Faces)
     3) Evaluate for behavioral indicators of pain, especially in pre-verbal child
     4) Have parents participate in assessment
   b. Use of pharmacologic control method
     1) Weight-appropriate (mg/kg) dosages
     2) Oral and IV routes preferred over IM; child will avoid "shot" and not be medicated
     3) Patient-controlled analgesia (PCA) is appropriate for children over age 7 (concrete operations) who understand cause and effect
   c. Use of non-pharmacologic control methods
     1) Distraction
     2) Relaxation
     3) Kinesthetic (rocking) stimulation
   d. Prevent pain with procedures
     1) Euteric mixture of local anesthetics (EMLA) cream (topic antimicrobial): applied in thick dollop at least 1–2 hours before procedure (venipuncture, biopsy), transparent dressing applied and removed just prior to procedure
     2) Conscious sedation: midazolam *(Versed)*, fentanyl citrate *(Sublimaze)*

Strategies for Health Promotion/Stress Reduction

A. Pre-Hospital Preparation (e.g., Preoperative Tour)

B. Specially Trained Pediatric Staff

C. Increased Use of Outpatient Facilities

D. Client Advocacy

E. Therapeutic Play
   1. Purposes
     a. Mastery
     b. Ego strengthening
     c. Test reality
     d. Deal with fears, anxieties, the unknown

   2. **NURSING INTERVENTIONS**
     a. Relate play to child's growth and development
     b. Allow child to proceed at own pace
     c. Provide a variety of materials, but let child choose media
     d. Reflect back child's feelings, behaviors

F. Communication

1. Appropriate for the situation
2. Clear, consistent
3. Communicate directly with child
   a. Verbally
   b. Nonverbally
4. Encourage parental verbalization concerning illness, hospitalization

G. Family

1. Support: comfort child
2. Encourage to stay with child
3. May use defense mechanisms to deal with hospitalization
   a. Anger
   b. Denial
   c. Projection
   d. Guilt
4. Encourage visitation by extended family members, peers (when appropriate)
5. Explain to parents that regressive behavior is normal and expected in hospitalized children
6. Explain to parents that separation anxiety behaviors are normal and expected in hospitalized children

SECTION III

NURSING CARE OF THE CHILD WITH CONGENITAL ANOMALIES

Congenital Heart Defects

A. Hemodynamics
1. Fetal circulation
   a. Ductus venosus: carries oxygenated blood from placenta to inferior vena cava; partially bypasses liver; closes by approximately 8th week of life
   b. Ductus arteriosus: by-passes flow of blood through lungs by shunting oxygenated and unoxygenated blood from pulmonary artery to aorta; closes 7–10 days after birth
   c. Foramen ovale: connects right and left atria; allows blood to flow from RA-LA, thereby bypassing RV and pulmonary circuit; closes by 2–3 months
2. Newborn circulation
   a. At first breath, lungs expand, which increases blood flow to pulmonary system
   b. Pulmonary vascular resistance decreased and systemic vascular resistance increased

B. Characteristics
1. Unknown etiology (always consider genetic factors in addition to intrauterine infection, radiation, or drugs)
2. Incidence is 1 in 1,000 live births (accounts for 50% of all deaths in first year of life); may be associated with other birth defects, syndromes
3. May not be diagnosed while hospitalized
4. Early manifestations indicate, more severe defect
5. Clinical signs include:
   a. Newborn and infant
      1) Cyanosis: especially circumoral and acrocyanosis; cyanosis on exertion (e.g., feeding, crying)
      2) Dyspnea: especially on exertion
      3) Failure to thrive
      4) Frequent upper respiratory infections
      5) Feeding difficulty

   b. Older child
     1) Cyanosis and dyspnea (as above)
     2) Impaired growth
     3) Fatigue
     4) Digital clubbing
     5) Squatting
     6) Polycythemia: increased RBC count to compensate for impaired gas exchange-increases oxygen-carrying capacity of blood
   c. Congestive heart failure
     1) Tachypnea, dyspnea
     2) Exercise intolerance
     3) Tachycardia (above 160 bpm)
     4) Diaphoresis
     5) Hepatomegaly and edema (late signs)
6. Increased risk of bacterial endocarditis

C. Diagnosis
1. Cardiac catheterization
2. Echocardiography

D. Pathology/Treatment
1. Acyanotic (see Table V-3.)
2. Cyanotic (see Table V-4.)

E. NURSING INTERVENTIONS
1. Correct knowledge deficit related to:
   a. Cardiac catheterization
     1) Consider developmental level of child when planning teaching strategies (e.g., preschooler)
     2) Child will be NPO 4–6 hours prior to procedure
     3) Procedure is done under conscious sedation
     4) Postoperative concerns include maintaining pressure dressing, keeping the extremity straight, palpating brachial or pedal pulse distal to the insertion site, no blood pressure on affected extremity, neurovascular checks, and hydration
   b. Anticoagulant therapy
     1) Usually seen with children who have prosthetic valves or increased blood viscosity
     2) Instruct parents to check for excessive bruising, epistaxis, hematuria, or bloody stools
     3) Child should wear MedicAlert bracelet
     4) Report any febrile illness, anorexia or bleeding to physician immediately
   c. Preoperative preparation
     1) Promote parental involvement
     2) Allow expression of fears through therapeutic play
     3) Include description of what child will feel during procedure, surgery
     4) Control parental anxiety through support, encouragement, and teaching

2. Altered cardiac output related to failure of the myocardium to meet the demands of the body
    a. Reduce energy expenditures by providing adequate rest periods, planning care to reduce interruptions, and recognizing signs of fatigue; infant seat very helpful; avoid temperature extremes
    b. Administer and monitor medications that will increase cardiac function
        1) Digoxin
            a) Check apical heart rate one full minute prior to administering (hold digoxin if heart rate is below: 100 for infants; 80 for toddlers and preschoolers; 60 for children and adolescents)
            b) Therapeutic effects include increased cardiac output, decreased heart rate, increased urine output
            c) Classic manifestations of toxicity include nausea (anorexia in infants), vomiting, lethargy and bradycardia; digoxin level greater than 2.1 may indicate toxicity
            d) Administer medication on an empty stomach; do not give with food or juice; do not repeat dose if child vomits
            e) Observe for hypokalemia (increases risk of digoxin toxicity)
        2) Diuretics: furosemide (*Lasix*), *Diuril*, ethacrynic acid (*Edecrin*)
            a) Reduce venous and systemic congestion
            b) Monitor potassium levels and supplement losses
            c) Include daily weights, intake/output, and respiratory assessment in daily care
3. Altered nutrition: less than body requirements related to congestive heart failure
    a. "Cardiac" infants usually have a weak suck, become cyanotic during feedings, tire easily, and may fall asleep while feeding
    b. Small, frequent feedings using soft nipple with large hole
    c. Administer 24 Kcal/oz formula in order to increase caloric intake
    d. Limit oral feedings to 20 minutes; gavage feed the remainder
4. Altered parenting related to chronic aspects of cardiac problems
    a. Discipline is the most difficult area of parenting due to feelings of guilt and powerlessness
    b. Parents need help remembering child should be treated as normally as possible
    c. Counsel family regarding possibility of developmental delays; include infant stimulation in teaching
    d. Involve all family members in child's care; siblings may feel left out, alienated, angry

TABLE V-3.
REVIEW OF ACYANOTIC CONGENITAL HEART ANOMALIES

ANOMALY	HEMODYNAMICS	CLINICAL MANIFESTATIONS	TREATMENT
Patent Ductus Arteriosus (PDA): A vascular channel between the L main pulmonary artery and the decending aorta, as a result of failure of the fetal ductus arteriosis to close	Shunt of oxygenated blood from the aorta into the pulmonary artery Increased left ventricular output and work load	Usually asymptomatic, but frequent impairment of growth or CHF "Machinery murmur" Wide pulse pressure	Medical: administration of indomethacin (Indocin) (prostaglandin inhibitor) is effective in some newborns and premature infants Surgical: ligation of patent ductus (in infancy)
Ventricular Septal Defect (VSD): Defect is in membranous muscular portion of the ventricular septum; may vary from small to large defect.	Shunt of oxygenated blood from L to R ventricle Leads to R ventricular hypertrophy Needs surgical repair Bi-directional shunting may occur with very large defect (Eisenmenger Syndrome)	May be asymptomatic Heart murmur is heard in 1st week of life (systolic) Growth failure, feeding problems during 1st year of life; FTT; frequent respiratory infections CHF is common	Some small defects may close spontaneously Open heart: direct closure suturing with plastic prosthesis (usually at preschool age, may be done earlier in infancy for large defects)
Atrial Septal Defect (ASD): Malfunctioning foremen ovale; or abnormal opening between the atria	Shunting of oxygenated blood from L to R atrium Increased R ventricular output and work load May develop pulmonary hypertension (in adulthood, if not surgically treated in childhood)	Acyanotic; assymptomatic Soft blowing systolic murmur Thin and asthenic Frequent episodes of pulmonary inflammatory diseases Poor exercise tolerance	Open heart with direct closure or suturing with plastic prosthesis (usually at pre-school age)
Coarctation of Aorta: Preductal constriction of the aorta between subclavian artery and ductus anteriosis Postductal constriction of aorta directly beyond the ductus	Obstruction of the flow of blood through the constricted segments Increased L ventricular pressure and work load Extensive collateral circulation bypasses coarcted area to supply lower extremities with blood	Hypertension in upper extremities with decreased BP in lower extremities Weak or absent pulsations in lower extremities CHF May be asymptomatic; occasionally fatigue, headaches, leg cramps, epistaxis	Surgical resection of coarctate area with direct anastomosis or use of a graft Correction usually done by 2 years of age to prevent premanent hypertension

TABLE V-4.
REVIEW OF CYANOTIC CONGENITAL HEART ANOMALIES

ANOMALY	HEMODYNAMICS	CLINICAL MANIFESTATIONS	TREATMENT
Tetralogy of Fallot: combination of four defects: 1) Pulmonary stenosis 2) Ventricular septal defect (VSD) 3) Overriding aorta 4) Hypertrophy of R ventricle	Obstruction to outflow of blood from R ventricle into pulmonary circuit and increased pressure in the R ventricle leads to R to L shunting of unoxygenated blood thru the VSD directly into the aorta Severity of defect depends on degree of pulmonary stenosis and size of VSD	Acute cyanosis at birth Cyanosis developing during early months that increases with physical exertion Clubbing of fingers and toes Systolic murmur Acute episodes of cyanosis and hypoxia called "tet spells" or hypercyanotic episodes occur if oxygen supply cannot meet demand (e.g., with crying, exertion, exercise, feeding) Squatting Growth retardation	Surgical: Blalock-Taussig Procedures: provides blood flow to pulmonary arteries from the L or R subclavian artery Repair: open heart closure of VSD and resection of stenosis Usually performed in first two years of life
Transposition of Great Vessels (TGV): the aorta originates from the R ventricle and the pulmonary artery from the L ventricle	Two separate circulations without mixture of oxygenated and unoxygenated blood except through shunts Mixture of blood may occur through one or more septal defects: - Ventricular septal defect (VSD) - Atrial septal defect (ASD) - Patent ductus arteriosus (PDA)	Usually deep cyanosis shortly after birth or after closing of ductus Early clubbing of toes and fingers Poor growth and development, FTT Rapid respirations; fatigue Congestive heart failure	Medical: administration of IV prostaglandin until surgical repair Repair: arterial switch is treatment of choice; must be done within first few days of life; great vessels reimplanted under complete circulatory arrest Several other types of repair are all multiple stage approaches

Neurological Defects

A. Hydrocephalus

1. Characteristics
   a. Definition: imbalance in either absorption or production of cerebrospinal fluid within intracranial cavity
   b. Classification: either congenital or acquired
   c. Usually diagnosed at birth or within two to four months of life of life
   d. Often associated with other neural tube defect (e.g., myelomeningocele)
   e. Clinical manifestations categorized by age
      1) Infant: increased head circumference, tense bulging anterior fontanel, distended scalp veins, high pitched cry, irritability, feeding problems, discomfort when held
      2) Older child: headache, vomiting (especially in the morning), diplopia, blurred vision, behavioral changes, decreased motor function, decreased level of consciousness, seizures

2. Diagnosis
   a. May be detected on prenatal sonogram
   b. Clinical signs
      1) Increasing intracranial pressure
      2) Increasing head circumference
   c. CT or MRI scan confirms diagnosis; shows excessive fluid in ventricles

3. Treatment
   a. Pressure relieved by surgical insertion of a shunting device
   b. Components of a shunt include: catheter, reservoir, pumping device with one-way valve, distal tubing with regulator valve
   c. Most common type of shunt is ventriculoperitoneal
   d. Complications include shunt failure and infection
   e. Shunt will require revision (lengthening of tubing) as child grows
   f. Early treatment necessary to prevent progressive mental retardation

4. **NURSING INTERVENTIONS**
   a. Risk for injury related to increased intracranial pressure
      1) Preoperatively, the nurse's focus should be on assessing neuro function; always measure head circumference by obtaining occipito-frontal measurement
      2) Postoperatively
         a) Neuro assessment with daily head circumference
         b) Position on non-operative site; check anterior fontanel to determine positioning of the head; do not pump shunt without physician's order.
      3) Control environmental stimuli; take seizure precautions
   b. Risk for infection
      1) Classic manifestations: elevated vital signs, decreased LOC, vomiting, feeding problems
      2) Assess incision site frequently for manifestations of inflammation or leakage

c. Additional interventions

       1) Alteration in nutrition (less than body requirements): frequent small feedings; planned rest periods after feeding; daily weight

       2) Knowledge deficit: instruct parents regarding manifestations of shunt failure; encourage infant stimulation to help maximize child's potential; use stress management techniques

B. Myelomeningocele (Neural Tube Defects)

  1. Characteristics

    a. Failure of posterior laminae to fuse with herniation of saclike cyst of meninges, CSF, and spinal nerves

    b. Usually associated with other neuro defects (e.g., hydrocephalus)

    c. Unknown etiology

    d. May be prevented by folic acid supplementation by women of child-bearing age prior to conception and through first trimester

  2. Pathology

    a. Partial to complete paralysis determined by location of defect (usually lumbosacral)

    b. Musculoskeletal problems such as club foot, scoliosis, congenital hip dysplasia

    c. Sensory disturbances parallel motor dysfunction

    d. Bowel and bladder problems including constipation, incontinence, neurogenic bladder

  3. Diagnosis

    a. Amniocentesis: 98% accurate; elevated AFP, confirmed by prenatal sonogram

    b. Apparent at birth: visible sac

  4. Treatment

    a. Decision to correct the defect or not is difficult as well as controversial

    b. Early surgical closure is advocated to preserve neural function, reduce risk of infection, control hydrocephalus

  5. **NURSING INTERVENTIONS**

    a. Risk for infection

      1) Preoperatively, the main goal is to prevent rupture of the sac, which would predispose the newborn to infection

        a) Prone position

        b) Cover sac with 4 x 4s moistened with sterile saline

        c) Check sac for tears or cracks

        d) Do not cover sac with clothing or diapers (places pressure on the sac)

        e) Perineal care to prevent contamination of sac

        f) Monitor for manifestations of meningitis (irritability, anorexia, fever, seizures)

      2) Postoperatively, the main goal is to promote healing and reduce neurological complications

        a) Prone position with head slightly lower than body

        b) Place protective barrier across incision to prevent contamination

3) Long-term problems of infection are related to urinary retention, reflux, chronic urinary tract infections
   a) Parents should be taught Crede's maneuver
   b) Intermittent self-catheterization can be performed as early as 5–6 years of age
   c) Stress hydration and early recognition of UTIs
   d) Urinary diversion procedures are often required

b. Risk for injury related to increased intracranial pressure secondary to hydrocephalus
   1) Neuro checks with daily head circumference
   2) Monitor for manifestations of increased intracranial pressure

c. Ineffective parental coping
   1) Parents will need help dealing with the issue of "chronic sorrow" as well as the long-term aspects of the condition
   2) Anger and denial are common defense mechanisms
   3) Assess family support and available resources
   4) Remember that every family's method of coping is different: offer options in non-judgmental manner; provide supportive environment that will help families make the most appropriate choices

d. Risk for injury related to latex exposure
   1) Children with neural tube defects are at increased risk for latex allergy
   2) Exposure to common medical products containing latex should be avoided (e.g., use of vinyl gloves)
   3) Environmental latex exposure (e.g., balloons) should be avoided

e. Additional nursing problems
   1) Risk for impaired skin integrity: frequent position changes, keep perianal area clean of dribbling urine and stool
   2) Impaired mobility: position changes, range-of-motion activities, physical therapy

Musculoskeletal Defects

A. Congenital Dysplasia of the Hip (CDH)

1. Characteristics
   a. Refers to imperfect development of the hip of varying degrees
   b. Etiology unknown; familial tendency; females are 8 times more likely to develop
   c. Manifestations: shortening of affected leg, asymmetrical gluteal folds, limited abduction, Ortolani's sign (audible click as examiner slips femoral head forward)
   d. Early detection critical: if untreated will lead to lordosis, scoliosis, "duck waddle"

2. Pathology
   a. The head of the femur must be properly located within the acetabulum for correct development of the hip joint
   b. As ossification proceeds, correcting the hip defect becomes more difficult
   c. Once child begins to walk, prognosis questionable
   d. Most common type is subluxation (incomplete dislocation of hip)

3. Diagnosis
   a. Assessment techniques with newborn (Ortolani's sign)
   b. X-rays difficult to read in early infancy because ossification of femoral head does not occur until 3–6 months of life

4. Treatment
   a. If diagnosed within first 2–3 months of life, the hip joint abduction is maintained via double diapering, Frejka pillow, splint, or Pavlik harness
   b. Once adductor muscles contract, traction and/or casting may be used; usually by 6 months (once the child is standing and walking) both methods are used in conjunction with surgery (Bryant's, traction if below 2 years)

5. **NURSING INTERVENTIONS**
   a. Risk for injury related to impaired neurovascular function
      1) Casts: support drying cast with pillow; turn with palms of hands; elevate extremity; reposition every 2–4 hours; neurovascular checks as needed; assess cast for drainage/infection; do not use abductor stabilizer bar when turning
      2) Traction: maintain weights and pulleys; correct body alignment; neurovascular checks as needed; pin care if appropriate
      3) Bryant's traction: legs at 90° angle to body, buttocks elevated off bed
   b. Risk for impairment of skin integrity: petal the cast; reposition (if appropriate); assess skin for irritation or pressure areas; do not allow child to play with small toys; supervise during eating; sheepskin or egg crate mattress; skin care with massage at least every 4 hours; active/passive range of motion (ROM) (if appropriate)
   c. Impaired physical mobility related to cast or traction: need to consider problems of immobility (e.g., pulmonary, renal eliminative, musculoskeletal); diet should include increased roughage, fluid, calcium, protein, carbohydrates

d. Knowledge deficit related to home care: Pavlik harness should be worn 24 hours/day; do not remove even when changing diaper, sponge bathing infant; check skin under harness at least daily; return demonstrations are most appropriate way to evaluate teaching effectiveness; assess parental attachment as well as infant's developmental progress; infant in hip spica cast will need specially designed car seat

B. Congenital Clubfoot (Talipes Equinovarus)
  1. Characteristics
    a. Forefoot adducted, heel tilted inward (varus), plantar flexion at ankle
    b. Important to differentiate between positional and true clubfoot
  2. Diagnosis and treatment
    a. Apparent at birth; longer treatment postponed, more soft tissue changes occur and correction more difficult
    b. Serial casting is employed to gradually manipulate the foot into normal position; casts are changed at weekly intervals; as each new cast is applied, the foot is re-manipulated and recasted
    c. Dennis-Brown splint may be used to maintain position once casting is completed
    d. Surgery may involve separating ligaments if casting ineffective

  3. **NURSING INTERVENTIONS**
    a. Risk for injury related to neurovascular impairment
    b. Knowledge deficit related to cast care or exercise regimen: compliance is critical if defect is to be corrected; encourage follow-up visits as well as meeting child's developmental needs within imposed limitations; parents must be able to perform neurovascular checks at home on casted limb due to infant's growth rate

---

Gastrointestinal Defects

A. Cleft Lip
  1. Characteristics
    a. Definition: failure of the maxillary processes to fuse with the nasal processes
    b. Etiology: unknown, but strong genetic and environmental factor
    c. Defect may be unilateral or bilateral
    d. More common in males
    e. May or may not be accompanied by cleft palate
  2. Pathology
    a. Prone to ear, nose, and throat infection
    b. Long-term problems include speech, hearing, and dentition problems
  3. Diagnosis and treatment
    a. Surgical repair initiated within first three months of life
    b. Staggered z-shaped suture line used to minimize scarring
    c. Logan bar may be applied to reduce tension on the suture line

4. **NURSING INTERVENTIONS**
   a. Alteration in nutrition: less than body requirements
      1) Preoperatively: feeding difficulties related to sucking problems; infants also swallow a great deal of air during feeding; burp frequently; use of adaptive feeding devices
         a) Large soft nipples
         b) Breck feeder (syringe with rubber tubing)
         c) Breast feeding
      2) Postoperatively: sucking places undue pressure on the suture line so feeding may present difficulties; use medicine dropper or Breck feeder; begin this type of feeding preoperatively
   b. Risk for injury related to trauma or pressure on the suture line
      1) Restrain infant to prevent pulling or tugging on the suture line (elbow restraints); remove periodically one at a time
      2) Do not position on abdomen
      3) Prevent crying as much as possible; pacifier cannot be used
      4) Physician may order a topical ointment such as *Neosporin* or bacitracin *(Baci-IM)* be applied to suture line as needed to prevent infection; if using cotton-tipped applicator, roll the applicator over the suture line; do not rub
   c. Ineffective airway clearance: infant is at risk for aspiration so positioning is very important; infant should be repositioned frequently to prevent stasis of secretions; side to side or infant seat only acceptable positions
   d. Ineffective family coping: birth of a child with "physical problems" elicits anger, disbelief, denial; parents will encounter "chronic sorrow"; be supportive and encouraging while helping parents overcome their concern; focus should be on bonding; convey attitude of acceptance; describe results of surgical correction; show photographs

B. Cleft Palate
   1. Characteristics
      a. Failure of palatine processes to fuse
      b. More common among females
      c. Defect may include both hard and soft palate
      d. Major problems are similar to cleft lip: feeding; aspiration; ear, nose, and throat infections
      e. May or may not be associated with cleft lip
   2. Diagnosis and treatment
      a. Repair usually completed by 12–18 months of age to prevent speech problems
      b. Surgery may be performed in stages

3. **NURSING INTERVENTIONS**
   a. Alteration in nutrition: less than body requirements
      1) Preoperatively: feeding difficulties related to sucking problems; infants also swallow a great deal of air during feeding (burp frequently); use of adaptive feeding devices
         a) large, soft nipples
         b) Breck feeder (syringe with rubber tubing)
         c) breast feeding
      2) Postoperatively: nothing can be placed in the child's mouth; child is fed liquified diet through a cup; spoon cannot be inserted into mouth as it can damage suture line; soft diet maintained until palate healed
   b. Risk for injury related to trauma or pressure on the suture line
      1) Use elbow restraints to keep the child's hands away from the mouth; remove periodically one at a time for ROM
      2) May position on abdomen
      3) Prevent crying as much as possible
      4) Child may not suck or place fingers in mouth; small toys or objects must be kept out of the child's reach; child may drink from a cup or sip from the side of a large spoon; oral hygiene after eating is essential to reduce problems with infection
   c. Ineffective airway clearance: child will be at risk for breathing problems during the first 48 hours; new breathing patterns must be established; croupette may be ordered
   d. Ineffective family coping (see cleft lip, p.265)

SECTION IV

NURSING CARE OF THE CHILD WITH AN ACUTE ILLNESS

Common Problems Associated with Acute Illness

A. Fever
1. Characteristics
   a. Defined as abnormal elevation of central body temperature
   b. Classified as temperature in excess of 100.4°F (38°C)
   c. Not always related to severity of illness; varies from child to child
   d. Always consider
      1) Age of child: below six months, more serious concerns;
      2) If child is immunosuppressed or receiving chemotherapy
   e. Most fevers in children are viral, self limiting, may play a role in recovery from infection
2. Diagnosis
   a. Feeling the child's skin for warmth is not an accurate indicator
   b. Always investigate family epidemiology
   c. Remember that diet, activity level, and behavioral changes are subtle diagnostic clues
   d. Laboratory tests ordered may include: CBC, Ua, chest film and blood cultures
3. Treatment
   a. Fever management is questionable because fever is considered a part of the body's defense mechanism
   b. Antipyretic, such as acetaminophen *(Tylenol)* or ibuprofen *(Motrin)*
   c. Do not give aspirin

4. **NURSING INTERVENTIONS**
   a. Altered body temperature related to infection
      1) Monitor child's temperature by checking it every 3–4 hours
      2) Employ environmental measures: remove excessive clothing, expose skin to air, encourage clear fluids if child not vomiting
   b. Risk for injury related to febrile seizures
      1) Usually seen in children between six months and three years old; related to sudden rise of temperature (above 102°F); child usually has a respiratory or gastrointestinal infection
      2) Therapeutic treatment includes diazepam *(Valium)*, antipyretics
      3) Nursing interventions: maintain a patent airway; protect the child from injury; observe the seizure

4) Do not attempt to restrain the child or put anything in mouth; remove all toys and sharp objects; if there is a history of seizures, the sides of the bed should be padded and emergency equipment (e.g., oxygen, suction) should be available; allow seizure to run its course (unless seizure lasts longer than five minutes); do not leave the child alone

c. Risk for fluid volume deficit related to dehydration:
1) Periodically assess the child for manifestations of dehydration (e.g., sunken eyes, depressed anterior fontanel, dry mucous membranes, poor tissue turgor); specific gravity will be elevated
2) Encourage clear fluids if child not vomiting
3) Check to make sure the child is voiding in adequate amounts

d. Knowledge deficit related to home care of child:
1) Parents need information regarding controlling the child's temperature, seizure precautions, preventing dehydration
2) If child is discharged on medications, parents need to know how the medication works, how long its to be given, common side effects
3) Parental fear is a major problem that should be addressed

B. Vomiting
1. Characteristics
   a. Assessment includes: amount, color, consistency, time of day emesis occurs, relationship to eating
   b. Vomiting causes a loss of hydrochloric (HCl) acid, which leads to metabolic alkalosis
2. Diagnosis
   a. Frequently the child is dehydrated and looks emaciated
   b. Diagnostic procedures include: upper GI (UGI), barium enema, abdominal ultrasound, CT of abdomen
   c. If gastroesophageal reflux is suspected, a Tuttle test (pH probe) and an esophagoscopy may be ordered
   d. Remember children with metabolic alkalosis are usually very lethargic, poorly perfused, and hyperventilating
3. Treatment
   a. It is essential to correct both the fluid and acid-base imbalance
   b. If the vomiting is predictable and of brief duration, antiemetics may be ordered to depress the vomiting center (e.g., promethazine HCl *[Phenergan]*, chlorpromazine HCl *[Thorazine]*, metoclopramide HCl *[Reglan]*); trimethobenzamide *(Tigan)* may also be ordered
   c. Gastroesophageal reflux is treated with drugs that promote gastric mobility and emptying, such as metochlorpramide *(Reglan)*, cisapride *(Propulsid)*, or omeprazole *(Prilosec)*; take gastroesophageal reflux precautions (e.g., positioning with HOB elevated, especially after meals or feeding)

4. **NURSING INTERVENTIONS**
   a. Risk for fluid volume deficit related to loss of fluid and electrolytes secondary to vomiting:
      1) Replacement therapy is determined by type (e.g., isotonic, hypotonic) and degree of dehydration (e.g., 5%, 10%)
      2) Monitor potassium (KCl) replacement closely
      3) Measure and record all fluid losses
      4) Assess for manifestations of dehydration
   b. Alteration in nutrition: less than body requirements related to persistent vomiting
      1) Any infant with a history of vomiting should be fed slowly while being held in an upright position; all activities such as bathing or medication administration, should be done prior to feeding.
      2) Refeeding following a period of NPO should be initiated slowly to observe response to PO fluids
      3) If gastroesophageal reflux is the cause of vomiting, feeding can be a unique challenge; since the lower esophageal sphincter matures throughout the first year of life, medical rather than surgical interventions may be the preferred route: elevating head of bed, maintaining infant with head elevated after all feeds (i.e., feed in infant seat); anti-reflux medications
   c. Additional nursing problems
      1) Risk for sensory-perceptual alterations: assess sensorium
      2) Risk for repeated injury related to aspiration: position on abdomen or side-supported; never position supine
      3) Ineffective parenting: parents need support regarding care and feeding
      4) Knowledge deficit: instruct parents regarding anti-reflux precautions

C. Gastroenteritis (Diarrhea)
   1. Characteristics
      a. Defined as an increase in fluid, frequency and volume of stool; usually results from increased rate of peristalsis; stools are watery, acidic, green in color, expelled forcefully; Na, K, and bicarbonate are also lost via the stool
      b. Diarrhea is serious in young children because:
         1) The extracellular space is larger so greater amounts of fluid will be lost
         2) Younger children have a greater body surface area and GI surface areas in relation to body weight
         3) Younger children have a higher basal metabolic rate (BMR) so the fluid and electrolyte balance is unstable
      c. Weight is a critical indicator of fluid loss in young children; 1 gram of weight equals 1 ml of body fluid, a weight loss or gain of 1 kg in a 24-hour period represents a fluid shift of 1,000 ml; the loss of fluid and electrolytes in the diarrhea stool results in dehydration and electrolyte depletion
      d. Dehydration associated with diarrhea is classified as mild: weight loss of 5% or less with loose, runny brownish-yellow stools
      e. Causative factors: bacteria (salmonella, shigella), viral (rotavirus), allergies, emotional disturbances, dietary and malabsorption problems

f. Chronic nonspecific diarrhea (CNSD) or irritable bowel syndrome is the most common form of chronic diarrhea in children:
   1) Diarrhea persists longer than 3 weeks
   2) Normal growth and development
   3) No evidence of enteric pathogens

2. Diagnosis
   a. Serum electrolytes, complete blood count, blood cultures may be ordered
   b. Antibiotic therapy is a common cause of diarrhea: (ampicillin *[Polycillin pediatric]*, tetracycline *[Achromycin]*, neomycin)
   c. Thorough history: dietary habits, travel, family patterns

3. Treatment
   a. Mild dehydration (2–9%) without hypernatremia; generally treated with oral rehydrating solutions (ORS); critical behaviors that demand immediate attention are persistent diarrhea, weight loss, bloody stools, or physiological changes such as deep breathing, listlessness, reduced urinary output
   b. A secondary lactose intolerance may occur following gastroenteritis; child may be maintained on temporary lactose-free diet
   c. Severe dehydration (greater than 10% weight loss) is an acute medical emergency; the child is NPO (12–48 hours), parenteral fluids are administered

4. **NURSING INTERVENTIONS**
   a. Risk for fluid volume deficit related to dehydration
      1) Periodically assess for manifestations of dehydration, weigh daily
      2) Monitor potassium replacement (KCl) closely; administer no more than 4 mEq/Kg/d to correct hypokalemia
      3) Carefully monitor intravenous infusions for correct infusion rate
      4) Monitor laboratory values: BUN/creatinine ratio, serum electrolytes, arterial blood gases; collect urine and stool specimens as needed
   b. Risk for infection related to diarrhea
      1) Isolate client; promote good handwashing
      2) Teach self-care precautions if child is old enough
   c. Alteration in nutrition (less than body requirements):
      1) Refeeding following a period of NPO should be initiated slowly to observe client's response to PO fluids; offer small amounts of fluid (usually clear) every 10 to 20 minutes; if vomiting occurs, increase time between feedings; if no vomiting, decrease time between feedings; initially offer oral rehydration solutions (ORS) such as *Pedialyte* as tolerated; progress to non-carbonated soft drinks (Gatorade); avoid Kool-Aid and Popsicles (they do not contain electrolyte); limit apple juice (it can cause diarrhea)

2) As diarrhea resolves, easily digested foods such a breast milk, half-strength soy based formula, applesauce, bananas, rice cereal (ABC diet), dry toast, and saltine crackers may be added; for older children try BRAT diet (bananas, rice cerea, applesauce and toast): after 48 hours, eggs, milk, cheese, and boiled meat; stay away from high-fat food; lactose intolerance may persist for several weeks following diarrhea; use soy-based formulas such as *Isomil*

   d. Additional nursing problems

      1) Risk for alteration in skin integrity: change diapers frequently; expose diaper area to air (unless explosive diarrhea) or heat lamp (no closer than 18 inches) for 20 minutes

      2) Knowledge deficit: instruct parents regarding fluid and dietary protocols

D. Respiratory Infections

  1. Acute otitis media

    a. Characteristics

      1) Middle ear infections are common in children under age 5:

        a) Eustachian tube is shorter, wider and straighter,

        b) Organisms from nasopharynx have easier access to middle ear,

        c) Tonsils and adenoids are usually enlarged,

        d) Young child has poorly developed immune mechanisms, and

        e) Infants and toddlers are supine a large portion of the day

      2) Usually follows an upper respiratory infection (URI) during which the swollen mucosa close off the eustachian tube; the growth of the organism along with the fluid retention in the ear combine to cause the infection

      3) Most frequently seen bacterial infection in young children; most serious long-term problem associated with otitis is conductive hearing loss

      4) Clinical manifestations: fever; irritability; pulling, tugging or rubbing the affected ear; anorexia; signs of a URI; older children may complain of earache or pain when chewing or sucking; purulent discharge may be present

    b. Diagnosis

      1) Otitis media: otoscopy reveals an intact tympanic membrane that appears inflamed, bulging, and without a light reflex

      2) Chronic otitis media: otoscopy reveals dull, gray membrane with visible fluid behind eardrum

    c. Treatment

      1) Oral antibiotics; therapy should last 10–14 days

      2) Oral decongestants such as sympathomimetics (vasoconstriction) or antihistamines (reduce congestion) may be used; analgesics may be ordered to reduce pain, discomfort

      3) Following completion of the antibiotic regimen, treatment effectiveness should be evaluated

      4) Children with recurrent otitis media should be tested for hearing loss

      5) Myringotomy (surgical incision of the ear drum) and insertion of PE (pressure equalizing) tubes may be ordered in cases of recurrent chronic otitis media

d. **NURSING INTERVENTIONS**
1) Pain
   a) Administer analgesics such as acetaminophen *(Tylenol)* as needed; apply warm compresses to affected ear; avoid foods that require chewing
   b) Be alert to non-verbal signs of discomfort; changes in behavior can be an early indicator of pain; humidity, clear PO fluids may also be helpful
2) Knowledge deficit
   a) Instruct parents regarding the importance of antibiotic compliance; medication should be taken for 10–14 days (even after manifestations have gone away)
   b) Instruct parents in feeding techniques to reduce the incidence of ear infection: upright when feeding; breast feeding offers protection against pathogens
   c) Eliminate tobacco smoke and known or potential allergens from environment
   d) Following myringotomy and PE (pressure equalizing) tubes insertion, ensure parents know some drainage from the ears is expected; report obvious bleeding and an abrupt rise in temperature; the ear should be kept dry; avoid activities that require submerging the head in water (use ear plugs for bathing)

2. Epiglottitis
   a. Characteristics
      1) Definition: acute bacterial infection of the supraglottic structures resulting in obstructive airway problems
      2) Seen primarily in children 3–7 years of age; considered a medical emergency, immediate treatment must be initiated
      3) Most common causitive organism: H. influenza, type B
      4) Clinical manifestations: abrupt onset with rapid progression to severe respiratory distress, sore throat, high fever (102°–104°F), drooling, dysphagia, muffled voice; tripod position (sit upright, lean forward with mouth open and tongue protruding)
   b. Diagnosis

      1) Throat is red, inflamed with a cherry-red epiglottis; under no circumstance should an inspection of the throat be initiated unless emergency equipment is available (e.g., trach setup, ET tube); do not take a throat culture
      2) Lateral neck film (i.e., soft-tissue x-ray) reveals swollen epiglottis
   c. Treatment
      1) Parenteral therapy with IV antibiotics is begun immediately; PO antibiotics for 10–14 days following IV therapy
      2) Steroid therapy: frequently used for anti-inflammatory effects
      3) Intubation or tracheostomy usually necessary to prevent obstruction; extubation may occur within 3–4 days
      4) Vaccine prevention: H influenza type B conjugate vaccine effective against H influenza epiglottitis; should be given at 2, 4, 6, and 15 months of age

d. **NURSING INTERVENTIONS**
1) Ineffective breathing patterns related to airway obstruction and pulmonary changes secondary to infection
   a) Respiratory assessment every 1–2 hours or prn; be alert for manifestations of increasing respiratory distress (e.g., increased retractions, stridor, cyanosis, irritability, nasal flaring, use of accessory neck muscles to breathe)
   b) Have oxygen and suction equipment at bedside; reposition every 2 hours
   c) Administer humidified air via trach collar or ET tube
   d) If client is in mist tent, be sure to keep warm and dry; have sides of tent tucked securely around tent, provide appropriate supportive care (e.g., toys, encourage rooming-in)
   e) Administer steroids, antibiotics as ordered
2) Other nursing problems
   a) Anxiety related to respiratory distress: do not leave child unattended; encourage parents to stay with child as much as possible
   b) Ineffective family coping: allow verbalization fears and concerns; assess current coping skills
   c) risk for fluid volume deficit: parenteral fluids while NPO; monitor for dehydration

3. Laryngotracheobronchitis (croup)
   a. Characteristics:
      1) Most common form of croup; peak age is below 5 years of age; because of smaller airway diameter, child is more prone to significant airway narrowing
      2) May begin as an upper respiratory infection, proceed to lower respiratory structures
      3) Most common causative organisms: parainfluenza viruses
      4) Clinical manifestations are the result of inflammation and subsequent narrowing of airway: hoarseness, barking or "seal-like" cough, inspiratory stridor, increasing respiratory distress
   b. Diagnosis
      1) Clinical manifestations are diagnostic
      2) Lateral or soft-tissue x-rays of neck may be ordered
   c. Treatment
      1) Humidity with cool mist provides relief by reducing inflamed mucosa
      2) Aerosol epinephrine *(Racepinephrine)* may also be used if client is hospitalized
      3) Corticosteroids may be used for their anti-inflammatory effect

d. **NURSING INTERVENTIONS**
  1) Ineffective breathing pattern related to inflammation
      a) Child usually is cared for at home: instruct parents in use of cool-mist humidifier; monitor for impending distress; nocturnal and spasmodic coughing episodes may be relieved by taking child into cool night air or humid, warm bathroom (shower running and door closed)
      b) If child hospitalized-continuous observation during periods of respiratory distress; be alert to signs of impending respiratory failure: nasal flaring, retractions, increased stridor; place client in cool-air mist tent, supplemental oxygen may be used
  2) Other nursing problems
      a) Anxiety related to respiratory distress: encourage rooming in
      b) Risk for fluid volume deficit: parenteral fluids if NPO

4. Bronchiolitis
  a. Characteristics
    1) Acute viral infection that primarily affects bronchioles; most commonly seen in infants between 1–12 months of age; occurs in winter and spring months
    2) Respiratory syncytial virus (RSV) is responsible for half of the documented cases of bronchiolitis; mode of transmission is hand to nose, droplet infections; reinfection common in all ages
    3) Bronchiolar obstruction leads to hyperinflation and air trapping
    4) The younger the client, the greater the chance of severe lower respiratory disease requiring hospitalization; infants at high risk for severe RSV infection include: premature infants, infants with underlying cardiac or respiratory conditions, immune deficient infants
    5) Clinical manifestations: initial manifestations of URI that progress to tachypnea; paroxysmal coughing, increased restlessness; nasal flaring, intercostal and substernal retractions, wheezing, and decreased breath sounds indicate severe lower respiratory tract disease
  b. Diagnosis
    1) Manifestations are clinically diagnostic
    2) RSV is diagnosed using ELISA-enzyme linked immunosorbent assay (nasal secretions)
    3) Chest film will reveal areas of consolidation that are difficult to differentiate from bacterial pneumonia; areas of hyperinflation
  c. Treatment
    1) Treated symptomatically; humidity, rest, adequate hydration are main therapeutic interventions; can be successfully treated at home in most cases
    2) Rationale for hospitalization: tachypnea (> 70 breaths/min), severe retractions, change in behavior, hydration problems; at-risk children with chronic or debilitating diseases should be hospitalized
    3) In serious cases, steroids and inhaled bronchodilators will be administered
    4) With severe RSV infection, ribavirin *(Virazole),* an anti-viral aerosol, may be administered via oxygen tent or hood; teratogenic effects have been reported, so pregnant caregivers are at-risk, strict guidelines exist for use

d. **NURSING INTERVENTIONS**
1) Ineffective airway clearance: respiratory assessment every two hours and as needed (should include respiratory rate, rhythm and depth, retractions, color, cough, chest auscultation for rales, rhonchi, wheezing); oxygen therapy via oxyhood or cool air mist tent; use ABGs and pulse oximetry to determine response to treatment; elevate head of bed; monitor for increased respiratory distress; NPO if tachypneic
2) Risk for fluid volume deficit related to insensible water loss secondary to tachypnea: monitor hydration status by daily weight, strict intake and output, urine specific gravity; assess for manifestations of dehydration; parenteral fluids if NPO
3) Anxiety related to parental fear and apprehension: include parents in infant's care as much as possible; encourage rooming in; assess current coping mechanisms; be alert for signs of parental anxiety (e.g., poor eye contact, fidgeting, repeating questions); encourage parents to ask as questions; use primary nursing to decrease parental anxiety
4) Additional nursing problems
   a) Impaired gas exchange: increased secretions in lower airway place infant at risk for hypoxia; be alert for manifestations of increasing distress
   b) Risk for infection: due to age of infant immune system poorly developed; increased risk for superimposed infection; risk for nosocomial spread is high: respiratory isolation and strict handwashing necessary; if RSV positive, child can only room with another child with RSV

E. **Urinary Tract Infection**
1 Characteristics
   a Infection may be lower (cystitis) or upper (pyelonephritis) urinary tract
   b. More common in girls, especially preschool and sexually active adolescents
   c. Predisposing factors
      1) Shorter female urethra
      2) Proximity of urethra to anus and vagina
      3) Hygiene (i.e., wiping back to front)
      4) Developmental factors ("holding" urine)
   d. Common organism is E. coli
2. Diagnosis
   a. Urine culture and sensitivity (clean catch or cath specimen)
   b. Radiology to check for structural abnormality or reflux
      1) Intravenous pyelogram (IVP)
      2) Voiding cystourethrogram (VCUG)
3. Treatment
   a. Antibiotics
   b. Hydration
   c. Surgical correction of structural abnormality

4. **NURSING INTERVENTIONS**
   a. Prevention: proper perineal hygiene; good hydration; not "holding" urine; cotton underwear; no bubble baths; voiding after intercourse
   b. Full course of antibiotics must be taken; prophylactic antibiotics may be given to children with recurrent infection or structural abnormalities

SECTION V
NURSING CARE OF THE SURGICAL CHILD

A. Preoperative Preparation
1. Assess parents' and child's level of understanding
2. Teaching based on developmental level
3. Involve parents and allow discussion
4. Gather baseline data

B. General Postoperative Care
1. Airway
2. Vital signs: q 15" x 4; q 30" x 2; q 1 hour until stable
3. NPO until awake, and bowel sounds and gag reflex return
4. Pain management
5. Check dressings
6. Monitor IVs, hydration
7. Provide parental support
8. General postoperative concerns
   a. Infections (3–5 days)
   b. Pulmonary complications (encourage early ambulation)
   c. Paralytic ileus
   d. Shock, hemorrhage

C. Common Surgical Problems
1. Tonsillectomy and adenoidectomy (T&A)
   a. Tonsils help protect body from infections; typically enlarged in children

b. Rationale for surgery
      1) Chronic tonsillitis (controversial)
      2) Massive hypertrophy that interferes with breathing
   c. Preoperative care
      1) Assess bleeding and coagulation time
      2) Confirm client is free from current infection
      3) Preparation

   d. **NURSING INTERVENTIONS** (postoperative)
      1) Hemorrhage: greatest risk first 48 hours, then 5–7 days later; manifestations: frequent swallowing or clearing of throat, bright red emesis, oozing from capillary bed, shock (late sign, indicates significant blood loss); prevention: avoid coughing, sneezing, sucking on straw
      2) Impaired swallowing related to inflammation and pain: advance diet as tolerated; cool liquid diet first 24 hours; no acidic foods, milk products, or red colored fluids; encourage soft, bland foods after 48 hours; advance to regular diet when tolerated
      3) Pain: administer analgesics regularly first 24 hours (acetaminophen *[Tylenol]*); may require rectal or parenteral route due to throat pain; may return to school in 1–2 weeks

2. Pyloric stenosis
   a. Congenital hypertrophy of pyloric sphincter
   b. Clinical manifestations
      1) Insidious vomiting occurring 2–3 weeks after birth, increasing in intensity until forceful and projectile (no bile) by about 6 weeks of age
      2) Small olive-size mass in right upper quadrant
      3) Peristaltic waves left to right
      4) Weight loss, dehydration
      5) Chronic hunger
   c. Diagnosis
      1) Upper GI series
      2) Barium swallow under fluoroscopy
   d. Treatment
      1) Correct dehydration, metabolic alkalosis
      2) Pylorus resected

   e. **NURSING INTERVENTIONS**
      1) Preoperative: fluid volume deficit related to persistent vomiting; NPO with parenteral fluid; daily weights; NG tube for gastric decompression; monitor intake, output and specific gravity; monitor emesis (amount and frequency)
      2) Postoperative: altered nutrition less than body requirements; position on right side to prevent aspiration; begin oral feedings 4–6 hours postoperatively after bowel sounds return; maintain in upright position after feeding in infant seat; start with small, frequent feeds of oral rehydration solution *(Pedialyte);* monitor for emesis; advance feeding as tolerated, reestablish breast feeding; monitor incision; provide parental support, teaching

3. Appendicitis
   a. Inflammation of vermiform appendix
   b. School-age problem

c. Characteristics
1) Periumbilical pain radiating to right lower quadrant; rebound tenderness
2) Low-grade temperature
3) Nausea and vomiting
4) White blood cells around 12,000–15,000
5) May perforate and lead to peritonitis; sudden relief of pain followed by increased pain and rigid abdomen; high fever

d. **NURSING INTERVENTIONS**
1) Preoperative
a) Pain: medicate, position for comfort
b) Risk for infection: obtain baseline vitals, monitor WBC, administer antibiotics, observe for peritonitis
c) Fluid volume deficit: NPO with parenteral fluids, monitor hydration; keep NPO until bowel sounds return postoperatively
2) Postoperative
a) Impaired skin integrity: if perforated, wound left to heal by secondary intention; dressing changes; administer antibiotics
b) Pain, risk for infection, fluid volume deficit: as preoperative

4. Intussusception
a. Telescoping of the bowel
b. Characterized by
1) Colicky pain with knees drawn up
2) Currant jelly stools
c. Treatment
1) Barium enema: diagnostic; may reduce intussusception by hydrostatic pressure
2) Bowel resection if barium enema does not reduce

d. **NURSING INTERVENTIONS**
1) Prepare for procedure
2) Routine postoperative abdominal surgery care

5. Hirschsprung's disease (megacolon)
a. Congenital absence of parasympathetic ganglion in distal colon
b. Bowel proximal to a ganglionic section becomes enlarged
c. Characterized by
1) In newborn: failure to pass meconium within 24 hours after birth
2) In older child: recurrent abdominal distension; chronic constipation with ribbon-like stools; diarrhea; bile-stained emesis
d. Treatment
1) Cleansing enemas with antibiotics preoperatively
2) Temporary colostomy
3) Bowel resection to remove aganglionic portion

e. **NURSING INTERVENTIONS**
   1) Colostomy care
      a) Check stoma for color
      b) Change dressings frequently (abdominal, perineal)
      c) Monitor accurate intake and output
      d) Avoid incision irritation (keep diapers low)
   2) Parent and child instruction
      a) Encourage independence of based on age of child
      b) Discuss diet and hydration

6. Hernias
   a. Most common: inguinal and umbilical
   b. Always consider developmental level (e.g., mutilation fears) when preparing child
   c. Usually repaired in ambulatory surgery setting

   d. **NURSING INTERVENTIONS:** instruct parents
      1) Surgical site care
      2) Manifestations of infection

SECTION VI

NURSING CARE OF THE PEDIATRIC ACCIDENT VICTIM

A. General Emergency Care
   1. ABCs
   2. Prevent and treat shock
   3. Monitor vital signs with neuro check
   4. Do systems review
   5. Continually reassess
   6. Provide parental support

B. Types of Accidents
   1. Burns (refer to burns in medical/surgical section)
      a. Characteristics
         1) Degree: 1st degree (superficial); 2nd degree (partial thickness); 3rd degree (full thickness)

2) Extent: rule of nines
   a) 19% head and neck
   b) 18% arms
   c) 36% trunk
   d) 26% legs
   e) 1% perineum
b. Pathophysiology
   1) Decreased cardiac output: hypovolemic shock
   2) Plasma: interstitial fluid shift
   3) Loss of plasma protein and fluid: shock
c. Treatment
   1) Support respiratory function
   2) Fluid and electrolytes to correct or prevent shock
   3) Treat burn
      a) Dressings: occlusive or open
      b) Topical agents
         (1) Silver nitrate *(Keratolytic)*
         (2) Silver sulfadiazine *(Flamazine)*
         (3) Nitrofurazone *(Furacin)*
      c) Primary excision
         (1) Debridement
         (2) Graft
      d) Antibiotics
      e) Analgesics
      f) Tetanus prophylaxis, if not current
   4) Hydrotherapy (whirlpool bath)
   5) Nutrition: hyperalimentation, enteral feedings to ensure high caloric intake
   6) Prevent complications
      a) Stress ulcer
      b) Infection
      c) Contractures

d. **NURSING INTERVENTIONS**
   1) Immediate
      a) Check airway
      b) Immerse in cool water (if burn small)
      c) Cover burns: sterile or clean cloth
      d) Don't use ointments, salve
   2) Emergency
      a) Check airway
      b) Monitor hyperthermia, vital signs
      c) Treat hypovolemic shock (burn shock) with parenteral fluids
      d) Insert Foley catheter to monitor output accurately
      e) Decompress gastrointestinal tract (NG tube)
      f) Control pain (IV narcotics)
      g) Tetanus prophylaxis

3) Acute hospital care
   a) Check airway
   b) Use aseptic technique, isolation
   c) Provide fluid replacement
      (1) Burn phase (24–48 hours); plasma: interstitial shift
         (a) Elevated potassium levels
         (b) Elevated hematocrit
         (c) Acid-base imbalance
         (d) Loss of protein
      (2) Post-burn phase (diuretic phase); interstitial: plasma shift
         (a) Low potassium
         (b) High sodium
         (c) Pulmonary edema
         (d) Hemodilution
4) Rehabilitative care
   a) Skin grafts
   b) Hydrotherapy
   c) Contracture
   d) Infection
   e) Supportive nutritional therapy
   f) Physical and occupational rehabilitation

2. Fractures
   a. Break in the continuity of the bone
   b. Frequently seen fracture: greenstick
   c. Complications include
      1) Osteomyelitis
      2) Compartment syndrome
      3) Injury to the epiphysis: growth failure
      4) Malunion
   d. Treatment
      1) Open reduction
      2) Closed reduction
      3) Cast
      4) Traction

e. **NURSING INTERVENTIONS**
1) Cast care
   a) Assess neurovascular function
   b) Assist with drying of cast
   c) Skin care, petal cast
   d) Reposition
   e) Safety concerning small objects
   f) Parent education
      (1) Activities of daily living (ADLs)
      (2) Skin care, reposition
      (3) Developmental needs
   g) Hip spica cast
2) Traction care
   a) Types of traction
      (1) Skin traction: major complication is skin breakdown
         (a) Buck's
         (b) Bryant's
      (2) Skeletal traction: major complication is osteomyelitis
         (a) 90–90 traction
         (b) External fixation device

   b) **NURSING INTERVENTIONS**
      (1) Monitor neurovascular status
         (a) Capillary refill
         (b) Temperature of extremity
         (c) Absence of numbness, tingling
         (d) Movement of fingers, toes
         (e) Peripheral pulses
      (2) Correct body alignment
      (3) Pin care
      (4) Skin care
      (5) Problems of immobility
         (a) Pulmonary
         (b) Renal
         (c) Osteoporosis
         (d) Constipation
         (e) Muscle atrophy, foot drop
      (6) Nutrition
      (7) Developmental needs
      (8) Parent, child education concerning application of cast
      (9) Home care of cast

3. Ingestions
    a. General information
        1) Emergency care: ABC's
        2) Identify substance, save evidence of poison
        3) Call poison control center for treatment advice
        4) Removal of substance
            a) Syrup of ipecac
                (1) Emetic
                (2) 15 ccs with 200–300 ccs of water
                (3) Save emesis
                (4) Contraindications
                    (a) Unconscious
                    (b) Convulsing
                    (c) Ingested hydrocarbon, lye, strychnine
            b) Activated charcoal
            c) Gastric lavage
            d) Administer specific antidote
        4) Provide supportive therapy
        5) Educate parents about childproof environment
        6) Provide anticipatory guidance
            a) Infants and toddlers: at risk because everything goes into the mouth
            b) Adolescents: at risk for intentional ingestion
    b. Types of ingestions (see Table V-5.)

TABLE V-5.
OVERVIEW OF COMMON ACCIDENTAL INGESTION

INGESTION	CLINICAL MANIFESTATIONS	TREATMENT	NURSING INTERVENTIONS
Salicylate (Aspirin)	Tinnitus Hyperpyrexia Seizures Bleeding	Emesis Hydration Vitamin K Activated charcoal	Anticipatory guidance Bleeding precautions Counseling if suicide attempt
Acetaminophen (Tylenol)	Liver necrosis in 2–5 days; nausea; vomiting; pain in R upper quadrant; jaundice; coagulation abnormalities	Emesis Mucomyst (antidote)	Counseling if suicide attempt Liver assessment

Lead (paint, also in soil near heavily trafficked roadways, households dust)	Developmental regression
	Impaired growth
		Chelation therapy:
		  EDTA
		  BAL
		  Child must be well hydrated
			Neuro assessment
			Diet high in calcium, iron
			Educate parents to wash child's hands, toys, frequently to remove lead dust
			Lead abatement

Hydrocarbons (kerosene, turpentine, gasoline)	Burning in mouth Choking and gagging CNS depression	DO NOT INDUCE EMESIS! Activated charcoal Gastric lavage	If vomiting, reduce aspiration
Corrosives (drain or oven cleaner, chlorine bleach, battery acid)	Burning in mouth White swollen mucous membranes Violent vomiting	DO NOT INDUCE EMESIS! Dilute toxin with water Activated charcoal	Keep warm and inactive

C. Child Abuse

1. Types
   a. Physical abuse: deliberate infliction of injury
   b. Physical neglect: failure to provide necessities of life
   c. Emotional abuse: deliberate assault on self-esteem
   d. Emotional neglect: failure to provide emotional nurturing
   e. Sexual abuse: use of child to meet adult's sexual needs
   f. Munchausen syndrome: fabrication of illness in child by parent to obtain medical cure
2. Risk factors
   a. Parental
      1) Poor self-esteem
      2) Abused as a child
      3) Lack of knowledge
      4) Lack of support system, poor coping skills
   b. Child
      1) Unwanted pregnancy or sex
      2) Difficult temperament, hyperactive
   c. Environmental
      1) Chronic stress
      2) Socioeconomic factors
3. Recognition of abuse and neglect
   a. Physical abuse
      1) Bruises: not on bony prominences; in varying degrees of healing; with patterns
      2) Burns: with immersion lines, in patterns
      3) Fractures: spiral, twisting injury
      4) Shaken baby: unconscious infant with retinal hemorrhage; no signs of external trauma
      5) Conflicting stories given by parents or others
      6) History incompatible with physical findings
      7) History developmentally improbable
      8) Delay in seeking treatment
   b. Physical neglect
      1) Failure-to-thrive: disruption in maternal-infant bonding; poor feeding behaviors; mother does not respond to infant's cues; weight less than 5th percentile; developmental delay
      2) Poor health care: lack of immunizations
      3) Failure to meet basic needs: malnutrition; poor hygiene
   c. Emotional abuse and neglect
      1) Failure-to-thrive: see above
      2) Extremes of behavior
      3) Poor self-esteem
   d. Sexual abuse
      1) Bruising of the genitalia
      2) Venereal disease
      3) Sudden change in behavior; regressive behavior

e. Munchausen syndrome
   1) Abusive parent has medical knowledge
   2) Illness only occurs in abuser's presence
   3) Parent "enjoys" hospital environment

4. **NURSING INTERVENTIONS**
   a. Risk for injury: prevent further abuse; report suspicions to child protective authorities; refer family to supportive services
   b. Anxiety: consistent caregiver; do not interrogate child; grieve loss of parents
   c. Altered parenting: role model parenting behaviors; teach appropriate discipline methods; teach normal growth and development

SECTION VII

NURSING CARE OF THE CHILD WITH CHRONIC OR LONG-TERM PROBLEMS

A. Allergic Disorders
1. Eczema
   a. Known as atopic dermatitis
   b. May be associated with bronchial asthma; often family history of asthma or atopy
   c. Due to hypersensitivity to:
      1) Food (e.g., milk, egg white)
      2) Pollen
      3) Environmental
      4) Psychological
   d. Characteristics
      1) Papules are red and oozing; predominantly on face and extensor surfaces in infants, flexural areas in children (i.e., knees, wrists, antecubital fossa)
      2) Lesions eventually become scaly
      3) Pruritus may lead to secondary infection
   e. Treatment
      1) Topical steroids: triamcinolone *(Kenalog);* avoid chronic use
      2) Diphenhydramine HCl *(Benadryl)* or hydroxyzine HCl *(Atarax):* reduces itching
      3) Elimination diet (e.g., milk, eggs, chocolate, wheat)
      4) Antibiotics if secondary infection occurs

f. **NURSING INTERVENTIONS**
   1) Impaired skin integrity:
      a) Control dry skin to minimize itching
         (1) Use non-soap cleanser such as *Cetaphil*
         (2) Apply lubricating creams such as *Eucerin*
      b) Clothing: cotton, long sleeves
      c) Clothing, sheets, towels washed with non-soap cleanser
      d) Fingernails and toenails should be cut (gloves, socks may help)
   2) Assess developmental needs; hypoallergenic diet
   3) Provide parental support and education

2. Bronchial asthma
   a. Also known as reactive airway disease (RAD)
   b. Usually begins before 5 years of age
   c. Pathology and etiology
      1) Chronic condition with acute exacerbations
      2) In response to allergen or trigger, acute hyperactive changes occur in reactive (lower) airways
         a) Spasm of smooth muscle
         b) Edema of mucous membranes
         c) Thick, tenacious mucous
      3) Potential triggers
         a) Foods
         b) Inhalants (e.g., second-hand smoke)
         c) Infection
         d) Vigorous activity
         e) Stress
         f) Allergens (e.g., pet dander, dust)
         g) Cold air
   e. Characterized by
      1) Abrupt or insidious onset (URI)
      2) Paroxysmal, hacking nonproductive cough
      3) Prolonged expiratory phase with expiratory wheeze
      4) Respiratory distress, anxiety
   f. Complications
      1) Pneumonia
      2) Atelectasis

g. Treatment
   1) Chronic (home) management
      a) Medications via nebulizer or metered dose inhaler
         (1) Bronchodilators: albuterol *(Proventil)* (useful for acute attack); serevent (for chronic daily use, not for acute attack)
         (2) Corticosteroids: effective in reducing airway hyperreactivity; for chronic daily use, not acute attack
         (3) Cromolyn sodium *(Intal):* mast call inhibitor; reduces allergic response; for chronic daily use, not acute attack

      b) **NURSING INTERVENTIONS**
         (1) Avoid allergens and triggers
         (2) Correct use of meter dose inhaler (with spacer device)
         (3) Activities requiring stop and start energy better tolerated
         (4) Use of a peak flow meter to monitor airway compliance
   2) Status asthmaticus: severe respiratory distress requiring hospitalization
      a) Bronchodilators
         (1) Epinephrine *(Epifrin):* subcutaneous
         (2) Aminophylline *(Phyllocontin):* IV drip
      b) Steroids: IV
      c) Inhalants: bronchodilators (albuterol *[Proventil]*, metaproterenol *[Alupent]*)
      d) Antibiotics: prophylactic
h. **NURSING INTERVENTIONS** (hospitalized child)
   1) Ineffective breathing pattern:
      a) Respiratory assessment; monitor oximetry
      b) Hydration
         (1) Monitor intake and output with specific gravity
         (2) Monitor IVs
      c) Monitor vital signs
      d) Oxygen therapy
      e) Semi-Fowler's or high-Fowler's
      f) Monitor medications
   2) Activity intolerance
      a) Provide diversional activities appropriate to child's ability to tolerate; promote rest

B. **Musculoskeletal Disorders**
   1. Scoliosis
      a. Lateral curvature of the spine
      b. Most common form is idiopathic seen (predominately) in adolescent females; unknown etiology
      c. Acquired scoliosis; associated with deformity resulting from other neuromuscular disorders
      d. Diagnosis
         1) Classic signs: truncal asymmetry; especially noted in hips and shoulders, posture
         2) Screening exam in school: child flexes at waist; one scapula more prominent
         3) Spinal x-ray

e. Treatment
  1) Mild scoliosis (< 20° curvature): observation, encourage physical exercise
  2) Moderate scoliosis (20°–40° curvature): Milwaukee brace (pelvis to neck), Boston brace (body jacket)
     a) Goal is to prevent worsening of curve; not a cure

     b) **NURSING INTERVENTIONS**
        (1) Risk for noncompliance: difficult for adolescent due to body image concerns; must wear 23 hours a day (one hour off for hygiene care); wears T-shirt under brace
        (2) Body image disturbance: Boston brace better accepted (can be completely hidden under clothing)
  3) Severe scoliosis (> 40° curvature): surgery
     a) Spinal fusion with instrumentation
     b) Requires prolonged immobilization in cast or body jacket
     c) **NURSING INTERVENTIONS**
        (1) High risk for injury related to spinal manipulation: log roll first 24 hours; neurovascular checks; advance activity as ordered; observe for paralytic ileus
        (2) Pain: adolescent good candidate for PCA pump

2. Juvenile rheumatoid arthritis (JRA)
   a. Autoimmune, inflammatory disease of the joints
   b. Toddler and school-age child more commonly affected
   c. Etiology unknown
   d. Early diagnosis essential due to long-term complications (blindness, contracture); early onset often associated with spontaneous permanent remission
   e. Classification
      1) Systemic (fever, rash, and organomegaly in addition to joint involvement)
      2) Polyarticular (many joints)
      3) Pauciarticular (few joints)
   f. Characterized by:
      1) Swelling, thickening of joint
      2) Pain, stiffness, impaired range of motion
      3) Lethargy, weight loss
   g. Treatment
      1) Medications
         a) Salicylates
         b) NSAID: tolmetin sodium *(Tolectin)*
         c) Gold compounds
         d) Immunosuppressants and steroids: used in severe cases that do not respond to other medications
      2) Supportive treatment to maintain joint mobility

h. **NURSING INTERVENTIONS**
   1) Impaired physical mobility related to inflamed joints
      a) Rest inflamed joints
      b) Assist with ADLs
      c) Provide heat, splints, passive range of motion
      d) Provide physical therapy
   2) Pain
      a) Administer medication
      b) Observe for side effects
   3) Risk for altered nutrition: less than body requirements
      a) Provide well-balanced diet
      b) Provide anticipatory guidance and parental support

C. Endocrine Disorders
1. Insulin dependent diabetes mellitus (IDDM)
   a. Etiology
      1) May be autoimmune response to environmental factors
      2) Genetic component: inherit tendency, not disease
      3) School-age child (5–7 years or at puberty)
   b. Characteristics
      1) Onset: rapid with progression to abrupt ketoacidosis
      2) Hypertrophy and hyperplasia of islet cells occur early
      3) Remission (honeymoon) phase
      4) Insulin replacement
      5) Exercise lowers blood sugar
      6) Management difficult due to
         a) Immaturity of child
         b) Lack of insight
   c. Clinical manifestations
      1) Polyuria
      2) Polyphagia
      3) Polydipsia
      4) Weight loss
      5) Enuresis
   d. Treatment
      1) Insulin
         a) Rapid: onset 1/2–1 hour; peaks 2–4 hours
         b) Intermediate: onset 2 hours; peaks 8–10 hours
         c) Long acting: onset 4–8 hours; peaks 14–20 hours
      2) Diet
      3) Exercise
   e. Complications (see Table V-6.)

f. **NURSING INTERVENTIONS**
   1) Teaching diabetic self care
      a) Blood glucose monitoring and urine testing
      b) Insulin injection technique and regimen
      c) Dietary management ("no concentrated sweets" diet)
      d) Recognition and treatment of hyperglycemia and hypoglycemia
      e) Need for regular exercise
   2) Periodic screening to prevent complications
   3) Assess developmental needs
   4) Assess self-care ability
   5) Evaluation of management by monitoring glycosylated hemoglobin levels every 2–3 months

TABLE V-6.
COMPARISON OF INSULIN SHOCK AND DIABETIC COMA GUIDE

	INSULIN SHOCK (HYPOGLYCEMIA)	**DIABETIC COMA (HYPERGLYCEMIA)**
Causes:	Too much insulin Not eating enough food Taking unusual amounts of exercise Delayed meals	Too little insulin Failure to follow diet Infection, fever, emotional stress
Clinical Manifestations:	Onset is abrupt, rapid Skin is pale, moist Vertigo (dizzy) Urine is normal Tachycardia Hungry (polyphagia) Normal urinary output Normal thirst Shallow respirations Breath normal Level of consciousness: inappropriate behavior, confused	Onset is slow, insidious Skin is hot, dry No vertigo Urine is positive for sugar and acetone Normal pulse Anorexia Polyuria Polydipsia Deep, labored respirations Acetone breath Level of consciousness: lethargic, drowsy
What to do:	Give fast-acting sugar (e.g., candy, orange juice) Call physician Do not give insulin Glucagon if unconscious	Call physician Encourage fluids without sugar Continue to check urine Give insulin as usual

D. Hematological Disorders
   1. Hemophilia
      a. Characteristics
         1) Impaired coagulation: deficiency of clotting factors
         2) Sex-linked recessive trait more common in males
         3) Factor VIII and IX are most common deficiencies
         4) Hemarthrosis (bleeding into joint cavities), bruises easily

  b. Treatment
    1) Cryoprecipitate (transfusion that replaces missing clotting factor)
    2) Supportive therapy

  c. **NURSING INTERVENTIONS**
    1) Control bleeding
      a) Immobilize joint
      b) Provide ice packs
      c) Administer cryoprecipitate
        (1) Prophylactic cryoprecipitate for invasive procedures
        (2) Risk for AIDS, hepatitis is decreased because of screening, but does still exist
    2) Safety directed toward developmental level to prevent injury, bleeding
      a) Avoid contact sports
      b) Childproof environment
      c) Avoid aspirin
    3) Provide parental support

2. Sickle cell anemia
  a. Characteristics
    1) Presence of hemoglobin S, which accounts for enlongated shape of red blood cells (RBC)
    2) Sickling occurs in response to
      a) Infection, stress
      b) Dehydration
      c) Decreased oxygen
      d) High altitude
    3) Sickling increases blood viscosity, which causes further sickling and RBC destruction
    4) Hemoglobin electrophoresis is definitive diagnostic test
    5) Types of crisis
      a) Vaso-occlusive: "hand-foot syndrome" caused by stasis of blood in capillaries; schema and infarction
      b) Sequestration: pooling of large amounts of blood in liver, spleen; hypovolemia and shock
  b. Treatment
    1) Eliminate cause of crisis
    2) Analgesics
    3) Blood transfusions
    4) Monitor complications
      a) Anemia
      b) Splenic sequestration
      c) Cerebrovascular accidents

c. **NURSING INTERVENTIONS**
1) Early recognition of crisis
   a) Increasing irritability
   b) Frequent infections
   c) Pallor
   d) Failure to thrive
2) Provide hydration
3) Administer analgesics, antibiotics as ordered
4) Oxygenation
5) Reduce stress of hospitalization
6) Provide parental support

E. Developmental Disorders
1. Cerebral Palsy
   a. Characteristics
      1) Motor function impairment
      2) Nonprogressive condition
      3) Due to prenatal, natal, postnatal trauma or hypoxic insult
      4) High-risk babies: Apgar below 5
   b. Classification
      1) Spastic: hypertonic muscles, persistent neonatal reflexes, positive Babinski, contractures
      2) Athetoid: hypotonic muscles, involuntary movements, drooling
      3) Ataxic: unsteady gait, uncoordinated voluntary movements
   c. Diagnosis
      1) Delayed motor development
      2) Persistent neonatal reflexes
      3) "Scissoring"
   d. Treatment
      1) Symptomatic
      2) Orthopedic surgery to release contractures
      3) Physical therapy to optimize development

e. **NURSING INTERVENTIONS**
1) Early detection
2) Dietary needs
   a) Feeding problems
      (1) Difficulty with sucking, swallowing
      (2) Persistent bite reflex
   b) Adequate nutrition
   c) Elimination and hydration
3) Joint and muscular integrity
   a) Contracture
   b) Skin breakdown
4) Mobility
5) Self-care
6) Parental and family education
7) Self image

2. Mental retardation
   a. Characteristics
      1) Classified by intelligence level or developmental potential
      2) Consists of both cognitive and socialization delays
      3) Due to metabolic, genetic (trisomy 21), or acquired problems

   b. **NURSING INTERVENTIONS**
      1) Early detection
      2) Promote optimal level of function
         a) Developmental stimulation, early infant stimulation programs
         b) Training, behavioral modification
      3) Consistent environment
      4) Education for family

F. Renal Disorders
   1. Glomerulonephritis (see Table V-7.)
   2. Nephrotic syndrome (see Table V-7.)

G. Metabolic Disorders
   1. Cystic fibrosis (see Table V-8.)
   2. Celiac disease (see Table V-8.)

TABLE V-7.
RENAL DISORDERS

	NEPHROTIC SYNDROME	ACUTE GLOMERULONEPHRITIS
Other names	Childhood nephrosis	Post-streptococcal glomerulonephritis
Etiology	Cause unknown; may follow the toxic effects of mercury or tridione exposure or bee sting	Antigen: antibody reaction secondary to infection elsewhere in the body; usually a Group A beta hemolytic streptococcal infection of the upper respiratory tract
Incidence	Average age of onset about 2-1/2 years; more common in boys	2/3 of cases in children under 4–7 years; more common in boys
Pathology	Increased permeability of the glomerular membrane to protein	Inflammation of the kidneys; damage to the glomeruli allows excretion of red blood cells
Clinical manifestations	Edema: appears insidiously; usually first noticed about the eyes and can advance to the legs, arms, back, peritoneal cavity and scrotum; massive proteinuria; anorexia; pallor	Periorbital edema: appears insidiously; tea-colored urine from heaturia; hypertension; oliguria
Blood pressure	Usually normal; transient elevation may occur early	Varying degrees of hypertension may be present; when blood pressure is elevated cerebral manifestations may occur as a result of vasospasm; these may include headache, drowsiness, diplopia, vomiting, convulsions
Laboratory findings	Urine shows heavy albuminuria	Urine contains red blood cells; has a high specific gravity
Blood	Involves reduction in protein (mainly albumin); gamma globulin is reduced; during the active stages of the disease, the sedimentation rate is greatly increased	Blood urea nitrogen value is elevated; anemia (reduction in circulating red blood cells, in hemoglobin or both) tends to develop rapidly
Course and prognosis	Characterized by remissions and relapses; with protection against infection and suppression of proteinuria by steriod therapy, most children can eventually expect a favorable outcome	Recovery from acute glomerulonephritis is to be expected in nearly all children; mild illnesses last as little as 2–3 weeks; in exceptional instances, the disease is progressive and takes on the characteristics of chronic nephritis
Treatments	1. Prednisone (Deltasone) 2. Furosemide (Lasix) 3. Salt-poor albumin	1. Antibiotics for strep infection 2. Anti-hypertensives and diuretics 3. Corticosteroids
Nursing interventions	Control edema; provide skin care; prevent infection; monitor nutrition: low sodium, high protein, high potassium; monitor urine for proteinuria; monitor for side effects from steriod therapy	Bedrest if hypertensive; restrict fluids; monitor neuro status; monitor blood pressure; provide low potassium diet, no added salt; prevent infection

TABLE V-8.

COMPARISON OF CYSTIC FIBROSIS AND CELIAC DISEASE

METABOLIC DISORDER	CYSTIC FIBROSIS	CELIAC DISEASE
Onset	0–6 months	6–18 months
Characteristics	Production of abnormally viscid secretions of: pancreas, respiratory, salivary, and sweat glands	Intestinal malabsorption: malnutrition; fat and gluten intolerance; dietary intolerance: fat, gluten
Etiology	Autosomal recessive: 25% chance	Inborn error of metabolism
Manifestations	Meconium ileus in newborn; large, fatty foul-smelling stools in older child; chronic respiratory disease; digestive problems; sweat abnormalities	Diarrhea: large bulky stools; anemia; retarded growth; frequent infections; malabsorption of vitamin D
Diagnosis	Sweat test; pancreatic enzymes	Bowel biopsy; sweat test; gluten-free diet
Treatment	Pulmonary: postural drainage, aerosol therapy, antibiotics; nutrition: pancreatic, enzymes with meals, high calorie, Vitamins A, D, E, K (water soluble) twice normal dose, free use of salt	Gluten free diet: meat, eggs, milk, fruit, vegetables, gluten-free bread, Vitamins A, D, E, K (water soluble) Avoid: BROW: barley, rice, oats, wheat
Nursing interventions	Avoid infection Respiratory toilet Frequent small feedings Pancreatic enzymes Developmental issues Anticipatory grieving	Avoid infection Instruct how to implement diet Developmental issues

SECTION VIII

NURSING CARE OF THE CHILD WITH AN ONCOLOGICAL DISORDER

A. **Leukemia**
1. Characteristics
   a. Most common childhood cancer
   b. Peak incidence: 3–5 years of age
   c. Etiology: unknown, may be related to environmental exposures (e.g., radiation)
   d. Characterized by proliferation of abnormal white blood cells
2. Pathology
   a. Bone marrow failure secondary to invasion of cancer cells
      1) Temperature and infection from decreased (normal) WBCs
      2) Anemia, pallor and fatigue from decreased RBCs
      3) Petechiae and epistaxis from decreased platelets
   b. Leukemic infiltrate
      1) Limb and joint pain
      2) Lymphadenopathy
      3) Central nervous system (CNS) involvement
      4) Hepatosplenomegaly
3. Classification
   a. Acute lymphocytic (ALL)
   b. Acute nonlymphoid (ANLL)
4. Complications
   a. Infection
   b. Intracranial hemorrhage
   c. Secondary cancer or relapse
5. Diagnosis: bone marrow aspiration reveals hypercellular marrow, abnormal cells
6. Treatments
   a. Terminology
      1) Induction, remission
      2) CNS prophylaxis, consolidation
      3) Maintenance
   b. Chemotherapy
      1) Purine antagonists: 6-mercaptopurine *(Purinethol)*
      2) Alkylating agents: cyclophosphamide *(Cytoxan)*
      3) Folic acid antagonists: methotrexate *(Folex)*
      4) Plant alkaloid: vincristine sulfate *(Oncovin)*
      5) Steroids: prednisone *(Prelone)*
      6) Enzymes: L-asparaginase *(Elspar)*

c. Radiation therapy for CNS involvement

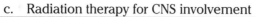

7. **NURSING INTERVENTIONS** (see Table V-9.)

B. Nephroblastoma (Wilms' Tumor)

1. Characteristics
    a. Most frequent type of renal cancer
    b. Peak age is 3 years
    c. Most common clinical sign: swelling, mass within the abdomen
    d. May also see: anemia, hypertension, hematuria
2. Pathology
    a. Arises from embryonal tissue
    b. Encapsulated
3. Diagnosis
    a. Intravenous pyelogram
    b. Computerized tomography
    c. Bone marrow to rule out metastasis
4. Treatment
    a. Nephrectomy and adrenalectomy
    b. Radiation and chemotherapy determined by staging

5. **NURSING INTERVENTIONS**
    a. Preoperative care
        1) Treatment begun quickly; support parents and keep explanations simple
        2) Monitor blood pressure due to excess renin production
        3) Prevent rupture of encapsulated tumor
            a) Post sign on bed: "DO NOT PALPATE ABDOMEN"
            b) Bathe and handle gently
    b. Postoperative care
        1) Problems related to radiation, chemotherapy (see Table V-9.)
        2) Large surgical incision
            a) Pain management
            b) Gentle handling
            c) Prepare parents
        3) Protect remaining kidney
            a) Monitor blood pressure
            b) Dipstick urine

C. Neuroblastoma

1. Characteristics
    a. Most frequently seen below 2 years of age
    b. Frequently called "silent" tumor because by the time of diagnosis, metastasis has occurred
    c. Clinical signs include: abdominal mass, urinary retention and frequency, lymphadenopathy, generalized weakness, malaise
    d. Primary site is abdomen, most often in flank area

2. Diagnosis
   a. Computerized tomography
   b. Bone marrow to determine metastasis
   c. Excessive catecholamine production
3. Treatment
   a. Surgery to remove as much of the tumor as possible, determine staging
   b. Chemotherapy and radiation determined by staging of tumor

4. **NURSING INTERVENTIONS** (see Table V-9.)

D. Hodgkin's Lymphoma
1. Characteristics
   a. Primarily affects adolescents and young adults
   b. Clinical signs include: painless enlargement of lymph nodes (cervical most common), metastasis related manifestations (persistent cough, abdominal pain), systemic problems (pruritus, night sweats, fever)
2. Pathology
   a. Malignancy originates in lymphoid system
   b. Metastasis may include spleen, liver, bone marrow, lungs
3. Diagnosis
   a. Computerized axial tomography
   b. Lymph node biopsy, exploratory laparotomy
4. Treatment
   a. Radiation and chemotherapy determined by clinical staging
   b. Surgical laparotomy
   c. Splenectomy

5. **NURSING INTERVENTIONS**
   a. See Table V-9.
   b. Instruct family on long-term care following splenectomy
      1) Increased susceptibility to infection
      2) Prophylactic long-term antibiotic therapy is necessary (compliance issues)

TABLE V-9.
NURSING CARE OF THE CHILD WITH CANCER

MANAGE PROBLEMS RELATED TO CHEMOTHERAPY	PREPARE CHILD/FAMILY FOR RADIATION THERAPY	TERMINAL PHASE—PROVIDE COMFORT CARE

Nausea and vomiting
  Administer antiemetic prior to treatment and regularly administer p.r.n. drugs
  Teach guided imagery
 	
Anorexia: difficult to handle with with children
 	
Mucosal ulceration
  Stomatitis: bland diet, soft tooth brush, oral hygiene
  Rectal ulcers: sitz baths, stool softeners, no rectal temperatures
 	
Neuropathy (vincristine related)
  Note bowel movements
  Instruct parents concerning foot-drop, weakness, numbness and jaw pain
 	
Hemorrhagic cystitis (cyclophosphamide related)
  1-1 and 2 times normal fluid intake
  Frequent voiding
  Administer drug early in day to allow for sufficient oral intake
	Meticulous skin care: avoid exposure to sun; limit use of soap and lotions; do not wash off markings
	
	Radiation to chest and abdomen frequently results in nausea & vomiting, weight loss, esophagitis
	
	Malaise is most frequent complaint of adolescents and prevents peer involvement
	
	Discuss effects radiation therapy has on puberty, fractures and spinal deformities
		If poor prognosis, assist family in dealing with life threatening illness
		
		Perception of death
		  Infant and toddler: different way of life (e g., "Mommy is sleeping"); major fear is separation
		
		Preschooler: reversible, cannot separate life and death
		
		School age child and preadolescent: similar to preschooler's reaction until 9-10 years, then adult concept of death; magical thinking may still be evident
		
		Adolescent: adult concept: of all age groups, has most difficulty dealing with death

SECTION IX

NURSING CARE OF THE CHILD WITH AN INFECTIOUS DISEASE

A. **Prevention**
  1. Immunizations
     a. Contraindications
        1) Acute febrile illness (temperature > 101°F)
        2) No live attenuated vaccines in the presence of:
           a) Pregnancy
           b) Malignancies
           c) Immunosuppressive therapy
           d) Immunodeficiency disorders
           e) Sensitivity to eggs, chicken, neomycin (MMR)
           f) Recent administration of immune serum globulin, plasma, blood
     b. Schedule (see Table V-10.)
  2. Communicability
     a. Most communicable diseases are most contagious prior to the onset of manifestations or rash and in the early prodromal period
     b. Most require respiratory isolation precautions if the child requires hospitalization
     c. Most are preventable through immunization or other measures
  3. Common childhood infections (see Table V-11.)

TABLE V-10.
RECOMMENDED IMMUNIZATION SCHEDULE

AGE	VACCINE	
2 months	DTP, OPV, HIB, Hep B	
4 months	DTP OPV, HIB, Hep B	**KEY:** **DTP:** diptheria, tetnus, pertussis **HIB:** H. influenza type B **MMR:** measles, mumps, rubella **DTaP:** acellular pertussis **Hep B:** hepatitis B **OPV:** trivalent oral polio **VZV:** varicella zoster vaccine **DT:** diptheria, tetnus *note: DTP and HiB can be given in combination injection: Tetrammune
6 months	DTP, (OPV) optional, HIB, Hep B	
12 months	VZV (optional)	
15 months	MMR, HIB	
18 months	DTaP, OPV	
4-6 years	DTaP, OPV, MMR	
11-12	MMR (if not given at preschool)	
14-16 years	DT (every 10 years), Hep B Series (if not given in infancy), VZV (if not given earlier and no history of chickenpox)	

TABLE V-11.
COMMUNICABLE DISEASES GUIDE

DISEASE	INFECTIOUS AGENTS	TRANSMISSION	INCUBATION	CLINICAL MANIFESTATIONS	TREATMENT and NURSING INTERVENTIONS	PREVENTION
Acquired immuno-deficiency syndrome (AIDS)	Human immuno-deficiency virus (HIV)	Blood and body fluids: in children: most common exposure is maternal-fetal; adolescents: at risk through sexual contacts or IV drug use	Months to years; in children average age of diagnosis is 18 months	In children: FTT, chronic candida, frequent URI, opportunistic infections (e.g., Pneumocystis carinii pneumonia [PCP])	Supportive and symptomatic care; antivirals and antiretrovirals; bactrim prophylaxis for PCP	AZT (Retrovir) given to HIV positive woman in pregnancy greatly reduces risks of prenatal transmission
Chicken pox	Varicella zoster virus	Direct contact, droplet spread, and contaminated objects or contact with skin lesions	2–3 weeks (usually 10–14 days)	Prodromal stage: slight fever, malaise and anorexia, first 24 hours; pruritic rash; macule to papule to vesicle to pustule; rash occurs in all different stages; lesions crust over and usually heal without scarring; client is communicable	Do not use aspirin; control itching; prevent secondary infection; acyclovir may lessen severity of outbreak and promote faster healing; strict isolation if child hospitalized	Varicella zoster immunoglobin (Zovirax)
Derma-tophytoses (tineas capitis) (ringworm)	Microsporum audouini (fungal injection)	Person to person Animal to person	N/A	Scaly circumscribed patches with alopecia; pruritic, flourescent green under woods light	Griseofulvin (Fulvicin-U/F) orally or topically; wash hair/hat	Caution children about sharing hair items
Enterobiases (pinworms)	Enterobius vermicularis	Ingested; inhaled; poor hygiene after toilet; reinfect self	Eggs hatch and mature in 2–4 weeks	Intense perianal itching; young child may present with general complaints (sleep problems, enuresis); tape test	Sanitize bedding; tight diapers and pants; family precautions; mebendazole (Vermox) prevent itching	Handwashing (especially after using toilet)
Fifth's disease (erythema infectiosum)	Human parvovirus 19	Respiratory secretions, blood	7–18 days	Red rash on cheeks—gives face a "slapped cheeks" appearance; followed by "lace-like" rash on extremes that may fade and reappear	Symptomatic treatment only; monitor for anemia	None
Impetigo	Group A beta strep or staph aureus	Direct contact with skin lesion or articles soiled with discharge	N/A	History of trauma or minor injury; honey-colored blisters that rupture and become crusted; lymphadenopathy; highly contagious	Soak lesions; topical ointment; communicability; prevent scratching; family precautions	Good hygiene; short fingernails
Lyme disease	Borrelia burgdorferi	Transmitted by bite of deer tick	3 days–1 month	Initially flu-like manifestations; red rash in bulls-eye pattern at bite site; later, joint pain, neurologic and cardiac involvement; may become chronic	Antibiotics; remove tick as soon as possible; symptomatic; analgesics; antipyretic	Avoid tick infested areas; dress appropriately in woods (tuck socks into jeans, long sleeves)

TABLE V-11.
COMMUNICABLE DISEASES GUIDE (CONTINUED)

DISEASE	INFECTIOUS AGENTS	TRANSMISSION	INCUBATION	CLINICAL MANIFESTATIONS	TREATMENT and NURSING INTERVENTIONS	PREVENTION
Meningitis	Viral or bacterial (H. Influenza: 3 months–3 years; menningococcal meningitis)	Direct invasion via otitis media, URI, head injury	2–10 days	Onset abrupt with fever, headache, irritability, altered LOC, nuchal rigidity, increased ICP; must do lumbar puncture to isolate organism	Isolate; reduce environmental stimuli; monitor hydration; seizure precautions; IV antibiotics	(Rifampin): given to contacts of client with menningococcal menningitis as prophylaxis
Mumps	Viral (paramyxovirus)	Saliva, direct contact or droplet	14–21 days	Prodromal stage: headache, malaise, anorexia, followed by earache; parotitis 3 days later with pain/tenderness	Symptomatic and supportive; analgesics; antipyretics; hydration	MMR
Pediculosis capitis (head lice)	Pediculus humanus capitis	Sharing of personal items, (e.g., hair ornaments, caps, hats)	Eggs hatch in 7–10 days	Intense itching; can visually see nits attached to base of hair shafts; differentiate from dandruff	Pediculocide: shampoo twice: immediately (Kwell, Rid); 7–10 days later; remove nits; spray furniture; family precautions	Caution children about sharing hair items
Pertussis (whooping cough)	Bordetella pertussis	Respiratory droplets and direct contact	7–21 days	Initially "cold" manifestations; progresses to spasms of paroxysmal coughing (whooping cough)	Antibiotics; corticosteroids; supportive care; isolation; stay with child during coughing spells	DTP, DTaP
Rabies	Viral	Contact with saliva of infected animal	1–3 months or as short as 10 days	Prodromal: malaise, sore throat followed by hypersensitivity, excitation, convulsions, paralysis; high mortality	Irrigate wound; psychologic follow-up	Avoid contact with wild animals; rabies shot (given after exposure)
Reye's syndrome	Viral	Unknown: proceded by viral infection and associated with use of aspirin	N/A	Prodromal: malaise cough, URI (upper respiratory infection); 1–3 days after: fever, decreased LOC, hepatic and cerebral dysfunction; high mortality	Monitor liver function; peak age 4–11 years; neuro assessments; intracranial pressure monitoring	Avoid use of aspirin in teens and children
Rheumatic fever	Group A beta-hemolytic strep	Nasopharynegal secretions; direct contact with infected person or droplet spread	1–3 weeks after acute infection, develops inflammatory disease	Carditis, arthritis, chorea (involuntary ataxic movements), subcutaneous nodules, erythema marginatum (rash)	Bed rest in acute phase to decrease cardiac workload; full course of antibiotics (penicillin/erythromycin); high dose aspirin therapy (monitor for toxicity, tinitis)	Adequate, prompt treatment of strep infection (Must finish entire course of therapy)

TABLE V-11.
COMMUNICABLE DISEASES GUIDE (CONTINUED)

DISEASE	INFECTIOUS AGENTS	TRANSMISSION	INCUBATION	CLINICAL MANIFESTATIONS	TREATMENT and NURSING INTERVENTIONS	PREVENTION
Roseola (exanthem subitem)	Viral (human herpes virus type 6)	Unknown (limited to children 6 months–2 years of age)	Unknown	Persistent high fever for 3–4 days; precipitous drop in fever with appearance of rash (rose-pink maculopapule on trunk, then spreading to neck, face and extremities); lasts 1–2 days	Antipyretics to control temperature and prevent febrile seizures; hydrate	None
Rubella (German measles)	Viral (rubella virus)	Nasopharyngeal secretions: direct contact, indirect via freshly contaminated nasopharyngeal secretions or urine	14–21 days	Prodromal phase; absent in children, present in adults; rash; first face and rapidly spreads downward to neck, arms, trunk, and legs; teratogenic to fetus	No treatment necessary; isolate child from pregnant women; women of childbearing years should have rubella titer drawn	MMR
Rubeola (measles)	Viral	Respiratory-droplets	10–21 days	Prodromal stage: fever and malaise, coryza, conjunctivitis, Koplik spots (spots with blue/white center on buccal mucosa opposite molars); rash: starts on face, spreads downwards, may desquamate (peel)	Antipyretics to control temperature and prevent seizures; dim lights if photophobia; respiratory precautions	MMR
Scarlet fever	Group A Beta hemolytic strep	Nasopharyngeal secretions, direct contact with infected person or droplet spread	2–4 days	Prodromal stage: abrupt high fever, pulse increased, vomiting, chills, malaise, abdominal pain; enanthema: tonsils enlarged, edematous reddened, covered with patches of exudate; strawberry tongue; exanthema: rash appears 12 hours after prodromal signs	Full course of antibiotics (penicillin/erythromycin); isolate; monitor for rheumatic fever, glomerulonephritis; hydrate	Adequate, prompt treatment of strep infection (Must finish entire course of therapy)
Tetanus	Clostridum tetany	Deep puncture, not contagious, "anaerobic"	7–14 days	Gradual stiffening of voluntary muscles until rigid (i.e., lockjaw, rigid abdomen); sensitive to stimuli; clear sensorium	Eliminate stimuli; monitor respirations, blood gases; muscle relaxants; monitor hydration	DTP, Td

APPENDICES

UNIT CONTENT

APPENDIX A
REVIEW OF CALCULATIONS AND CONVERSIONS

A. Metric System

> 1 kg = 1,000 gm
> 1 gm = 1,000 mg
> 1 mg = 1,000 mcg
> 1 L = 1,000 ml
> 1 ml = 1 cc
> 1 cm = 10 mm

B. Apothecary System

> 1 dram = 60 grains
> 1 ounce = 8 drams
> 1 dram = 60 minims
> 1 fluid ounce = 8 fluid drams

C. Household System

> 1 pound = 16 ounces
> 1 tablespoon = 3 teaspoons
> 1 ounce = 2 tablespoons
> 1 cupful = 6 ounces
> 1 glassful = 8 ounces
> 1 pint = 16 ounces
> 1 quart = 2 pints
> 1 gallon = 4 quarts

D. Conversions Between Systems

> 1 grain = 60 mg
> 1 gm = 15 grains
> 4 gm = 1 dram = 60 grains
> 1 tablespoon = 4 fluid drams = 15–16 ml
> 2 tablespoons = 1 ounce = 30–32 ml
> 1 cupful = 6 ounces = 180 ml
> 1 glassful = 8 ounces = 240–250 ml
> 2 glassfuls = 1 pint = 500 ml
> 1 inch = 2.54 cm
> 1 pound = 2.2 kg
> 1 minim = 1 drop
> 1 ml = 15 minims = 15 drops
> 60 drops = 1 teaspoon = 1 fluid dram

E. Temperature Conversions

$$98.6°F = 37.0°C$$
$$C = (F - 32) \times 5/9$$
$$F = (C \times 9/5) + 32$$

F. Calculations for IV Administration

1. $\# \text{ of hours} = \dfrac{cc/hour}{total\ volume}$

2. $\text{gtts per min} = \dfrac{total\ volume \times gtts/cc\ in\ administration\ set}{total\ number\ of\ minutes}$

G. Calculations for Dosage

$$\dfrac{Dosage\ on\ hand\ (H)}{cc} = \dfrac{Dosage\ desired\ (D)}{cc}$$

Test Questions

1. **A client has the following served for lunch: one glass of tea, one cup of coffee, and 240 cc of milk. The client drinks all of the tea and coffee and half of the milk. What was the total intake for lunch is:**
   a. 470 cc
   b. 480 cc
   c. 540 cc
   d. 660 cc

2. **A client has an order for 0.25 mg of digoxin. You have 0.5 mg tablets of digoxin. How many tablets should you give the client?**
   a. 1/4 tablet
   b. 1/2 tablet
   c. 1 tablet
   d. 2 tablets

3. **A client's IV infusion rate is 75 cc per hour. How many hours will a 500 cc bag of IV fluid last?**
   a. 5.5 hours
   b. 6.0 hours
   c. 6.6 hours
   d. 7.2 hours

4. **When the IV rate is 100 cc per hour and the administration set is 15 drops per cc, how many drops per minute should the IV run?**
   a. 15 drops
   b. 18 drops
   c. 25 drops
   d. 28 drops

5. A 4 year old client is taking 5 cc of ampicillin *(Polycillin Pediatric)* for otitis media every six hours. In preparing for the client's discharge, the nurse should tell the client's mother to give how much ampicillin every six hours at home?
   a. 1/2 teaspoon
   b. 1 teaspoon
   c. 2 teaspoons
   d. 3 teaspoons

6. A client has an order for heparin *(Heparin Sodium)* 7,000 units IV. The vial contains 10,000 units/cc. How many cc of heparin should be administered?
   a. 0.5 cc
   b. 0.7 cc
   c. 1.0 cc
   d. 1.4 cc

7. The nurse is preparing 300,000 units of procaine penicillin *(Wycillin)*. The vial contains 1,500,000 units per 2 cc. How many cc will the nurse administer?
   a. 0.2 cc
   b. 0.4 cc
   c. 2.5 cc
   d. 5.0 cc

8. A client weighs 180 pounds and has an order for 0.5 cc of medication per kilogram of body weight. How many cc of medication should he receive?
   a. 20 cc
   b. 41 cc
   c. 56 cc
   d. 90 cc

9. A client is receiving D5W at 50 cc per hour in one IV and D5NS 75 cc per hour in another IV. The client also receives IVPB medication every 8 hours prepared in 100 cc of fluid. How much IV fluid will the client receive in 8 hours?
   a. 700 cc
   b. 1,000 cc
   c. 1,100 cc
   d. 1,300 cc

10. When the IV administration set delivers 10 drops per cc, the rate of flow in drops per minute for 1,000 cc D5NS to infuse in 8 hours is:
   a. 15 drops per minute
   b. 20 drops per minute
   c. 50 drops per minute
   d. 125 drops per minute

11. While measuring a client's output, the nurse has measured 300 cc urine at 8:00 AM, 450 cc liquid stool at 11:30 AM, 225 cc urine at 1:00 PM, and 35 cc emesis at 2:30 PM. What is the client's total output for this shift?
   a. 785 cc
   b. 975 cc
   c. 1,010 cc
   d. 1,100 cc

12. A client receiving an IV infusion has an order for 1,000 cc in 12 hours. Using a micro drip system that delivers 60 micro drops per cc, the nurse should adjust the infusion for how many drops per minute?
   a. 45 drops
   b. 68 drops
   c. 83 drops
   d. 96 drops

13. A client's temperature is 100°F. What is this temperature in degrees Centigrade?
   a. 36.0° C
   b. 37.0° C
   c. 37.7° C
   d. 38.3° C

14. The nurse has a tubex marked Demerol 50 mg per cc. To give 35 mg of Demerol, the nurse should give how many cc?
   a. 0.7 cc
   b. 0.9 cc
   c. 1.2 cc
   d. 1.5 cc

15. A client on fluid restriction may have 800 cc in 8 hours. The IV is running at 50 cc per hour. How much fluid may the client have by mouth?
   a. 2 glasses
   b. 2 glasses and 1 cup
   c. 1 glass and 1 cup
   d. 4 cups

Test Answers

1.	C	9.	C
2.	B	10.	B
3.	C	11.	C
4.	C	12.	C
5.	B	13.	C
6.	B	14.	A
7.	C	15.	C
8.	B		

APPENDIX B

NUTRITION

Therapeutic Diets

A. Nutrient Modification

1. Low-protein diet
   a. Indicated for renal impairment, hepatic coma, and advanced cirrhosis
   b. Controls end products of protein metabolism by limiting protein intake
   c. Encourage high carbohydrate foods
   d. Limit foods high in protein such as eggs, meat, milk and milk products

2. High-protein diet
   a. Used for tissue building, burns, correction of malabsorption syndromes, mild to moderate liver disease, undernutrition, and pregnancy
   b. Corrects protein loss and/or maintains and rebuilds tissues
   c. Encourage high-protein foods such as fish, fowl, organ and meat sources, and dairy products
   d. May include protein supplements such as Sustagen or Meritene

3. Abnormalities in amino acid metabolism
   a. Use for phenylketonuria (PKU), galactosemia, and lactose intolerance
   b. Reduce or eliminate the offending enzyme
   c. Avoid milk and milk products for all three diets
   d. Use substitutes

4. Low-cholesterol diet
   a. Indicated for cardiovascular diseases, diabetes mellitus, high serum cholesterol levels
   b. Controls cholesterol levels by limiting cholesterol intake
   c. Limit high-cholesterol foods such as egg yolks, shellfish, organ meats, bacon, pork, avocado, olives
   d. Encourage low-cholesterol foods such as vegetable oils, raw or cooked vegetables, fruits, lean meats, and fowl

5. Modified-fat diet
    a. Indicated for malabsorption syndromes, cystic fibrosis, gallbladder disease, obstructive jaundice and liver disease, and obesity
    b. Fat content in the diet is lowered
        1) To stop contractions of the diseased organs
        2) When there is inadequate absorption of fat
        3) To decrease fat storage in the body
    c. To reduce fat intake, avoid gravies, fatty meat and fish, cream, fried foods, rich pastries, whole milk products, cream soups, salad and cooking oils, nuts, and chocolate; allow 2–3 eggs per week, lean meat, butter and margarine
    d. For a fat-free diet, restrict all fatty meats and fat; allow vegetables, fruits, lean meats, fowl, fish, bread, and cereal

6. High polyunsaturated fat diet
    a. Indicated for cardiovascular diseases
    b. Reduce saturated fats by avoiding foods from animal sources, peanuts, olives, avocados, coconuts, chocolate, and cashew nuts
    c. Increase polyunsaturated fats by including vegetable sources, margarine, corn/soybean/safflower oil

7. Carbohydrate modification (diabetic diet or ADA diet)
    a. Principles of diabetic diet management
        1) Attain or maintain ideal body weight
        2) Ensure normal growth
        3) Maintain plasma glucose levels as close to normal as possible
        4) Provide 30 calories per kg of ideal body weight
        5) Provide 25% of calories at each meal and 25% for snacks
        6) Provide 20% of calories as protein, 55–60% as carbohydrates, and 20–30% as fats
        7) Include unsaturated fats, high fiber, and complex carbohydrates
    b. Develop meal plans designed for individual needs using exchange lists
        1) Milk exchanges
        2) Vegetable exchanges
        3) Fruit exchanges
        4) Bread exchanges
        5) Fat exchanges
        6) Combination foods

B. Mineral Alterations

1. Potassium-modified diets
   a. Increase potassium intake for diabetic acidosis, thiazide diuretics, 48 hours after burns, vomiting, fevers
   b. Reduce potassium intake for kidney failure
   c. Foods high in potassium include: fruits and fruit juices, (e.g., orange, grapefruit, banana, apple); avocados, prunes, dried apricots; dried beans, soy beans, lima beans, kidney beans, squash, baked potatoes, milk and broiled meats
   d. Foods low in potassium include: breads, cereals, sugar, fats, cranberry and grape juice

2. Sodium-restricted diets
   a. Sodium is restricted in hypertension, congestive heart failure, myocardial infarction, hepatitis, adrenal cortical diseases, kidney disease, lithium carbonate therapy, cystic fibrosis, and conditions such as cirrhosis of the liver and preeclampsia, which cause persistent edema
   b. Mild restriction is 2–3 gm of sodium
   c. Moderate restriction is 1,000 mg of sodium
   d. Strict restriction is 500 mg of sodium
   e. Severe restriction is 250 mg of sodium
   f. Limit foods high in sodium, such as: potato chips and other salted snack foods; canned soups and vegetables; baked goods that contain baking powder or baking soda; cereals; seafood; beef; processed meats such as bologna, ham, and bacon; dairy products, especially cheese; pickles, olives, and condiments such as soy sauce, steak sauce, Worcestershire sauce, and salad dressings
   g. Encourage low-sodium foods such as fresh fruits and vegetables, chicken, salt substitutes, and low-sodium products

3. Iron alterations
   a. Increased iron intake is indicated for correction or prevention of iron deficiency anemia, which is most likely to occur in infants, toddlers, adolescents, and pregnant women
   b. Food sources high in iron include: fish; meats (particularly organ meats); green leafy vegetables; enriched breads, cereals, and macaroni products; whole grain products; dried fruits, such as raisins and apricots; and egg yolks
   c. Vitamin C enhances absorption of iron from the gastrointestinal tract
   d. Administration of iron supplements
      1) Oral administration with a straw
      2) Maximum absorption occurs when administered between meals
      3) Fewer GI side effects occur when administered with meals
      4) Injectable iron administered deep IM with Z track

4. Calcium alterations
   a. Increased calcium intake is indicated for growing children and adolescents, pregnant and lactating women, and postmenopausal women
   b. Decreased calcium intake is indicated for kidney stones composed of calcium
   c. Food sources high in calcium include: milk and milk products like yogurt and cheese; dark green vegetables, such as collard greens, kale, broccoli; dried beans and peas; and shellfish and canned salmon
   d. Some antacids contain calcium
   e. Vitamin D enhances absorption of calcium from the gastrointestinal tract

D. Consistency Modifications
1. Clear-liquid diet
   a. Indicated for resting the gastrointestinal tract, maintaining fluid balance; immediately postop; for diarrhea, nausea, and vomiting
   b. Includes water, tea, broth, jell-o, apple juice
   c. Not nutritionally adequate

2. Full-liquid diet
   a. When clear liquids are tolerated well, progress to full liquids
   b. Include clear liquids plus milk and milk products, such as custard, pudding, creamed soups, ice cream, sherbet, fruit juices
   c. Can be nutritionally adequate

3. Soft diet
   a. Include full liquids plus pureed vegetables, eggs that are not fried, tender meats, potatoes, cooked fruit

4. Bland diet
   a. Used to promote healing of gastric mucosa by eliminating chemically and mechanically irritating food sources
   b. Indicated for gastric and duodenal ulcers and postoperative stomach surgery
   c. Given in small, frequent feedings to assist in diluting or neutralizing stomach acid; protein foods are good at neutralizing; fat has some ability to inhibit the secretion of acid and delays stomach emptying
   d. Foods usually introduced in stages with gradual addition of foods
   e. Foods allowed include milk; butter; eggs that are not fried; custard; vanilla ice cream; cottage cheese; cooked refined or strained cereal; enriched white bread; jell-o; homemade creamed, pureed soups; baked or broiled potatoes

5. Low-residue diet
   a. Indicated for ulcerative colitis, postoperative colon and rectal surgery, prep for X-rays and colon surgery, diarrhea, and regional enteritis
   b. Encourage ground meat, fish, skinless broiled chicken, creamed cheeses, warm drinks, refined strained cereals and white bread
   c. Foods high in carbohydrates are usually low in residue
   d. Avoid high-residue foods that have skins and seeds

APPENDIX C
POSITIONING CLIENTS

POSITION	DESCRIPTION	INDICATIONS
Semi-Fowler's	Head of bed elevated to 30°	Head injury; postop cranial surgery; respiratory diseases with dyspnea; postop cataract removal; increased intracranial pressure
Fowler's	Head of bed elevated to 45°	Head injury; postop cranial surgery; postop abdominal surgery; respiratory diseases with dyspnea; cardiac problems with dyspnea; bleeding esophageal varices; postop thyroidectomy; postop cataract removal; increased intracranial pressure
High Fowler's	Head of bed elevated to 90°	Respiratory diseases with dyspnea: emphysema, status asthmaticus, pneumothorax; cardiac problems with dyspnea; feeding, meal times; hiatus hernia, during and after meals
Supine (dorsal recumbent)	Lying on back, head, and shoulders; usually slightly elevated with a small pillow	Spinal cord injury (no pillow); urinary catheterization
Prone	Lying on abdomen, legs extended and, head turned to the side	Immobilized client; amputation of lower extremity; unconscious client; post lumbar puncture 6–12 hours; post myelogram 12–24 hours (oil-based dye); postop T&A
Lateral (side lying)	Lying on side with most of body weight borne by the lateral aspect of lower scapula and the lateral aspect of the lower ilium	Post abdominal surgery; unconscious client; seizures (head to side); postop T&A; postop pyloric stenosis (right side); post liver biopsy (right side); rectal irrigations
Sims (semiprone)	Lying on side with most of body weight borne by the anterior aspect of the ilium, humerus, and clavicle	Unconscious client; rectal irrigations
Lithotomy	Lying on back with hips and knees flexed at right angles and feet in stirrups	Perineal procedures; rectal procedures; vaginal procedures
Trendelenburg	Head and body are lowered while feet are elevated	Shock
Reverse Trendelenburg	Head elevated while feet are lowered	Cervical traction
Elevate one or more extremities	Elevate legs/feet or arms/hands by adjusting bed or supporting with pillows	Thrombophlebitis; application of cast; edema; postop surgical procedure on extremity

APPENDIX D
PSYCHIATRIC TERMS

ACTING OUT: The active expression of emotions through actions, not words, that occurs when the client relives the feelings, wishes or conflicts that are operating unconsciously

AFFECT: The emotion or mood an individual shows as a response, such as flat affect or inappropriate affect

AMBIVALENCE: The simultaneous presence of strong, but contradictory or opposite, feelings or ideas about something or someone

ANXIETY: Fear or apprehension caused by an unknown or unrecognized threat

AUTISM: A syndrome involving abnormal sensory perception and developmental (usually language and psychosocial) issues

BODY IMAGE: One's perception of one's body

CATATONIC STATE: Immobility

COHESIVENESS: Group togetherness

COMPULSION: Emotional urge or need to act

CONFABULATION: A compensatory mechanism for memory loss; filling in the memory gaps with imaginary stories the teller believes to be true

CONFUSION: Mental bewilderment from disorientation

CRISIS: A conflict that cannot readily be resolved by using usual coping mechanisms

DEFENSE MECHANISMS: Mental strategies used to help cope with areas of conflict

DELIRIUM TREMENS: Alcohol withdrawal syndrome, including restlessness continuing to disorientation, hallucinations, and convulsions

DELUSION: A fixed false idea

DENIAL: Unconscious refusal to acknowledge that which is anxiety provoking

DESENSITIZATION: Gradual systematic exposure of the client to feared situations under controlled conditions

ECHOLALIA: Repetition by one person of what is said by another

ECHOPRAXIA: A meaningless imitation of movement

EMPATHY: Objective and insightful awareness of another's feelings

EXTRAPYRAMIDAL REACTION: A reversible side effect of some psychotropic drugs characterized by muscle rigidity, drooling, restlessness, shuffling gait, and blurred vision

FAMILY THERAPY: Treatment that involves the family and explores the relationships among the members

FANTASY: Daydreams

FLIGHT OF IDEAS: Rapid shift from an idea to another before the first idea has been concluded

GRIEF: An emotional response to a recognized loss

GROUP THERAPY: Application of psychotherapy techniques by a skilled leader to a group of clients

HALLUCINATION: False sensory perceptions involving any of the senses

HOSTILITY:	Feeling similar to anger but of longer duration
IDEAS OF REFERENCE:	Ideas stemming from the incorrect interpretation of incidents as referring directly to self
ILLUSIONS:	Misinterpretation of a real, external sensory experience
INSIGHT:	Self understanding
INTRAPSYCHIC:	Within the mind
LABILE:	Rapidly changing emotions
LIMIT SETTING:	Clear statement of rules with consistent reinforcement
LOOSENESS OF ASSOCIATION:	Ideas appear unrelated or only slightly related
MANIA:	Elated, excited mood state
MANIPULATION:	Control of another's behavior for one's own purposes
NEOLOGISM:	Coined word with special meaning to the user
OBSESSION:	Repetitive, uncontrollable thought
PARANOID:	Suspicion, mistrust, without a basis in reality
PHOBIA:	Irrational fear
PREMORBID:	Occurring before development of a disease
PSYCHOSIS:	State in which there is impairment in a person's ability to recognize reality, communicate and relate to others appropriately
RESISTANCE:	Opposition to uncovering unconscious material
ROLE:	Pattern of behavior
SECONDARY GAINS:	Benefits from being ill, such as attention
SELF ESTEEM:	The degree of feeling worthwhile or valued
SELF IMAGE:	One's thoughts about one's own self
SOMATIC THERAPY:	Treatment of the emotionally ill by physiological means
STEREOTYPED BEHAVIOR:	Persistent mechanical repetition of speech or motor activity
TRANSFERENCE:	Unconscious phenomenon in which feelings, attitudes, and wishes toward significant others in one's early life are linked to and projected onto others, usually a therapist in one's current life
WAXY FLEXIBILITY:	The extremities remain in a fixed position for a long period of time
WORD SALAD:	Words and phrases having no apparent meaning or logic

APPENDIX E

PHARMACOLOGY

Antimicrobial Agents

PENICILLINS

DRUG: GENERIC/TRADE

amoxicillin *(Polymox)*   dicloxacillin *(Dycill)*   penicillin G *(Bicillin L-A)*
ampicillin *(D-Amp)*   nafcillin *(Unipen)*   penicillin V *(Beepen-VK)*
cloxacillin *(Cloxapen)*

ACTION
Bacteriocidal against microbes by inhibiting cell wall synthesis during cell division

ADVERSE EFFECTS
Hypersensitivity: rash, urticaria, anaphylaxis

INDICATIONS
Infections due to gram-positive cocci and some gram-negative cocci

NURSING INTERVENTIONS
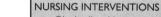
- Observe for hypersensitivity
- Teach client to call physician if rash, fever, or chills
- Teach client to take medications as ordered until entire amount taken
- Give 1–2 hours before meals or 2–3 after meals for best absorption

OTHER INFORMATION
Resistant strains of bacteria may develop

CEPHALOSPORINS

DRUG: GENERIC/TRADE
cefazolin sodium *(Ancef, Kefzol)*   cephalexin monohydrate *(Keflex)*   cephalothin sodium *(Keflin)*

ACTION
Bacteriocidal or bacteriostatic
Inhibits cell wall synthesis

ADVERSE EFFECTS
Hypersensitivity
Local irritation at injection site

INDICATIONS
Infections due to gram-positive cocci and some gram-negative cocci
Prophylactically before certain operative procedures

NURSING INTERVENTIONS
- Obtain client history
- Use *Clinistix, Diastix* or *Tes-Tape*, but not *Clinitest* for urine glucose test
- Change IV sites after 3 days
- Use with caution in clients with renal impairment

OTHER INFORMATION
Structurally related to penicillin
May cause false positive urine glucose test
Excreted unchanged in urine

SULFONAMIDES

DRUG: GENERIC/TRADE
sulfamethoxazole-trimethoprim *(Bactrim, Septra)*
sulfisoxazole *(Gantrisin)*

ACTION
Broad spectrum bacteriostatic

ADVERSE EFFECTS
Hypersensitivity
Blood dyscrasia-agranulocytosis, aplastic anemia
Toxic to kidney when output is low
GI manifestations: nausea, vomiting, diarrhea

INDICATIONS
Urinary tract infections
Otitis media

NURSING INTERVENTIONS

* Obtain client history
* Teach client to report skin rash, sore throat, fever or mouth sores
* Increase fluid intake to maintain output of 3,000–4,000 cc
* Give 1 hour before or 2 hours after meals for best absorption

AMINOGLYCOSIDES

DRUG: GENERIC/TRADE
gentamicin sulfate *(Garamycin)*
kanamycin sulfate *(Kantrex)*
neomycin sulfate *(Mycifradin Sulfate)*
streptomycin sulfate
tobramycin sulfate *(Nebcin)*

ACTION
Bacteriostatic or bacteriocidal
Inhibits protein synthesis

ADVERSE EFFECTS
Nephrotoxicity
Ototoxicity (tinnitus, vertigo, hearing loss)

INDICATIONS
Serious bacterial infections
Promote bowel sterility prior to GI surgical procedures

NURSING INTERVENTIONS

* Weigh client and obtain baseline renal function studies prior to therapy
* Monitor output for specific gravity, urinalysis, BUN, creatinine, and creatinine clearance
* Encourage fluids
* Evaluate client's hearing before and during hearing loss therapy

ANTITUBERCULARS

DRUG: GENERIC/TRADE
ethambutol *(Myambutol)*

ACTION
Impairs RNA synthesis

ADVERSE EFFECTS
Vision loss and loss of color discrimination

INDICATIONS
Pulmonary tuberculosis

NURSING INTERVENTIONS
* Evaluate client's visual acuity and color discrimination before and during therapy

ANTITUBERCULARS

DRUG: GENERIC/TRADE
rifampin *(Rifadin)*

ACTION
Impairs RNA synthesis

ADVERSE EFFECTS
Hepatotoxicity
Red-orange color to urine and feces
Drowsiness

INDICATIONS
Pulmonary tuberculosis

NURSING INTERVENTIONS
*   Monitor liver function studies
*   Teach client about urine color change
*   Teach client to avoid activities that require alertness

OTHER INFORMATION
May require increased doses of warfarin corticosteroids and oral hypoglycemics

---

ANTITUBERCULARS

DRUG: GENERIC/TRADE
isoniazid *(INH)*

ACTION
Interferes with DNA synthesis

ADVERSE EFFECTS
Hepatotoxicity
Peripheral neuropathy

INDICATIONS
Infection due to tubercle bacilli

NURSING INTERVENTIONS
*   Monitor liver function studies
*   Teach client to notify physician for loss of appetite, fatigue, malaise, jaundice, and dark urine
*   Teach client to avoid alcohol
*   Give pyridoxine *(Beesix)* to prevent peripheral neuropathy

---

ANTITUBERCULARS

DRUG: GENERIC/TRADE
para-aminosalicylic acid *(PAS)*

ACTION
Inhibits folic acid synthesis

ADVERSE EFFECTS
Hepatotoxicity
GI symptom: nauseaa, vomiting

INDICATIONS
Tuberculosis

NURSING INTERVENTIONS
*   Monitor liver function studies
*   Teach client to notify physician of loss of appetite fatigue, malaise, jaundice, and dark urine
*   Give with meals or antacid

ANTIFUNGALS

DRUG: GENERIC/TRADE
amphotericin B *(Fungizone)*

ACTION
Alters fungal cell permeability

ADVERSE EFFECTS
Fever, chills, nauseaa, vomiting, and headache
Thrombophlebitis
Hypokalemia

INDICATIONS
Systemic fungal infections

NURSING INTERVENTIONS

- Give acetaminophen *(Tylenol)* and diphenhydramine *(Benadryl)* 1 hour before infusion
- Add hydrocortisone to infusion
- Observe for signs of hypokalemia
- Large doses of potassium may be needed

ANTIFUNGALS

DRUG: GENERIC/TRADE
Nystatin *(Mycostatin)*

ACTION
Alters fungal cell permeability

ADVERSE EFFECTS
Rash, urticaria, stinging, burning

INDICATIONS
Infections due to Candida in the mouth, GI tract, or vagina

NURSING INTERVENTIONS
- Medical asepsis (hand washing) before, after application

Agents for Fluid and Electrolyte Balance

THIAZIDES AND THIAZIDE-LIKE DIURETICS

DRUG: GENERIC/TRADE
chlorothiazide *(Diuril)*
hydrochlorothiazide *(Hydro Diuril)*
chlorthalidone *(Hygroton)*
quinethazone *(Hydromox)*

ACTION
Inhibit sodium reabsorption in the kidney
Increase excretion of sodium and water

ADVERSE EFFECTS
Hypokalemia
Altered glucose metabolism

INDICATIONS
Hypertension
Edema

NURSING INTERVENTIONS
* Monitor intake and output, weight, and potassium level
* Teach client to increase dietary potassium intake
* Observe for signs of hypokalemia: muscle weakness, cramps
* Monitor blood sugar
* Observe for signs of hyperglycemia

OTHER INFORMATION
Give in the morning to prevent nocturia
High risk of digitalis toxicity due to potassium depletion

LOOP DIURETICS

DRUG: GENERIC/TRADE
furosemide *(Lasix)*
ethacrynate sodium *(Sodium Edecrin)*
ethacrynic acid *(Edecrin)*

ACTION
Inhibit sodium and chloride reabsorption in the kidney
Increase excretion of sodium and water

ADVERSE EFFECTS
Fluid and electrolyte imbalances   Hypocalcemia
Hypokalemia   Dehydration
Hyponatremia   Orthostatic hypotension
Hypochloremia

INDICATIONS
Edema
Pulmonary edema

NURSING INTERVENTIONS
* Monitor intake and output, weight, and serum electrolytes
* Teach client to increase dietary potassium intake
* Observe for signs of hypokalemia: muscle weakness, cramps
* Teach clients to stand up, take the stairs, and move around slowly

OTHER INFORMATION
Give in the morning to prevent nocturia
High risk of digitalis toxicity due to potassium depletion
Lasix is similar in appearance to digoxin

CARBONIC ANHYDRASE INHIBITOR DIURETICS

DRUG: GENERIC/TRADE
acetazolamide *(Diamox)*

ACTION
Promote urinary excretion of sodium, potassium, bicarbonate, and water

ADVERSE EFFECTS
Acidosis
Hypokalemia

INDICATIONS
Edema
Glaucoma

NURSING INTERVENTIONS
- Use for short-term treatment or use intermittent administration schedule
- Monitor intake and output, weight, and serum electrolytes
- Teach client to increase dietary potassium intake
- Observe for signs of hypokalemia: muscle weakness, cramps

MISCELLANEOUS DIURETICS

DRUG: GENERIC/TRADE
spironolactone *(Aldactone)*
triamterene *(Dyrenium)*

ACTION
Increased excretion of sodium and water
Reduces potassium excretion

ADVERSE EFFECTS
Hyperkalemia

INDICATIONS
Edema
Hypertension

NURSING INTERVENTIONS
- Monitor intake and output, weight, and serum electrolytes
- Teach clients to avoid excessive dietary potassium

OTHER INFORMATION
May be used in combination with potassium depleting diuretics

MISCELLANEOUS DIURETICS

DRUG: GENERIC/TRADE
mannitol *(Osmitrol)*

ACTION
Increases osmotic pressure of glomerular filtrate
Increases excretion of water and electrolytes

ADVERSE EFFECTS
Fluid and electrolyte imbalances
Transient plasma volume increase
Pulmonary edema
Cellular dehydration

INDICATIONS
Oliguria
Edema
Increased intraocular pressure
Increased intracranial pressure

NURSING INTERVENTIONS
- Monitor vital signs hourly, including central venous pressure
- Insert Foley, record urine output hourly
- Monitor weight, intake and output, serum sodium and potassium

OTHER INFORMATION
IV solution may crystallize; redissolve before infusing by warming bottle and shaking

ELECTROLYTE REPLACEMENT DRUGS

DRUG: GENERIC/TRADE
potassium chloride

ACTION
Necessary for cardiac contraction, renal function, and transmission of nerve impulses

ADVERSE EFFECTS
Cardiac arrhythmias, heart block, cardiac arrest
GI distress

INDICATIONS
Hypokalemia

NURSING INTERVENTIONS
- Give IV infusions as dilute solution infuses slowly
- Monitor EKG and serum potassium levels
- Give oral dose with meals and plenty of fluids

Cardiovascular Drugs

CARDIOTONIC GLYCOSIDES

DRUG: GENERIC/TRADE
digitoxin *(Crystodigin)*
digoxin *(Lanoxin)*

ACTION
Increases the force of cardiac contraction
Decreases heart rate

ADVERSE EFFECTS
Bradycardia, arrhythmias
Fatigue, muscle weakness, agitation
Hallucinations
Anorexia, nausea, yellow-green halos around visual images

INDICATIONS
Congestive heart failure
Tachyarrhythmias

NURSING INTERVENTIONS
- Take apical pulse for full minute; record and report significant changes in rate or rhythm
- Monitor serum levels of potassium and drug and monitor EKG
- Assess for these manifestations
- Teach how to take pulse and what signs to report

OTHER INFORMATION
Narrow range between therapeutic and toxic doses
Calcium salts are contraindicated

CORONARY VASODILATORS

DRUG: GENERIC/TRADE
nitroglycerin *(Nitrostat)*   diltiazem *(Cardizem)*
nifedipine *(Procardia)*

ACTION
Dilate coronary arteries
Decrease cardiac workload

ADVERSE EFFECTS
Headache   Flushing
Orthostatic hypotension   Palpitations
Tachycardia

INDICATIONS
Angina

NURSING INTERVENTIONS
- Treat with acetaminophen *(Tylenol)*
- Tolerance usually develops
- Monitor vital signs
- Teach to stand up, move slowly
- Teach client to lie down if dizzy

OTHER INFORMATION
Protect this drug from light, moisture and heat
Sublingual tablet taken at the first sign of anginal pain
Client should sit or lie down
May repeat tablet every five minutes times three if needed
Call physician if no relief
Topical drug measured on ruled application paper and applied to non-hairy area

ANTIARRHYTHMICS

DRUG: GENERIC/TRADE
lidocaine (*Xylocaine*)

propranolol hydrochloride (*Inderal*)

procainamide hydrochloride (*Pronestyl*)

quinidine gluconate (*Dura-Tabs*)

ACTION
Decreases cardiac conduction

ADVERSE EFFECTS
Bradycardia

Tachycardia

Hypotension

INDICATIONS
Prevention or treatment of atrial or ventricular

Arrhythmias including those secondary to MI and digitalis toxicity

NURSING INTERVENTIONS
- Remain with client during infusion, tachycardia
- Monitor EKG, BP, and heart rate and rhythm

OTHER INFORMATION
Narrow therapeutic index

Do not confuse lidocaine with epinephrine used for local or topical anesthesia

IV dose of Inderal much smaller than PO dose

ANTIARRHYTHMICS

DRUG: GENERIC/TRADE
verapamil (*Calan, Isoptin*)

ACTION
Calcium blocker

Decrease cardiac conduction

ADVERSE EFFECTS
Headache   Dizziness

Constipation   Heart failure

INDICATIONS
Atrial arrhythmias

NURSING INTERVENTIONS
- Treat with acetaminophen (*Tylenol*)
- Increase dietary fiber, fluid intake, and exercise

ANGIOTENSION-CONVERTING ENZYME INHIBITORS (ACE)

DRUG: GENERIC/TRADE
captopril (*Capoten*)   benazepril (*Lotensin*)

enalapril (*Vasotec*)

ACTION
Prevents production of angiotension II, causing system vasodilations

ADVERSE EFFECTS
Dry cough

Drop in BP during first 1–3 hours following first dose

Dizziness, orthostatic hypotension

INDICATIONS
Hypertension   Management of CHF

NURSING INTERVENTIONS
- Advise patient to change positions slowly
- Monitor BP, weight, signs to CHF resolution

ANTIHYPERTENSIVES

DRUG: GENERIC/TRADE
hydralazine hydrochloride (Apresoline)
prazosin hydrochloride (Minipress)

ACTION
Relaxes smooth muscle

ADVERSE EFFECTS
Tachycardia, palpitation
Orthostatic hypotension
Headache, dizziness
Nausea, vomiting, diarrhea, anorexia
Weight gain

INDICATIONS
Hypertension; congestive heart failure

NURSING INTERVENTIONS

- Monitor heart rate and rhythm
- Teach client to stand up, take stairs, and move around slowly
- Treat with acetaminophen (Tylenol); teach client to lie down if dizzy
- Give with meals
- Weigh daily
- Give diuretic if needed

OTHER INFORMATION
Compliance is biggest problem because side effects are worse than the disease
Side effects can be minimized by adjusting dose or changing drugs
Compliance may be increased by giving drugs QD rather than several times daily

---

ANTIHYPERTENSIVES

DRUG: GENERIC/TRADE
methyldopa (Aldomet)

ACTION
Sympatholytic

ADVERSE EFFECTS
Drowsiness, sedation
Orthostatic hypotension
Nausea, vomiting
Dry mouth
Edema, weight gain

INDICATIONS
Hypertension

NURSING INTERVENTIONS

- Teach client that drug may cause drowsiness and to stand up, take stairs, and move around slowly
- Give with meals
- Provide fluids, hard candy
- Weigh daily
- Give diuretic if needed

Central Nervous System Drugs

NON-NARCOTIC ANALGESICS

DRUG: GENERIC/TRADE
aspirin

ACTION
Analgesic, antipyretic, anti-inflammatory

ADVERSE EFFECTS
Prolonged bleeding time
Nausea, vomiting, GI distress

INDICATIONS
Arthritis
Mild pain, fever

NURSING INTERVENTIONS
- Teach client who takes large doses for a long time to watch for signs of bleeding
- Give with meals, milk, or antacids

OTHER INFORMATION
Contraindicated for children under 18 years old because use has been linked to Reye's syndrome

NON-NARCOTIC ANALGESICS

DRUG: GENERIC/TRADE
acetaminophen *(Tylenol)*

ACTION
Analgesic antipyretic

ADVERSE EFFECTS
Hepatotoxicity only with very large doses

INDICATIONS
Mild pain, fever

NURSING INTERVENTIONS
- Teach client not to exceed recommended dosage

NON-NARCOTIC ANALGESICS

DRUG: GENERIC/TRADE
ibuprofen *(Motrin)*

ACTION
Anti-inflammatory analgesic

ADVERSE EFFECTS
GI distress, occult bleeding

INDICATIONS
Arthritis, gout
Pain

NURSING INTERVENTIONS
- Give with meals, milk, or antacids

NARCOTIC ANALGESICS

DRUG: GENERIC/TRADE
codeine sulfate
meperidine hydrochloride *(Demerol)*
morphine sulfate

ACTION
Alter perception of pain

ADVERSE EFFECTS
Respiratory depression
Hypotension, bradycardia
Sedation, clouded sensorium, euphoria
Nausea, vomiting, constipation

INDICATIONS
Moderate to severe pain

NURSING INTERVENTIONS
- Monitor respirations before and during treatment
- Monitor BP and pulse
- Teach client to avoid activities that require alertness

OTHER INFORMATION
naloxone *(Narcan)* is used to reverse narcotic-induced respiratory depression

---

ANTICONVULSANTS

DRUG: GENERIC/TRADE
phenytoin sodium *(Dilantin)*

ACTION
Inhibits spread of seizure activity

ADVERSE EFFECTS
Ataxia

INDICATIONS
Grand mal seizures

NURSING INTERVENTIONS
- Determine if ataxia is a manifestation of the disease or a toxic effect of the drug
- Teach client to avoid activities that require alertness
- Use only clear solutions for infusion
- Good oral hygiene and regular dental care required

OTHER INFORMATION
Do not mix with 5% dextrose because precipitation will occur

Autonomic Nervous System Drugs

CHOLINERGIC BLOCKERS

DRUG: GENERIC/TRADE
benztropine mesylate *(Cogentin)*

biperiden hydrochloride *(Akineton)*

procyclidine hydrochloride *(Kemadrin)*

trihexyphenidyl hydrochloride *(Artane)*

ACTION
Parasympatholytic

ADVERSE EFFECTS
Anticholinergic

Blurred vision

Dry mouth

Constipation

Urinary retention

Orthostatic hypotension

Drowsiness

INDICATIONS
Parkinson's disease

Extra-pyramidal manifestations associated with antipsychotics

NURSING INTERVENTIONS
* Provide fluids, hard candy, ice chips
* Increase dietary fiber, fluid intake and exercise
* Monitor intake and output
* Monitor BP; teach client to stand up slowly
* Teach client to avoid activities that require alertness

OTHER INFORMATION
Elderly patients particularly sensitive to side effects

Can produce euphoria and have abuse potential

Amantadine *(Symmetrel)* is newer agent for treating Parkinson's disease; is not a cholinergic blocker

Gastrointestinal Drugs

ANTACIDS

DRUG: GENERIC/TRADE
aluminum hydroxide *(Amphojel)*
aluminum and magnesium hydroxide *(Maalox)*
calcium carbonate *(Tums)*

aluminum and magnesium hydroxide and simethicone Mylanta
aluminum magnesium complex *(Riopan)*

ACTION
Reduce acid in GI tract
Decrease pepsin activity

ADVERSE EFFECTS
Constipation
Hypernatremia
Hypermagnesemia
Hypophosphatemia

INDICATIONS
Peptic ulcers

NURSING INTERVENTIONS

- Record amount and consistency of stools
- Increase dietary fiber, fluid intake, and exercise
- Use laxatives and stool softeners
- Give Riopan, which has very low sodium content
- Do not give magnesium containing antacids to clients with renal disease
- When giving aluminum containing antacids, observe for anorexia, malaise, muscle weakness

ANTIEMETICS

DRUG: GENERIC/TRADE
prochlorperazine maleate *(Compazine)*
trimethobenzamide hydrochloride *(Tigan)*

ACTION
Acts centrally by blocking chemoreceptor trigger zone, which acts on vomiting center

ADVERSE EFFECTS
Drowsiness, dizziness

INDICATIONS
Nausea and vomiting

NURSING INTERVENTIONS

- Teach client to avoid activities that require alertness

ANTIEMETICS

DRUG: GENERIC/TRADE
dimenhydrinate *(Dramamine)*
scopolamine *(Transderm V)*

ACTION
Acts centrally by blocking chemoreceptor trigger zone, which acts on vomiting center

ADVERSE EFFECTS
Drowsiness, dizziness

INDICATIONS
Prevention of nausea and vomiting associated with motion sickness

NURSING INTERVENTIONS
- Teach client to avoid activities that require alertness

ULCER MEDICATIONS

DRUG: GENERIC/TRADE
propantheline bromide *(Pro-Banthine)*

ACTION
Anticholinergic

ADVERSE EFFECTS
Drowsiness, dizziness

INDICATIONS
Peptic ulcer

NURSING INTERVENTIONS

* Teach client to avoid activities that require alertness

ULCER MEDICATIONS

DRUG: GENERIC/TRADE
cimetidine *(Tagamet)*
sucralfate *(Carafate)*
omeprazole *(Prilosec)*

ACTION
Tagamet is GI antihistamine; reduces gastric acid secretion
Carafate coats and protects surface of ulcer
Omeprazole blocks acid production

ADVERSE EFFECTS
Abdominal cramps, diarrhea
Agranulocytosis, increased pro-time

INDICATIONS
Short-term treatment of duodenal and gastric ulcers, gastroesophageal reflux disease (GERD)

NURSING INTERVENTIONS

* Give with meals for prolonged drug effect
* Avoid OTC preparations such as aspirin, cough medications
* Report bruising
* Do not crush, chew, or open capsules *(Prilosec)*

OTHER INFORMATION
Short-term treatment only
Separate administration of these medications from administration of antacids by one hour

Hormonal Agents

STEROIDS

DRUG: GENERIC/TRADE
cortisone acetate *(Cortone)*
dexamethasone *(Decadron)*
prednisone *(Meticorten)*

ACTION
Anti-inflammatory

ADVERSE EFFECTS
Euphoria, insomnia, psychotic behavior
Hypokalemia
Hyperglycemia and carbohydrate intolerance
Peptic ulcer
Cushingoid symptoms with long-term therapy
Withdrawal symptoms

INDICATIONS
Adrenal insufficiency
Allergic inflammation, edema, immunosuppression

NURSING INTERVENTIONS

- Assess behavior, especially with high doses
- Potassium supplement may be needed
- High-protein diet rich in potassium
- Diabetics may require higher doses of insulin
- Give with meals
- Teach client manifestations
- Reduce dose gradually, not abruptly

INSULINS

DRUG: GENERIC/TRADE
Semilente regular insulin (Rapid acting)
Lente NPH (Intermediate acting)
Ultralente protamine (Long acting)

ACTION
Facilitates transport of glucose into cells
Lowers serum glucose level

ADVERSE EFFECTS
Hypoglycemia
Hyperglycemia

INDICATIONS
Diabetes Mellitus

NURSING INTERVENTIONS
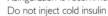
- Give orange juice or candy PO
- Give rapid-acting insulin

OTHER INFORMATION
Refrigeration is recommended for long-term storage
Do not inject cold insulin

SULFONYLUREAS

DRUG: GENERIC/TRADE
tolbutamide (Orinase)
chlorpropamide (Diabinese)
tolazamide (Tolinase)

ACTION
Increases insulin release from the pancreas

ADVERSE EFFECTS
Hypoglycemia
Hepatotoxicity

INDICATIONS
Adult onset, non-insulin dependent
Diabetes mellitus

NURSING INTERVENTIONS
- Teach client to take in morning to avoid hypoglycemic reaction at night
- Avoid OTC medications and alcohol

Hematologic Agents

HEMATONICS

DRUG: GENERIC/TRADE
ferrous sulfate (Slow-Fe)

ACTION
Source of iron replacement

ADVERSE EFFECTS
Nausea, constipation, black stool

INDICATIONS
Iron deficiency anemia

NURSING INTERVENTIONS
- Absorption best if given between meals
- For GI upset, give with meals or orange juice
- Teach client to increase dietary fiber, fluid intake, and exercise

OTHER INFORMATION
Vitamin C may increase absorption

ANTICOAGULANTS

DRUG: GENERIC/TRADE
heparin sodium *(Hep Lock, Hepalean)*

ACTION
Prevents conversion of fibrinogen to fibrin and prothrombin to thrombin

ADVERSE EFFECTS
Hemorrhage

INDICATIONS
Thrombosis
Pulmonary embolism
Myocardial infarction (MI)

NURSING INTERVENTIONS
- Monitor platelet count
- Monitor partial thromboplastin time (PTT)
- Avoid salicylates
- Observe for bleeding gums, bruises, nosebleeds, and petechiae

OTHER INFORMATION
IV absorption is more regular than subcutaneous injection
PTT should be 1.5–2 times control value
Antagonist is protamine sulfate

ANTICOAGULANTS

DRUG: GENERIC/TRADE
warfarin sodium *(Coumadin)*

ACTION
Interferes with blood clotting

ADVERSE EFFECTS
Hemorrhage

INDICATIONS
Pulmonary embolism
Thrombosis, MI, heart valve damage

NURSING INTERVENTIONS
- Monitor PT
- Avoid salicylates
- Observe for bleeding gums, bruises, nosebleeds and petechiae
- Teach client to use soft toothbrush and electric razor

OTHER INFORMATION
Oral administration PT should be 1.5–2 times control value
Antagonist is Vitamin K

ANTINEOPLASTICS

DRUG: GENERIC/TRADE
methotrexate (Folex, Rheumatrex)
cisplatin (Platinol)
bleomycin (Blenoxane)

ACTION
Act by many different mechanisms, most affect DNA synthesis or function

ADVERSE EFFECTS
Many cause bone marrow depression, thrombocytopenia, nausea, vomiting, mouth ulcers

INDICATIONS
Cancer
Chemotherapy

NURSING INTERVENTIONS
- Assess for signs of infection
- Monitor platelet count
- Monitor IV site carefully, ensure patency; follow protocols for infiltration to prevent tissue ulceration/necrosis
- Wear gloves, masks, gowns while handling or preparing medication; discard equipment in designated containers

Eye Medications

MIOTICS

DRUG: GENERIC/TRADE
pilocarpine hydrochloride (Carpine)

ACTION
Pupillary constriction

ADVERSE EFFECTS
Myopia
Blurred vision

INDICATIONS
Glaucoma
Surgical procedures on the eye

NURSING INTERVENTIONS
- Usually disappears after 10–14 days of treatment

OTHER INFORMATION
Press inner canthus for a minute or two to decrease systemic absorption

MYDRIATICS

DRUG: GENERIC/TRADE
atropine sulfate *(Atropisol)*

ACTION
Pupillary dilatation, cycloplegia

ADVERSE EFFECTS
Blurred vision
Photophobia

INDICATIONS
Acute inflammation of the eye
Diagnostic procedure

NURSING INTERVENTIONS

- Warn client about temporary blurring of vision
- Dark glasses
- Teach client not to drive until vision is clear

MYDRIATICS

DRUG: GENERIC/TRADE
phenylephrine hydrochloride *(Neo-Synephrine)*

ACTION
Pupillary dilatation

ADVERSE EFFECTS
Hypertension
Blurred vision

INDICATIONS
Diagnostic procedure

NURSING INTERVENTIONS
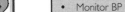
- Monitor BP
- Avoid use in clients with hypertension
- Teach client not to drive until vision is clear

Antianxiety Agents (Minor Tranquilizers)

BENZODIAZEPINE COMPOUNDS

DRUG: GENERIC/TRADE
chlordiazepoxide *(Librium)*   clorazepate *(Tranxene)*
diazepam *(Valium)*   lorazepam *(Ativan)*
oxazepam *(Serax)*   alprazolam *(Xanax)*
clonazepam *(Clonopin)*

ACTION
CNS depression
Muscle relaxation
Anticonvulsant

ADVERSE EFFECTS
Drowsiness, sedation

LONG TERM ADVERSE EFFECTS
Tolerance
Dependency
Rebound insomnia/anxiety

INDICATIONS
Anxiety disorder
Detoxification alcohol dependence disorder
Skeletal muscle relaxation
Premedication operative procedures
Seizures

NURSING INTERVENTIONS
- Teach client to avoid activities that require alertness, such as driving
- Caution to avoid falls
- Discourage social isolation
- Observe carefully, offer support
- Short-term use only
- Avoid alcohol or other CNS depressant
- Discontinue by slowly tapering off

OTHER INFORMATION
Avoid during pregnancy and lactation
Elderly more vulnerable to side effects

SEDATING ANTIHISTAMINES

DRUG: GENERIC/TRADE
hydroxyzine *(Vistaril, Atarax)*

ACTION
CNS depressant (subcortical levels)

ADVERSE EFFECTS
Convulsions
Tremors, fatigue
Dizziness, confusion, depression
Headache
Dry mouth

INDICATIONS
Preoperative medication
Anxiety disorders

NURSING INTERVENTIONS
- Observe closely, may lower seizure threshold
- Teach client to avoid activities that require alertness

ANXIOLYTICS

DRUG: GENERIC/TRADE
buspirone *(BuSpar)*

ACTION
Unknown

ADVERSE EFFECTS
Depression, stimulation, insomnia
Tremors
Hypotension
Tachycardia, palpitations

INDICATIONS
Relief of short-term anxiety

NURSING INTERVENTIONS
- Teach 2–3 week lag time before therapeutic effect achieved
- Monitor BP, pulse

OTHER INFORMATION
No sedative/hypnotic properties or muscle relaxation properties
Do not use with MAIOs

BETA-BLOCKERS

DRUG: GENERIC/TRADE
propranolol *(Inderal)*
clonidine *(Catapres)*

ACTION
Non-selective B-blocker

ADVERSE EFFECTS
Dizziness, confusion
Hypotension, bradycardia
Dry mouth
Drowsiness, sedation

INDICATIONS
Anxiety disorders
Narcotic withdrawal
Convulsions

NURSING INTERVENTIONS
- Observe carefully
- Monitor when out of bed
- Monitor BP, pulse
- Increase fluids

SEDATIVE-HYPNOTICS

DRUG: GENERIC/TRADE
flurazepam *(Dalmane)*
temazepam *(Restoril)*
triazolam *(Halcion)*

ACTION
Produces CNS depression and sedation

ADVERSE EFFECTS
Drowsiness
Dizziness, lightheadedness

OVERDOSE
Somnolence
Confusion
Impaired coordination
Coma

INDICATIONS
Sleep disturbance of anxiety
Short-term use only

NURSING INTERVENTIONS
- Observe carefully
- Advise caution when out of bed
- Suicide assessment
- Obtain emergency medical treatment

Antipsychotic Agents (Major Tranquilizers)

ANTIPSYCHOTICS

DRUG: GENERIC/TRADE
chlorpromazine (Thorazine)
mesoridazine (Serentil)
perphenazine (Trilafon)
chlorprothixene (Taractan)
haloperidol (Haldol)
loxapine (Loxitane)
risperidone (Risperdal)

thioridazine (Mellaril)
fluphenazine (Prolixin)
trifluoperazine (Stelazine)
thiothixene (Navane)
molindone (Moban)
clozapine (Clozaril)

ACTION
Depresses cerebral cortex, which controls activity aggression

ADVERSE EFFECTS
Sedation
Extrapyramidal effects
  dystonia
  akathisia
  tardive dyskinesia
Anticholinergic symptoms
  dry mouth
  constipation
  urinary retention
  blurred vision
  nasal congestion
  Hypotension

Photosensitivity
Agranulocytosis (esp. Clozaril)
Neuroleptic malignant syndrome
Weight gain

INDICATIONS
Schizophrenic disorders
Bipolar disorder, manic phase
Agitated organic disorders

NURSING INTERVENTIONS
- Ask physician if entire dose can be given at bedtime
- Report parkinsonian symptoms, dystonia to physician
- Medication may be changed
- Antiparkinsonian medication may be given
- Discontinue at first sign
- Fluids, sugarless candies, gum
- Laxatives, diet
- Monitor intake, output
- Will disappear within a week
- Increase humidity
- Monitor BP, sitting and standing
- Caution to stand up slowly
- Sunscreen, protective clothing
- Observe and report signs of infection, discontinue
- Observe and report signs: altered consciousness, unstable BP&P, muscle rigidity, diaphoresis, tremors
- Discontinue medication if present
- Monitor diet, increase physical exercise

OTHER INFORMATION
Drug Interactions: CNS depressants have additive effects; antacids inhibit absorption
Lowers seizure threshold
Clozapine (Clozaril) requires weekly WBC
Use low doses only for elderly
Avoid thioridazine (Mellaril) in sexually active males
Risperidone (Risperdal) also effective on negative manifestations

Antidepressant Agents

TRICYCLIC ANTIDEPRESSANTS

DRUG: GENERIC/TRADE
imipramine *(Tofranil)*   clomipramine *(Anafranil)*
desipramine *(Norpramin)*   doxepin *(Sinequan)*
amitriptyline *(Elavil)*   protriptyline *(Vivactil)*
nortriptyline *(Aventyl, Pamelor)*   trimipramine *(Surmontil)*

ACTION
Blocks re-uptake of norepinephrine and serotonin into nerve endings

ADVERSE EFFECTS
Agranulocytosis
Hypotension
Paralytic ileus
Cardiovascular

INDICATIONS
Major depressive disorders
Agoraphobia
Panic disorders
Obsessive compulsive disorder
Psychogenic pain disorder

NURSING INTERVENTIONS

- Monitor CBC
- Caution to stand up slowly
- Observe for nausea and vomiting
- Use cautiously in clients with known heart disease

TETRACYCLIC ANTIDEPRESSANTS

DRUG: GENERIC/TRADE
amoxapine *(Asendin)*
maprotiline *(Ludiomil)*

ACTION
Blocks re-uptake of norepinephrine and serotonin into nerve endings

ADVERSE EFFECTS
Agranulocytosis
Hypotension
Paralytic ileus

INDICATIONS
Depression

NURSING INTERVENTIONS
- Monitor CBC
- Caution to stand up slowly
- Observe for nausea and vomiting

NEWER ANTIDEPRESSANTS

DRUG: GENERIC/TRADE

trazodone *(Desyrel)*

fluoxetine *(Prozac)*

bupropion *(Wellbutrin)*

sertraline *(Zoloft)*

paroxetine *(Paxil)*

Venlafaxine hydrochloride *(Effexor)*

ACTION

Inhibits serotonin and potentiates behavioral changes

ADVERSE EFFECTS

Anticholinergic effects
  Dry mouth
  Constipation
  Urinary retention
  Blurred vision
  Aggravates glaucoma
Cardiovascular effects
  Postural hypotension
  Tachycardia, arrhythmias
Allergic reactions
  Rashes
  Photosensitivity
  Tremors
CNS
  Insomnia
  Stimulation
  Sedation
  Delirium
  Myoclonic twitches
  Seizures (especially high doses)

INDICATIONS

Depression

NURSING INTERVENTIONS

- Increase fluids
- Good oral hygiene
- Bulk diet, exercise, stool softeners
- Monitor intake and outflow, lower dose
- Corrective lenses, large print, change to another antidepressant
- Ophthalmic consult
- Take BP regularly, sitting and standing
- Use smaller divided doses in conduction defects clients with known heart disease
- Avoid in clients with conduction defects or recent MI
- Do pretreatment EKG
- Sunscreen, protective clothing
- Observe carefully
- Advise to avoid caffeine
- Observe and report; may have to discontinue
- High doses usually, reduce dose
- Start at low dose and gradually increase (maprotiline and bupropion) to monitor weight gain (except bupropion and fluoxetine)

OTHER INFORMATION

- Response rate varies but often takes 3–4 weeks for therapeutic effect
- Allow 14 days waiting period before changing from antidepressant to MAOI and vice versa
- Tricyclics can be fatal with overdose; do suicide assessment
- Drug Interactions:
  - Antihypertensives (unable to control BP)
  - Antacids inhibit absorption
  - Antipsychotics
  - Antiarrhythmics

MAO INHIBITORS

DRUG: GENERIC/TRADE
isocarboxazid *(Marplan)*
phenelzine *(Nardil)*
tranylcypromine *(Parnate)*

ACTION
Acts on CNS by increasing concentration of epinephrine, serotonin, and dopamine, thereby reducing depression   effective

ADVERSE EFFECTS
Excessive perspiration
Erection/orgasm difficulty preparation
Anxiety, restlessness
Hypertensive crisis
Anticholinergic manifestations
CNS effects: drowsiness, fatigue, headache, restlessness, insomnia, constipation
Orthostatic hypotension
Insomnia *(Parnate)*
Weight gain

INDICATIONS
Because of dietary restrictions, use as second line antidepressant if other antidepressants not effective

NURSING INTERVENTIONS
- Observe, report, provide comfort measures
- Lower dose or switch to a less anticholinergic preparation
- Teach clients to avoid foods with high tyramine content such as aged cheese, fava or Italian green beans, fermented foods, liver, yeast extracts, bologna, beer, Chianti and red wines; limit sour cream, yogurt
- Teach clients to avoid OTC cold preparations
- See antipsychotic medications
- Some side effects can be expected for a short period
- Treat symptoms medically if not severe
- Monitor BP, sitting and standing
- Single AM dose

OTHER INFORMATION
Drug Interactions:
Tricyclic antidepressants cause hypertensive crisis
Cocaine and amphetamines potentiate the action
Asthma inhalants
Narcotics, especially meperidine
Local anesthetics with epinephrine
Sinus and nasal decongestants

Mood Stabilizers

MOOD STABILIZERS

DRUG: GENERIC/TRADE
lithium carbonate (*Eskalith, Lithonate, Lithotabs, Lithobid*)

ACTION
Alters Na, K, and ion transport in nerve; interferes with balance of epinephrine and serotonin in CNS, thereby affecting emotional responses

ADVERSE EFFECTS
Fine tremor
Transient nausea
Drowsiness, lethargy
Diarrhea, abdominal discomfort
Polyuria
Thirst
Weight gain
Signs of toxicity:
  Vomiting
  Diarrhea
  Lethargy
  Muscle twitching
  Ataxia
  Slurred speech
  Coma
  Seizure
  Cardiac arrest

INDICATIONS
Bipolar disorder, manic phase
Major depression
Aggressive conduct disorder

NURSING INTERVENTIONS

- Teach client that side effects are short of duration
- Observe carefully for changes in manifestations
- Check blood levels
- Advise to avoid caffeine
- Keep side rails up
- Teach client to avoid activities that require alertness
- Give with meals
- Increase fluid intake
- Restrict calories, increase physical exercise
- Assess for edema
- Careful observation for manifestations and monitoring of blood levels as Na decreases and lithium levels increase
- Hold next dose and report STAT
- Pretreatment medical exam with thyroid and kidney function testing and EKG
- Nonsteroidal anti-inflammatory drugs may lead to lithium toxicity

OTHER INFORMATION
Narrow therapeutic index
  .5- 1.5 meg/liter: therapeutic
  Above 1.5 meg/liter: toxic
  2.0 meg/liter: lethal

Drug Interactions:
Diuretics increase the risk of lithium toxicity
Antipsychotics may cause neurotoxicity, especially in the elderly
Ingestion of excessive Na increases lithium excretion
D/C prior to elective surgery or ECT
Do not take if pregnant

MOOD STABILIZERS

DRUG: GENERIC/TRADE
carbamazepine *(Tegretol)*

ACTION
Affects mood by inhibiting nerve impulses, by limiting Na exchange

ADVERSE EFFECTS
Skin rash
Sore throat, mucosal ulcerations
Low-grade fever
Drowsiness, ataxia, vertigo
Diplopia, blurred vision
Nausea and vomiting, hepatotoxicity

INDICATIONS
Acute mania and prevention of manic episodes with lithium ineffective
Temporal lobe epilepsy

NURSING INTERVENTIONS
- Caution when used with lithium and haloperidol (Haldol)

MOOD STABILIZERS

DRUG: GENERIC/TRADE
valproic acid *(Depakote)*

ACTION
Increases levels of GABA in brain

ADVERSE EFFECTS
GI complaints
Tremor, sedation, ataxia
Increased appetite, weight gain
Pancreatitis
Severe hepatic dysfunction
Thrombocytopenia

INDICATIONS
Manic episodes when lithium ineffective (better tolerated)

NURSING INTERVENTIONS
- Administer with food or milk
- Teach client to avoid activities that require alertness
- Monitor liver function test and hematology levels

Drugs Used in the Obstetrics Setting

OXYTOCICS

DRUG: GENERIC/TRADE
oxytocin *(Pitocin)*

ACTION
Stimulates contractions of the uterus

ADVERSE EFFECTS

Hypotension	Fetal bradycardia or tachycardia
Tachycardia	Decreased urine output

INDICATIONS
Induction of labor

NURSING INTERVENTIONS
- Monitor uterine contractions, blood pressure, maternal heart rate and fetal heart rate
- Monitor intake and output

OTHER INFORMATION
Use only when pelvis is adequate, vaginal delivery is indicted, fetus is mature, and fetal position is favorable

---

OXYTOCICS

DRUG: GENERIC/TRADE
methylergonovine maleate *(Methergine)*

ACTION
Stimulates motor activity of the uterus

ADVERSE EFFECTS

Headache	Chest pain
Nausea	Palpitations

INDICATIONS
Postpartum hemorrhage due to uterine atony

NURSING INTERVENTIONS
- Assess uterine contractions following administration
- Monitor vital signs and vaginal bleeding

OTHER INFORMATION
Contraindicated prior to the fourth stage of labor

UTERINE RELAXANTS

DRUG: GENERIC/TRADE
isoxsuprine hydrochloride *(Vasodilan)*

ACTION
Vasodilator

ADVERSE EFFECTS
Hypotension
Tachycardia

INDICATIONS
Premature labor
Labor contractions too frequent or uncoordinated

NURSING INTERVENTIONS
- Monitor blood pressure and pulse

OTHER INFORMATION
Contraindicated in immediate postpartum period

UTERINE RELAXANTS

DRUG: GENERIC/TRADE
ritodrine hydrochloride *(Yutopar)*

ACTION
Inhibits contraction of uterine smooth muscle

ADVERSE EFFECTS
Hypotension
Hypertension

INDICATIONS
Premature labor

NURSING INTERVENTIONS
- Monitor blood pressure; maternal heart rate and fetal heart rate

UTERINE RELAXANTS

DRUG: GENERIC/TRADE
terbutaline sulfate *(Brethine)*

ACTION
Relaxes uterine smooth muscle

ADVERSE EFFECTS
Nervousness
Tremors
Headache

INDICATIONS
Premature labor

NURSING INTERVENTIONS
- Monitor blood pressure and pulse
- Monitor maternal heart rate and fetal heart rate

OTHER INFORMATION
Use cautiously in clients with diabetes, heart disease, and hypertension

ANTICONVULSANTS

DRUG: GENERIC
magnesium sulfate

ACTION
Anticonvulsant

ADVERSE EFFECTS
Respiratory depression
Heart block
Circulatory collapse
Increased magnesium

INDICATIONS
Primary intracerebral hemorrhage (PIH)

NURSING INTERVENTIONS
- Hold drug if respirations less than 16
- Monitor for arrhythmias
- Monitor intake and output
- Observe for neuromuscular or respiratory depression

OTHER INFORMATION
Antidote is calcium gluconate

ANTIDOTES

DRUG: GENERIC/TRADE
calcium gluconate

ACTION
Needed for nervous musculoskeletal enzyme reactions, cardiac contraction, blood coagulation, and endocrine and exocrine secretions

ADVERSE EFFECTS
Bradycardia
Arrhythmias
Venous irritation

INDICATIONS
Hypermagnesemia

NURSING INTERVENTIONS
- Monitor pulse
- Monitor for arrhythmias
- Assess IV site

OTHER INFORMATION
Contraindicated in digitized clients

ESTROGENS

DRUG: GENERIC/TRADE
estradiol *(Estrace)*

ACTION
Hormone needed for adequate functioning of female reproductive system; inhibits ovulation
Promotes calcium use in bone structure

ADVERSE EFFECTS
Hypoglycemia
Dizziness, hypotension
GI: nausea, vomiting
Appetite increase, weight gain
Embolism

INDICATIONS
Prevent postpartum breast engorgement

NURSING INTERVENTIONS
- Observe glucose in diabetics
- Monitor weight
- Report headache, chest pain

NARCOTIC ANTAGONISTS

DRUG: GENERIC/TRADE
naloxone *(Narcan)*

ACTION
Interferes with narcotic absorption at narcotic receptor sites

ADVERSE EFFECTS
Rapid pulse
Drowsiness, nervousness
Nausea, vomiting

INDICATIONS
Treatment of narcotic induced depression of neonate

NURSING INTERVENTION
- Monitor respiratory rate and depth of neonate

ANTI-INFLAMMATORY DRUGS

DRUG: GENERIC TRADE

betamethasone (*Celestone*)

ACTION

Corticosteroid

ADVERSE EFFECTS

GI distress, hemorrhage, pancreatitis
Poor wound healing
CNS depression, flushing, sweating
Thrombocytopenia
Hypertension, circ. collapse, embolism

INDICATIONS

Stimulate lung development in infant

NURSING INTERVENTIONS

* Monitor temperature
* Monitor blood pressure, report chest pain

OTHER INFORMATION

Do not discontinue abruptly; adrenal crisis can occur

APPENDIX F
NURSING MANAGEMENT

I. Management
A. Concepts of Management
1. Leadership
   a. Definition: A way of behaving that influences others to respond, not because they have to, but because they want to. Leaders help others to identify and focus on goals and the achievement of them. Think of leadership as a personal interaction that focuses on the personal development of the members of the group.
   b. Essential components of leadership
      1) Knowledge
      2) Self-awareness
      3) Communication
      4) Energy
      5) Goals
      6) Action

2. Management
   a. Definition: A problem-oriented process with a focus on the activities needed to achieve a goal. Supplying the structure, resources, and direction for the activities of the group. Management involves personal interaction but the focus is on the group's process. The most effective managers are also effective leaders.
   b. Essential components of management
      1) Planning/organization
      2) Direction
      3) Monitoring
      4) Recognition and reward
      5) Development of staff
      6) Representation
   c. Management styles
      1) Autocratic
      2) Laissez-faire
      3) Democratic

3. Power
   a. Definition: Power is the ability to take action, having the strength to accomplish goals. Power can be both inherent and acquired. Everyone has power, in different ways and to different degrees.
   b. Types of power
      1) Legitimate
      2) Referent
      3) Reward
      4) Expert
      5) Information
      6) Coercive

4. Group Dynamics/Teamwork
   a. Definition: A team is a group of individuals working together toward a common goal. Members of the team engage in varying roles supporting achievement of these goals. Each team member's contribution is valued and important to the success of the team as a whole. Think collaboration, coordination, communication. Group dynamics are the underlying process that the group engages in during their work as a team. Some of these facilitate and some hinder the progress of the group.
   b. Team roles
      1) Task roles
         a) Initiating
         b) Seeking information
         c) Giving information
         d) Clarifying
         e) Coordinating
         f) Summarizing
      2) Group maintenance roles
         a) Supporting
         b) Mediating
         c) Gate keeping
         d) Following
         e) Tension reducing
         f) Standard setting

5. Change
   a. Definition: Planned change involves working through a process that closely reflects the nursing process: Assessing and diagnosing a problem that needs to be solved; planning and implementing ways to institute changes to solve or minimize the problem; and evaluating or monitoring the progress of the changes made and modifying these changes as needed. After change occurs, the changed behaviors, attitudes or processes have to be supported and reinforced until they become a natural, comfortable response.
   b. Catalysts for change
      1) System or process
      2) Management
      3) Clients
      4) Individuals
   c. Stages of change
      1) Resistance
      2) Uncertainty
      3) Assimilation
      4) Transference
      5) Integration
   d. Lewin's phases of change
      1) Unfreezing
      2) Changing
      3) Refreezing

6. Communication
   a. Definition: Communication involves sending, receiving, and interpreting both verbal and non-verbal information between at least two people
   b. Components of communication
   c. Basic elements of effective communication
   d. Assertive communication

7. Conflict
   a. Definition: conflict arises when there are two opposing views, feelings, expectations and many other issues. It can occur within the individual, between individuals, or between groups and organizations. Conflict can be managed.
   b. Sources of conflict
   c. Conflict resolution
      1) Avoidance
      2) Accommodation
      3) Compromise
      4) Competition
      5) Collaboration
   d. Process of negotiation
   e. Sexual harassment

B. Continuity of Care
1. Definition: Continuity of care focuses on the experience of the client as the client moves through the health care system. Moving the client through this experience requires coordination, integration, and facilitation of all the events along the continuum.
2. Nursing's role
3. Factors impacting the continuum of care

C. Quality Improvement
1. Definition: A planned process to evaluate the delivery of care and to develop ways to address any problems or difficulties.
2. Continuous versus Total Quality Improvement
3. Types of quality indicators
   a. Structure
   b. Process
   c. Outcome
4. Data collection

D. Variances/Incidence Reports
1. Definition: A variance or incident is an event that occurs outside the usual expected, "normal" events or activities of the client's stay, unit functioning or organizational processes
2. Purpose
3. Documentation standards

E. Resource Management
1. Health care delivery
   a. Retrospective versus prospective payment
   b. Health maintenance organizations
2. Budgeting
   a. Types of budgets
   b. The budget process
      1) Planning
      2) Preparation
      3) Modification and approval
      4) Monitoring
3. Nurse's role in resource management

F. Case Management
1. Definition: Case management involves the development of a partnership with the client with a goal of managing declines in health and/or function that are due to serious, chronic and persistent illness and disability.
2. Types of case management
   a. Independent
   b. Hospital based
   c. Physician based
   d. Insurance based

G. Consultation and Referral

1. Definitions
   a. Consultation: To ask for help in solving a problem or meeting a need of an individual or group. This help is then applied and monitored by the nurse. Often, it is a request for information from someone with specialized knowledge, including peers.
   b. Referral: A request for assistance from someone with specialized knowledge or skills to help in the management of the client's problems. Most often, it is a request for intervention from another professional who has the needed skills and knowledge. The intervention becomes that specialist's responsibility, but the nurse continues to be responsible for the monitoring of the client's response and progress.

2. Common nursing consultation and referral situations
3. Appropriate use of consultation and referral

II. Delegation
A. Delegation/Supervision

1. Definitions
   a. Delegation: The act of asking another to do some aspect of care, assignment or work that needs to be accomplished. Delegation can be horizontal to peers, upwardly vertical to management, or downwardly vertical to subordinate.
   b. Supervision: Monitoring the progress towards completion of delegated tasks. The amount of supervision required depends on the direction of the delegation, the abilities of the person being delegated to, and the location of the ultimate responsibility for outcomes.

2. Accountability
3. Components
   a. Tasks
   b. Person
   c. Communication
   d. Feedback

III. Ethical Issues
A. Ethical Practice

1. Basic ethical principles
   a. Nonmaleficence
   b. Beneficence
   c. Autonomy/self-determination
   d. Fidelity
   e. Justice
   f. Confidentiality
2. ANA Code for Nurses
3. Ethical dilemmas
4. Ethical decision making

B. Organ Donation

1. Determination of death
2. Nursing role
3. Family needs
4. Criteria for donation

C. Advanced Directives
1. Definition: A document in which a competent person is able to express wishes regarding futures acceptable health care and/or designate another person to make decisions for the client if the client is physically or mentally unable.
2. Legislative action
3. Living will
   a. Definition: Declaration of what the person finds acceptable or would refuse under identified situations that may occur in the future
   b. Legal standing
   c. Content
4. Durable power of attorney
   a. Definition: Designation of another person to make decisions for the client when the client become unable to make decisions independently
   b. Legal issues
   c. Purpose
5. Challenges

IV. Legal Issues
A. Informed Consent
1. Definition: Consent given by the client that is based on adequate information to consider the risks and benefits of the offered service
2. Elements of informed consent
3. Nursing roles and responsibilities

B. Client Rights
1. Client Bill of Rights
2. Americans with Disabilities Act
3. Nursing role, responsibilities
4. Legal implications

C. Legal Responsibilities
1. Types of law
2. Nurse Practice Act
3. Good Samaritan Law
4. Mandatory Reporter of Abuse
5. Malpractice/Negligence

D. Advocacy
1. Definitions: A process by which the nurse assists other to grow and develop towards self-actualization
2. Nursing role as advocate

INDEX

carbon dioxide narcosis, 27
carcinomas, 120
cardiac catheterization, 80
cardiac problems
  in pregnancy, 207
cardiopulmonary resuscitation (CPR), 90-91
cardiovascular system, failure of, 79
casts, 57
cataract, 118
catheterization, 94
celiac disease, 294, 296
central venous pressure, 79
cerebral arteriogram, 105
cerebral palsy, 293
cerebrovascular accident (CVA), 110
cesarean section, 202
Chadwick's sign, 190
chemical dependence/abuse, 167-172
chemotherapy, 31-32, 297-298. *See also* cancer
chest physiotherapy (chest PT), 35
chest tube
  removal of, 30
  systems, 29
chicken pox, 302
child abuse, 180-181, 285-286
children, hospitalized
  developmental factors in, 252-253
  reaction to pain in, 253-254
  reactions of, 252
  regression in, 252
  strategies for health promotion for, 254-255
children, school age
  developmental stages of, 247
  health deviations of, 248-249
  health maintenance of, 248
  language development of, 246
  motor skills of, 246
  nutritional needs of, 246
  physical characteristics of, 245-246
  play of, 247
  sleeping patterns of, 246
cholangiogram, 43
cholecystitis, 52
cholecystogram, 42
cholelithiasis, 52
chronic airflow limitation (CAL). *See* chronic obstructive
  pulmonary disease
chronic obstructive pulmonary disease (COPD), 24-28,
  33, 83
  complications of, 26-28
clean catch, 93
cleft lip, 265-266
cleft palate, 266-267
closed chest drainage, 28
  types of, 29
clubfoot, congenital, 265
colonoscopy, 42
colostomy, 49
coma scale, Glasgow, 107
coma, diabetic, 291
communication, tools of, 142-143
community mental health model, 137
computed tomography (CT scan), 106
congenital dysplasia of the hip (CDH), 264-265
congestive heart failure, 83

Conn's syndrome, 67
continuous ambulatory peritoneal dialysis (CAPD), 100
contraceptives, types of, 228-229
COPD. *See* chronic obstructive pulmonary disease
cor pulmonale, 26-27
CPR (cardiopulmonary resuscitation), 90-91
cretinism, 68
crisis intervention, 137-138
Crohn's disease, 48, 76
croup, 274-275
cryptococcosis, 125
CT scan (computed tomography), 106
Cushing's syndrome, 65-66
cystic fibrosis, 294, 296
cystitis, 95
cystoscopy, 94, 101
cytology, 42

D

deep breathing exercises, 40
defense mechanisms
    definition of, 140
    types of, 140-141
delirium tremens (DTs), 168-169
depression, 157-159
    treatments for, 160
dermatophytosis, 302
development
    characteristics of, 233
    Erikson's stages of, 135
developmental disabilities, 178-179
diabetes insipidus, 63
diabetes mellitus, 72-74
    in children, 290-291
    pregnancy and, 207
dialysis, 97-99
diarrhea, in children, 270-272
diffuse toxic goiter, 69
diffusion, 16
digitalis therapy, 83
dissociative disorders (hysterical neurosis), 148. *See also*
    anxiety disorders
diuretics
    potassium depleting, 87
    potassium sparing, 87
drug abuse, 170-172
DTs (delirium tremens), 168-169
duodenal ulcer, 46-47
dwarfism, 63
dysplasia of the hip, congenital (CDH), 264-265

E

ECG (electrocardiogram), 80
eclampsia, 210
ECT (electroconvulsive therapy), 164
eczema, 286-287
EEG (electroencephalogram), 106
elation. *See* mania
electrocardiogram (ECG), 80
electroconvulsive therapy (ECT), 164
electroencephalogram (EEG), 106

nephroblastoma, 298
nephrotic syndrome, 96
　in children, 294-295
neuroblastoma, 298-299
neurological assessment, 104-105
　neuro checks, 107
neurological defects. See individual defects
newborn
　initial assessment of, 217-218
　initial care of the, 200
　jaundice (hyperbilirubinemia) in, 222
　postmature, 222
　premature, 220
　substance abuse and the, 222-223
non-stress test, 215
nurse-client relationship, 141-143

O

operative obstetrics
　cesarean section, 202
　episiotomy, 201
　forceps delivery, 201-202
　vacuum extraction, 202
organic mental disorders
　delirium, 173
　dementias (See individual types)
normal aging, 173
osmosis, 16
osteoarthritis, 55
ostomies, intestinal, 49, 54
otitis media, acute, 272-273
oxygen toxicity, 27

P

pacemakers, 85, 91
pancreas, disorders of the, 72-74
pancreatitis, 53
paracentesis, 43
paraplegia, 111
parathyroid gland, 70-71
Parkinson's disease, 114
patch graft, 86
pediculosis capitis, 303
PEG, 45
pelvic inflammatory disease (PID), 226
percutaneous endoscopic gastronomy, 45
percutaneous radiofrequency
　trigeminal gangliolysis, 116
personality disorders, 165-166
pertussis, 303
pH, regulation of body, 17
pheochromocytoma, 67
pinworms, 302
pituitary gland, 61
placenta
　abruptio, 211
　development of the, 188
　previa, 211-212
　transfer of material to fetus from, 189
pleural space, disorders of the, 35
Pneumocystis carinii pneumonia, 124
pneumonia, 32-33

pneumothorax, 27-28
posterior pituitary, disorders of the, 63
postoperative care
　for children, 277
　general, 39-40
postoperative complications, common, 40
postpartum
　puerperium, 203-204
postpartum complications
　hemorrhage, 214
　infection, 214
　thromboembolic disease, 214
postpartum nursing
　client education, 205-206
　physical assessment of client, 205
　psychological adaptation of client, 204
postural drainage, 35-36
preeclampsia, 210
pregnancy, 187-189. See also prenatal care
　discomforts of, 192-194
　ectopic, 209
　emotional adaptations to, 195
　high-risk, 206-208
　hyperemesis gravidarum, 208
　incompetent cervix, 210
　induced hypertension (PIH), 210-211
　molar (hydatidiform mole), 209
　physical adaptations to, 192-194
　polyhydramnios, 208
　signs of, 190-191
　terminology of, 189
prenatal care, 195-196
preoperative care
　for children, 277
　general, 38-39
preschoolers
　developmental stages of, 244
　health maintenance of, 245
　language development of, 243-244
　motor skills of, 243
　nutritional needs of, 242
　physical characteristics of, 242
　play of, 244-245
　sleeping patterns of, 242-243
prostatectomy, 101-103
prostatitis, 101-102
psychiatric nursing. See also individual treatment
　models
　legal aspects of, 183-184
　overview of, 133
psychoanalytical model, 134
psychosexual stages (of Freud), 134
psychosocial development model, 134
psychosomatic disorders, 148. See also anxiety disorders
pulmonary edema, 83
pulmonary emphysema, 24
pulmonary toilet, 36
pyloric stenosis, 278

Q

quadriplegia, 111

R

rabies, 303
radiation. See cancer
radiologic tests, 93
radionuclide uptake, 42
rape, 182, 227
Raynaud's phenomenon, 86
reactive airway disease
  in children, 287-288
renal
  angiography, 93
  disease, 75
  failure, 97-98
  function tests, 93
respiratory infections, 272-276. See also
  individual infections
respiratory system disorders, 23-37
retina, detached, 117-118
Reye's syndrome, 303
rheumatic fever, 303
rheumatoid arthritis, 55
ringworm, 302
roseola, 304
rubella, 304
rubeola, 304

S

sarcomas, 120
scarlet fever, 304
Schilling's test, 76
schizophrenia
  medications for, 154-156
  overview of, 150
  paranoid personality disorders, 152
  pervasive development disorders, 153
  schizophrenic disorders, 150-151
scoliosis, 288-289
secretions, analysis of, 42
Sengstaken-Blakemore tube, 52
sexual abuse
  of children, 285
shock
  89-90
SIADH (syndrome of inappropriate secretion
  of antidiuretic hormone), 63-64
sickle cell anemia, 77, 292-293
sigmoidoscopy, 42
somatoform disorders, 147. See also anxiety disorders
spinal board, 112
spinal cord injury, 111-112
sputum examination, 24
stools, analysis of, 42
stress, characteristics of, 137
Stryker frame, 112
suctioning
  pulmonary, 37
suicide, 159
surgical carotid endarterectomy, 111
syndrome of inappropriate secretion of
  antidiuretic hormone (SIADH), 63-64
systemic lupus erythematosus, 60

T

talipes equinovarus, 265
test-taking tips, 11
tetanus, 304
thermosclerectomy, 119
thoracentesis, 24
thoracic cavity, 23
thromboangiitis obliterans, 86
thrombophlebitis, 88
thymectomy, 115
thyroid gland, 68-70, 74
thyroidectomy, 69, 70
Tic douloureux, 116
toddlers
  developmental stages of, 240
  health deviations of, 242
  health maintenance of, 241-242
  language development of, 240
  motor skills of, 239-240
  nutritional needs of, 239
  physical characteristics of, 239
  play of, 241
  sleeping patterns of, 239
tonsillectomy, 277-278
tooth eruption
  permanent, 246
  primary, 233
total parenteral nutrition (TPN), 45
trabeculectomy, 119
traction, 56
transient ischemic attacks, 111
trigeminal nerve, microvascular decompression of, 116
trigeminal neuralgia, 116
tuberculosis, 30-31, 125
tumors
  classification of, 120
  staging of, 120-121

U

ulcerative colitis, 48
ulcers, 46-47
umbilical cord compression, 212
urinalysis, 92
urinary antiseptics, 101
urinary tract infection
  in children, 276-277
urinary tract surgery, 100
urolithiasis, 96-97
uterine disorders
  endometriosis, 226
  myomas, 226

V

vaginal infections
  candidiasis (yeast), 224
  condyloma, 224
  trichomoniasis, 224
vagotomy, 47
valvular disorders, 84

valvulotomy, 84
varicose veins, 89
vascular disorders, 87-88
vascular graft, 86
vasodilators, 88
venous disorders, 88-89
ventricular failure, 83
vomiting, in children, 269-270

W

Wernicke-Korsakoff's syndrome, 51, 168, 174-175
western blot, 125
whooping cough, 303
Wilms' tumor, 298

X

x-ray
  chest, 24
  KUB, 93

Y

yeast infection, 224

Additional Study Materials for Nursing Students

B O O K S

FOR NURSING EXAMS AND THE NCLEX . . . MAXIMIZE YOUR TIME

TEST-TAKING BOOKS (WITH DISK)

BECOME TEST SMART, REDUCE TEST ANXIETY & INCREASE CONFIDENCE

Successful Problem Solving and Test Taking for Beginning Nursing Students
2nd ed, 252 pp., 75 figures, test-taking tips highlighted.
ISBN#: 1-56533-026-9
#BK9 $29.95

Successful Problem Solving and Test Taking for the Advanced Student and the NCLEX-RN
4th ed, 165 pp., 130 figures, 150 test-taking tips highlighted.
ISBN#: 1-56533-027-7
#BK1 $29.95

Successful Problem Solving and Test Taking for the NCLEX-PN
2nd ed, 166 pp., 130 figures, 75 test-taking tips highlighted.
ISBN#: 1-56533-029-3
#BK4 $29.95

- User-friendly format walks you through the maze of answering multiple-choice test questions.
- Pass exams easier and learn how to get to the right answer.
- Increase confidence with the test-taking strategies and problem-solving skills. Gain the skills needed to master complex nursing questions in any area.

Essential NCLEX books in a format students can easily understand!

NCLEX REVIEW BOOKS (WITH DISK)

ELIMINATE OVER-STUDYING . . . FOCUS ON ESSENTIAL INFORMATION

The Comprehensive NCLEX-RN Review 2000
9th ed, 384 pp., 33-pg pharm outline charts/tables/figures, nursing interventions highlighted, quick-access index.
ISBN#: 1-56533-032-3
#BK2 $29.95

The Comprehensive NCLEX-PN Review
3rd ed, 379 pp., 33-pg pharm outline, charts/tables/figures.
ISBN#: 1-56533-023-4
BK#5 $29.95

Now on CD-ROM!
See Page 371 for details.

- Easy-to-use outline format focuses on essential NCLEX information.
- Eliminate over studying with this all-in-one outline review of all clinical areas.
- Increase nursing knowledge with highlighted nursing interventions and inviting graphics & charts.
- Become test wise with up-to-date information about the computerized exam & exclusive test-taking strategies.
- Locate topics instantly and maximize your study time.

Q&A BOOKS (WITH DISK)

TEST DRIVE THE NCLEX—PRACTICE MAKES PERFECT

The Complete Q&A for the NCLEX-RN
2nd rev. ed, 522 pp., test-taking tips highlighted, quick-access index.
ISBN#: 1-56533-024-2
#BK3 $29.95
Book with 10 accompanying audio tapes
#LP4 $139.00

The Complete Q&A for the NCLEX-PN
1st rev. ed, 522 pp., test-taking tips highlighted, quick-access index.
ISBN#: 1-56533-028-5
BK#6 $29.95

- Test-drive the NCLEX with over 1,000 up-to-date, challenging test questions.
- Learn more from the most complete rationales for all options.
- Hundreds of test-taking tips, strategy alerts highlighted in all rationales.
- Save valuable study time with quick-access index that locates topics instantly.
- Boost pharmacology retention with special exam.
- Disk with simulated NCLEX questions included allows you to chart your progress & assess test success.

SOFTWARE

COMPREHENSIVE PHARMACOLOGY SERIES

BOOST PHARMACOLOGY RETENTION

With this powerful solution for managing the complex subject of pharmacology, students will easily access key information on the most commonly prescribed drugs for each major body system, learn common attributes of major drug categories and instantly assess their critical-thinking skills with test questions embedded throughout the programs. Students can quickly access over 800 medical terms and drugs—and master their correct pronunciation with MEDS new audio glossary. And, with one click of the mouse, students navigate directly to each drug category for information on pharmacokinetics, drug use, contraindications, nursing interventions, client teaching and more! Each title in the series also includes a complete exam covering all drug categories used in each body system.

PSYCHIATRIC DRUGS

Antiparkinsonian and Antianxiety (Anxiolytic) Drugs,
Antipsychotic and Antidepressant Drugs,
Mood-Stabilizing Drugs

CD-ROM	FLOPPY
CDP-19	F-19

DRUGS USED IN LABOR AND DELIVERY

Oxytoxic, Uterine Relaxant, and Anticonvulsant Drugs,
Electrolyte Replacement, Narcotic Antagonists,
and Corticosteroid Drugs

CD-ROM	FLOPPY
CDP-22	F-22

ANTIMICROBIAL AND ANTI-INFECTIVE DRUGS

Penicillins, Cephalosporins, Macrolides,
Lincomycins, Aminoglycosides, Tetracyclines,
Quinolones, and Sulfonamides,
Antitubercular and Antifungal Drugs

CD-ROM	FLOPPY
CDP-26	F-26

RESPIRATORY DRUGS

Bronchodilators, Anti-inflammatories, Antihistamines,
Antitussives

CD-ROM	FLOPPY
CDP-53	F-53

CARDIOVASCULAR DRUGS

Antihypertensives, Antianginal Drugs,
Cardiac Glycosides, Antiarrhythmic Drugs

CD-ROM	FLOPPY
ICDP-54	F-54

ANALGESIC DRUGS

Narcotics (inc. Opiates), Non-narcotics, other pain relieving medications

CD-ROM	FLOPPY
ICDP-8	F-8

ENDOCRINE DRUGS

Drugs affecting the Pituitary Gland, the Parathyroid and Thyroid Glands, the Adrenal Cortex, and the Pancreas

CD-ROM	FLOPPY
ICDP-1	F-1

GI DRUGS

Drugs that affect the Mouth, Stomach, Gallbladder;
Laxatives; Antidiarrheals

CD-ROM	FLOPPY
ICDP-2	F-2

GU DRUGS

Diuretics, Antimicrobials for UTIs, Renal System Disfunction Therapies

CD-ROM	FLOPPY
ICDP-3	F-3

ONCOLOGY DRUGS

Antimetabolites, Alkylating Agents, Antibiotic Antitumor Agents, Mitotic Inhibitors

CD-ROM	FLOPPY
ICDP-4	F-4

PHARM PROGRAM 11:
VITAMINS

Fat-Soluble Vitamins, Water-Soluble Vitamins, Minerals

CD-ROM	FLOPPY
ICDP-5	F-5

DOSAGE & CALCULATIONS

Conversions Between the Metric, Apothecary and Household Systems; Calculations for Dosage and IV Administration

CD-ROM	FLOPPY
ICDP-6	F-6

HEMATOLOGIC DRUGS

Anticoagulants, Thrombolytics, Blood Components,
Antihyperlipidemic Drugs

CD-ROM	FLOPPY
ICDP-7	F-7

All Software Programs

CD-ROM	FLOPPY
$79.00	$69.00

TEST-TAKING SUCCESS SERIES

BECOME TEST SMART & TO GET TO THE RIGHT ANSWER

NCLEX-RN Test Taking 2000 (ver.1.0)

CD-ROM	FLOPPY
#CDTT42	#FTT42

Increase critical thinking skills, make the most of your nursing knowledge, and maximize your NCLEX scores.

Beginning Test Taking 2000 (ver. 1.0)

CD-ROM	FLOPPY
#CDTT32	#FTT32

Designed to enhance test-taking and problem-solving skills. Teaches MEDS' exclusive methods for passing beginning nursing exams. An essential resource for new and ESL nursing students.

NCLEX-PN Test Taking 2000 (ver. 1.0)

CD-ROM	FLOPPY
#CDTT36	#FTT36

Provides MEDS' exclusive test-taking strategies and problem-solving methods for the PN student. Maximize your NCLEX-PN scores. A required learning resource for all PN students.

PSYCHIATRIC NURSING

MASTER DIFFICULT PSYCHIATRIC NURSING CONCEPTS

Comprehensive Review of Psychiatric Nursing

CD-ROM	FLOPPY	
#CD43	#F43139	$149.00

Reviews psychiatric nursing concepts. Special nurse-alert screens highlight essential nursing interventions. Assessment test provided for each unit. Defense mechanisms, anxiety, schizophrenia, mood disorders, chemical abuse, comprehensive exam, and more.

Q&A COMPUTERIZED TESTING

MASTER CHALLENGING, HIGH-LEVEL NURSING EXAM QUESTIONS RIGHT IN YOUR OWN HOME

NCLEX Q&A SOFTWARE SUCCESS SERIES

TEST-DRIVE THE NCLEX!

Updated for the 1998 Test Plan!

Go for the NCLEX-RN Gold 2000!

The Guaranteed Stand-Alone Review— PASS or Your Money Back!

NCLEX-RN GOLD 2000: Q&A Software Review—Success Guaranteed
Learn more from each of the perfectly crafted practice exams with over **2,100** NCLEX-simulated test questions. **Become test smart with: integrated exams, pre-test, final exam, and tests in all clinical areas: medical/surgical, psychiatric, women's health, pediatrics, nursing management, and pharmacology.** Reinforce nursing content with quick access to 800 medical terms and drugs. Problem-solving ability increased with highlighted key words. Test-taking strategies identified in all rationales. Comes with *The Comprehensive NCLEX-RN Review* book and *The MEDS NCLEX-RN 30-Day Planner* & a money-back guarantee for first-time NCLEX candidates. The only program where you can test in all clinical areas.

| Floppy | #F57 | $225.00 |
| CD-ROM | #CT57-CD | $259.00 *ALL NEW!* |

FEATURES OF ALL MEDS PUBLISHING'S NCLEX Q&A PROGRAMS:

- ✔ One Button, One Finger, One Mouse, Total Control
- ✔ All key words highlighted with the "Hint Button"
- ✔ Get started in three minutes
- ✔ Quick access to 800 definitions of medical terms and drugs
- ✔ Powerful test-taking strategies highlighted
- ✔ Instant review of incorrect answers with detailed rationales
- ✔ NCLEX key stroke, screen design, test plan

NCLEX-PN GOLD: Q&A Software Review

Students learn more from the 10 practice exams with the most challenging test questions. Incorporates NCLEX threads and nursing process. An instant review of all incorrect questions reinforces learning. More than 200 powerful test-taking tips identified in rationales. Provides 15 hours of interactive, self-paced learning. *The Comprehensive NCLEX-PN Review* book included.

| Floppy | #CT72F | $169.00 |
| CD-ROM | #CT72-CD | $179.00 |

Building Test Success for Beginning Nursing Students

Maximize your test-taking skills and increase nursing test success. Features test questions in 11 fundamental nursing categories. Enhance confidence as you answer questions and quickly access the definitions of 400 medical terms, rationales, and test-taking strategies. A superb learning tool that is essential for ESL students. Get yourself off to a great start!

| Floppy | #CT68F | $99.00 |
| CD-ROM | #CT68-CD | $99.00 |

NCLEX Pharmacology 2000:

A Comprehensive Review of Essential Medical Terms & Drugs
Everything a nursing student needs to know to pass the pharmacology portion of the NCLEX with confidence! Software features a glossary with over 800 medical terms & drugs, plus practice exams with hundreds of NCLEX-style pharmacology questions.
Audio tape contains the most comprehensive pharmacology review available—designed for students on the go!

(Windows Version 1.0)

| Floppy Disk | ISBN# 1-56533-311-X | $69.00 |
| CD-ROM | ISBN# 1-56533-310-1 | $79.00 |

All MEDS computer programs come with free technical support.

Windows Specifications:
IBM-compatible 386 processor (486 recommended); 8 MB RAM (12 recommended); Windows 3.1 or higher; VGA display or better, set at 16-bit color; sound card (optional)

R N   A U D I O S

PROVIDE AN OVERALL REVIEW AS YOU PREPARE FOR YOUR NURSING EXAMS AND THE NCLEX-RN

EVERYTHING YOU NEED TO KNOW ABOUT THE NCLEX-RN

(Tapes 1-32)	**Only $249**	**#RAC1**
Save $197 when ordering the set		
Individual tapes	$13.95	

FEATURES OF ALL MEDS AUDIOTAPES:

✔ Up-to-date info

✔ Featuring dynamic nurse experts

✔ Designed for students on the go

✔ Learning made easy

✔ Approximate running time: 45 to 60 minutes

Tape 1: **How to Study for the NCLEX-RN Exam**
Essential information about the computerized NCLEX exam. Teaches what and how to study.

Tape 2: **Assessing Lab Values**
CBC, electrolytes, urinalysis, spinal fluid, renal, and liver function tests.

Tape 3: **Nutrition**
Organizes the essential material such as therapeutic diets.

Tape 4: **Growth and Development**
Organizes information in an easy-to-remember outline.

Tape 5: **Fluids and Electrolytes**
Makes this difficult content about the acid/base easy-to-learn.

Tape 6: **Cardiovascular Disorders** (M/S Pt 1)
Cardiac catheterization procedure, angina, myocardial infarction, CHF, pacemakers, cardiac surgery, and vascular diseases.

Tape 7: **Respiratory Disorders** (M/S Pt 2)
Pulmonary diseases such as a COPD, asthma, pneumothorax, TB and AIDS. Also includes chest tubes and pneumonectomy.

Tape 8: **Endocrine Disorders** (M/S Pt 3)
Endocrine diseases, treatments, nursing measures and drugs. Examples of these disorders are Addison's and Cushing's.

Tape 9: **Blood Disorders** (M/S Pt 4)
Blood disorders, nursing measures and drugs. Includes sickle cell, hemophilia, and leukemia.

Tape 10: **GI, Hepatic and Pancreatic Disorders** (M/S Pt 5)
Information about these disorders, nursing care and drugs. Includes hepatitis, ostomies, and liver transplants.

Tape 11: **Renal Disorders** (M/S Pt 6)
Renal disorders, nursing measures and drugs. Includes renal failure, dialysis and renal transplants.

Tape 12: **Musculoskeletal Disorders** (M/S Pt 7)
Arthritis, lupuserythematosus, fractures, osteomyelitis and complications of immobility.

Tape 13: **Neurological Disorders - Pt. 1** (M/S Pt 8)
Assesses the functions of the cranial nerves, neurological diagnostic tests, and seizure disorders.

Tape 14: **Neurological Disorders - Pt. 2** (M/S Pt 9)
Degenerative neuromuscular disorders such as myasthenia gravis, spinal cord, and head injury.

Tape 15: **Questions & Answers**
Specific strategies to use when answering the NCLEX-RN Exam multiple choice test questions and other nursing exams. Learn how to get to the right answer.

Tape 16: **Psycho-Social Component - Pt. 1** (PSY Pt 1)
Communication tools, nurse-client relationships, common neurotic behaviors, and 14 coping mechanisms.

Tape 17: **Psychiatric Disorders - Pt. 2** (PSY Pt 2)
Anxiety disorders, schizophrenia, organic brain syndrome, eating disorders, aggression, rape, and drugs.

Tape 18: **Psychiatric Disorders - Pt. 3** (PSY Pt 3)
Paranoid behavior, depression, manic depressive, addiction, antisocial personality, and drugs.

Tape 19: **Normal Pregnancy** (OB Pt 1)
Signs of pregnancy, prenatal care, stages of labor and delivery, and the postpartum period.

Tape 20: **Complications of Pregnancy** (OB Pt 2)
Complications of pregnancy (such as the high-risk mother with cardiac or diabetic problems) and abortions.

Tape 21: **Complications of Pregnancy** (OB Pt 3)
Complications of pregnancy such as dystocia, fetal distress, premature labor, and cesarean section.

Tape 22: **The Newborn** (OB Pt 4)
Initial assessment of the newborn and the high-risk newborn (such as prematurity, LGA, jaundice, and the addicted infant).

Tape 23: **Pharmacology**
Key information about common drugs. Includes their actions, side effects, and nursing implications.

Tape 24: **Math and Calculations**
Concepts on how to calculate fractional dosage, IVB drip rates, intake and output, and pediatric dosages.

Tape 25: **Emergencies**
Fractures, choking, poisoning, chest wounds, multiple trauma, and burns.

Tape 26: **Pediatric Bacterial Communicable Diseases** (PED Pt 1)
Treatment and nursing measures related to such diseases as meningitis, rheumatic fever, and glomerulonephritis.

Tape 27: **Pediatric Viral Communicable Diseases** (PED Pt 2)
LTB, URI, otitis, chicken pox, mumps, Rocky Mountain spotted fever, and infestations.

Tape 28: **Pediatric Chronic Illness** (PED Pt 3)
Down's syndrome, cystic fibrosis, spina bifida, failure to thrive, and child abuse.

Tape 29: **Pediatric Surgical Conditions** (PED Pt 4)
Tonsillectomy, pediatric reactions to illness, common pediatric procedures, tracheotomy care, and tube feeding.

Tape 30: **Postoperative Positioning and Tubes**
Describes the positions (prone, side-lying, Sims', semi-Fowler's) and tubes such as oxygen, tracheostomy, port-vac, water-seal chest drainage, NG, CVP, TPN, and superpubic.

Tape 31: **The Aging Client**
Communication techniques for clients with altered thought processes; physiological changes such as TIA, CVA, hypertension, osteoporosis and fractured hip.

Tape 32: **Communicable Diseases** (M/S Pt10)
Key information about TB, infectious hepatitis, and AIDS.

RN VIDEOS

THE COMPREHENSIVE NCLEX-RN VIDEO REVIEW

(Tapes 1-35 with book)	Only $595	#RVC5
Save $453 when ordering the set		
Individual tapes	$29.95	

RN Medical-Surgical Nursing — MODULE 1

(Tapes 1-14 with book)	Only $249 (save $70)	#RVC1

Video 1: Fluids and Electrolytes (M/S Pt 1)
Respiratory and metabolic acidosis and alkalosis, and blood gases.

Video 2: Respiratory Disorders-Pt. 1 (M/S Pt 2)
Most frequently tested disorders such as COPD, pneumothorax, asthma and chest tubes disorders.

Video 3: Respiratory Disorders-Pt. 2 (M/S Pt 3)
TB, pneumonia, chronic bronchiectasis, chest PT and AIDS.

Video 4: Pre- and Postoperative Care (M/S Pt 4)
Informed consent, pre- and postop drugs, assessment and complications.

Video 5: GI, Hepatic, and Pancreatic Disorders-Pt. 1 (M/S Pt 5)
Diagnostic procedures such as upper and lower GI, sigmoidoscopy liver biopsy, paracentesis and TPN. Presents information about peptic ulcers, gastric resection, ulcerative colitis, colostomy and ileostomy.

Video 6: GI, Hepatic, and Pancreatic Disorders-Pt. 2 (M/S Pt 6)
Disorders that frequently occur on the exam such as hepatitis A, hepatitis B, cirrhosis, esophageal varices, cholecystectomy and pancreatitis.

Video 7: Musculoskeletal Disorders (M/S Pt 7)
Rheumatoid and osteoarthritis, skeletal and skin traction, fractures, crutch walking, amputation, and Lupus.

Video 8: Blood Disorders (M/S Pt 8)
Iron deficiency, aplastic anemia, pernicious anemia, hemolytic anemia, and blood transfusions.

Video 9: Endocrine Disorders (M/S Pt 9)
Functions of each hormone and includes acromegaly, Addison's disease, Cushing syndrome, Grave's disease, thyroidectomy, hyperparathyroidism, diabetes mellitus, and insulin therapy.

Video 10: Cardiovascular Disorders (M/S Pt 10)
Dynamics of the CV system in failure, CVP, ECG and cardiac catheterization. Additional topics included are myocardial infarction, CHF, heart block, pacemakers, ASO, hypertension, venous disorders, shock, and CPR.

Video 11: Genitourinary System Disorders (M/S Pt 11)
Diagnostic exams such as renal function tests, KUB, IVP, cystoscopy, kidney biopsy. Includes glomerulonephritis, nephrotic syndrome, urolithiasis, chronic renal failure, peritoneal and hemodialysis, prostatectomy, and kidney transplants.

Video 12: Neurological Disorders-Pt. 1 (M/S Pt 12)
Diagnostic procedures such as lumbar puncture, CAT, myelogram, ECT, and neuro checks. Describes conditions such as ICP, seizures, CVA, and TIA.

Video 13: Neurological Disorders-Pt. 2 (M/S Pt 13)
Spinal cord, head injuries, laminectomy, multiple sclerosis, Parkinson's disease, myasthenia Gravis, cataracts, and glaucoma.

Video 14: Oncology Nursing and Burns (M/S Pt 14)
Neoplastic diseases, types of cancer therapy, chemotherapy, and radiation.

RN Psychiatric Nursing — MODULE 2

(Tapes 15-21 with book)	Only $159 (save $51)	#RVC2

Video 15: Introduction to Psychiatric Nursing (PSY Pt 1)
Psychiatric nurse, models of treatment, Erikson, Maslow, behavior modification, crisis intervention and self-help groups.

FEATURES OF ALL MEDS VIDEOS:

✔ Study at your own pace, in your own home

✔ Expert instructors make learning easy

✔ The most complete NCLEX review

✔ Approximate running time: 45-90 minutes

Great supplements for nursing exams, and NCLEX preparation.

SPECIAL

The Comprehensive NCLEX-RN Review book (with disk) is included FREE (a $29.95 value) with the purchase of one or more modules.

Video 16: **Defense Mechanisms** (PSY Pt 2)
Nurse-client relationships, communication skills, defense mechanisms.

Video 17: **Anxiety Disorders** (PSY Pt 3)
Anxieties: panic disorders, obsessive compulsiveness, phobics, hypochondriacs and anti-anxiety drugs.

Video 18: **Schizophrenia/Paranoid Behavior** (PSY Pt 4)
Treatment and nursing interventions for schizophrenia, paranoid behavior and anti-psychotic drugs.

Video 19: **Mood Disorders** (PSY Pt 5)
Depression and elation. Reviews moods, suicide, antidepressant agents, antimania agents and ECT therapy.

Video 20: **Chemical Dependency** (PSY Pt 6)
Chemical and substance abuse. Includes withdrawal, delirium tremens, treatment and rehabilitation.

Video 21: **Eating Disorders, Developmental Disabilities, Personality Disorders, Family Violence, Child Abuse, Rape and Legal Aspects** (PSY Pt 7)
Anorexia/ bulimia, retardation, signs of abuse, rape, and the legal aspects of psychiatric nursing.

RN Maternity Nursing   MODULE 3

(Tapes 22-27 with book)	Only $149 (save $31)	#RVC3

Video 22: **Female Reproductive Nursing** (OB Pt 1)
Anatomy and physiology, fetal development, teratogenic effects, signs of pregnancy, and emotional adaptations.

Video 23: **Labor and Delivery** (OB Pt 2)
Signs of impending labor, stages of labor, and operative obstetrics.

Video 24: **Postpartal Adaptation and Nursing Assessment** (OB Pt 3)
Postpartal changes, both physical and psychological.

Video 25: **Reproductive Risk** (OB Pt 4)
High-risk pregnancy, cardiac, diabetics, ectopic pregnancy, pregnancy induced hypertension, abruptio placentae, fetal distress, and postpartum and fetal assessment.

Video 26: **Newborn/High-Risk Newborn** (OB Pt 5)
Initial assessment of the newborn. Defines prematurity (SGA), postmature infants (LGA), jaundice, substance abuse, and AIDS in the newborn.

Video 27: **Gynecology** (OB Pt 6)
Vaginal infections, cancer, uterine disorders, menopause, battering/abuse, and rape.

RN Pediatric Nursing   MODULE 4

(Tapes 28-35 with book)	Only $159 (save $51)	#RVC4

Video 28: **Growth and Development-Pt. 1** (PED Pt 1)
Stress of hospitalization and G&D for infancy through toddler.

Video 29: **Growth and Development-Pt. 2** (PED Pt 2)
Growth and development for toddler through adolescent.

Video 30: **Nursing Care of the Child with Congenital Anomalies** (PED Pt 3)
Congenital heart defects, hydrocephalus, myelomeningocele, CDH, congenital clubfoot, cleft lip, and cleft palate.

Video 31: **Nursing Care of the Child with an Acute Illness** (PED Pt 4)
Vomiting, gastroenteritis, and respiratory infections.

Video 32: **Child Surgical Care** (PED Pt 5)
Pre- and postop care and common surgical problems.

Video 33: **Children as Accident Victims** (PED Pt 6)
General emergency care, burns, fractures, and ingestions.

Video 34: **Children with Chronic Problems** (PED Pt 7)
Allergies, asthma, rheumatic fever, JRA, diabetes, sickle cell, cerebral palsy, nephritis, and cystic fibrosis.

Video 35: **Oncological/Infectious Diseases** (PED Pt 8)
Leukemia, nephroblastoma (Wilm's tumor), neuroblastoma, and Hodgkin's lymphoma.

Video 36: **Nutrition** $29.95   #RV36
Outlines the foods included in and excluded from different therapeutic diets.

Video 37: **Pharmacology** $29.95   #RV37
Organizes the drugs that are most likely to appear on the NCLEX-RN Exam. Clarifies the actions, side effects, and nursing implications.

370

PN AUDIOS/ VIDEOS

SET YOUR SIGHTS ON A GREAT SUPPLEMENT FOR NURSING EXAMS, CLINICALS, AND THE NCLEX!

PN Medical/Surgical Nursing — PACKAGE #1
(Tapes 1-10 with book)   Only $175 (save $124)   #PVC1

Video 1: Fluids and Electrolytes (M/S Pt 1)
Respiratory and metabolic acidosis and alkalosis, and blood gases.

Video 2: Respiratory Disorders-Pt. 1 (M/S Pt 2)
Frequently tested disorders such as COPD, pneumothorax, asthma, and chest tubes.

Video 3: Respiratory Disorders/Pre- & Postoperative Care-Pt. 2 (M/S Pt 3)
TB, pneumonia, chronic bronchiectasis, chest PT and AIDS. Reviews informed consent, pre- and postop drugs and complications.

Video 4: Gastrointestinal Disorders (M/S Pt 4)
Diagnostic procedures such as upper and lower GI, sigmoidoscopy, liver biospy, paracentesis and TPN. Presents information about peptic ulcers, gastric resection, ulcerative colitis, colostomy, and ileostomy.

Video 5: Hepatic, Pancreatic Disorders (M/S Pt 5)
Disorders that frequently occur on the exam such as hepatitis A, hepatitis B, cirrhosis, esophageal varices, cholecystectomy, and pancreatitis.

Video 6: Musculoskeletal & Endocrine Disorders (M/S Pt 6)
Skeletal and skin traction, fractures, amputation and Lupus. Reviews function of each hormone and includes Addison's disease, Cushing's disease, Grave's disease, thyroidectomy, hyperparathyroidism, diabetes mellitus, and insulin therapy.

Video 7: Blood and Cardiovascular Disorders (M/S Pt 7)
Key information about iron deficiency, asplastic anemia, pernicious anemia, and blood transfusions. Begins by clarifying the dynamics of the CV systems in failure, CVP, and cardiac catheterization. Topics included are: myocardial infarction, CHF, pacemakers, hypertension, shock, and CPR.

Video 8: Genitourinary System Disorders (M/S Pt 8)
Diagnostic exams such as renal function tests, KUB, IVP, cystoscopy and kidney biopsy. Includes glomerulonephritis, nephrotic syndrome, urolithiasis, chronic renal failure, peritoneal and hemodialysis, and prostatectomy.

Video 9: Neurological Disorders (M/S Pt 9)
Diagnostic procedures such as lumbar puncture, CAT, myelogram, ECT and neuro checks. Describes conditions such as ICP, seizures, CVA. Includes spinal cord, head injuries, laminectomy, multiple sclerosis, Parkinson's disease, myasthenia gravis, cataracts and glaucoma.

Video 10: Oncology Nursing and Burns (M/S Pt 10)
Neoplastic disease, including the manifestations, types of cancer therapy, chemotherapy, and radiation.

PN Psychiatric Nursing — package #2
(Tapes 11-14 with book)   Only $89 (save $31)   #PVC2

Video 11: Intro to Psychiatric Nursing/Defense Mechanisms (PSY Pt 1) Role of the nurse in treatment models: Erikson, Maslow, behavior modification, crisis intervention and self-help groups. Reviews nurse-client relationships, defense mechanisms, and communications skills.

Video 12: Anxiety Disorders and Schizophrenia (PSY Pt 2)
Panic disorders, obsessive compulsive, phobic, hypochondriacs, and anti-anxiety drugs. Defines the major characteristics, treatment, and nursing interventions associated with schizophrenia and suspicious patterns of behavior. Includes the antipsychotic drugs.

Video 13: Mood Disorders/Chemical Dependency (PSY Pt 3)
Depression and elation. Reviews range and severity of moods, suicide, anti-depressant agents, anti-mania agents, and ECT therapy. Reviews chemical and substance abuse, alcohol dependency, withdrawal, delirium tremens, and rehabilitation.

Video 14: OMD, Eating Disorders, Developmental Disabilities, Personality Disorders, Family Violence, Child Abuse, Rape and Legal Aspects (PSY Pt 4) Anorexia/bulimia, signs of abuse, rape & the legal aspects of psychiatric nursing.

PN Maternity Nursing — package #3
(Tapes 15-19 with book)   Only $115 (save $35)   #PVC3

Video 15: Female Reproductive Nursing (OB Pt 1)
Anatomy and physiology, fetal development, teratogenic effects, signs of pregnancy and emotional adaptations.

Video 16: Labor and Delivery-Pt. 1 (OB Pt 2)
Signs of impending labor, stages of labor, analgesia/anesthesia for labor and delivery, and operative obstetrics.

Video 17: Labor and Delivery-Pt. 2 (OB Pt 3)
Continuation of the topics described in Labor and Delivery - Part 1.

Video 18: Postpartal Adaptation and Reproductive Risks (OB Pt 4)
Physical and psychological changes. High-risk pregnancy, cardiac, diabetics, abortion, ectopic pregnancy, incompetent cervix, pregnancy induced hypertension, placenta previa, fetal distress, premature labor, emergency childbirth, postpartum and fetal assessment.

Video 19: Newborn/High Risk Newborn/Gynecology (OB Pt 5)
Initial assessment of the newborn. Defines prematurity (SGA), postmature infants (LGA), jaundice, substance abuse, and AIDS in the newborn. Vaginal infections, cancer, uterine disorders, tubal disorders, menopause, battering/ abuse and rape, infertility, family planning and medications.

PN Pediatric Nursing — PACKAGE #4
(Tapes 20-24 with book)   Only $115 (save $35)   #PVC4

Video 20: Growth and Development (PED Pt 1)
The stress of hospitalization and characteristics of development for infancy.

Video 21: Nursing Care of the Child with Congenital Anomalies (PED Pt 2)
Congenital heart defects, hydrocephalus, cleft lip and cleft palate.

Video 22: Nursing Care of the Child with an Acute Illness/Child Surgical Care (PED Pt 3)
Fever, vomiting, gastroenteritis and respiratory infections. Reviews pre- and post-care and common surgical problems.

Video 23: Children as Accident Victims and with Chronic Problems (PED Pt 4)
General emergency care, burns, fractures and ingestions. Allergies, asthma, rheumatic fever, diabetes, sickle cell, cerebral palsy, nephritis, and cystic fibrosis.

Video 24: Oncological/Infectious Diseases (PED Pt 5)
Leukemia, Wilms' tumor, Hodgkin's disease, immunizations, and common infectious diseases

Video 25: Pharmacology $29.95
Drugs that are most likely to appear on the NCLEX-PN Exam. Clarifies the actions, side effects and nursing implications of using these drugs.

Video 26: Medical Terms $29.95
Medical terms and abbreviations most frequently used in nursing.

The Comprehensive NCLEX-PN Audio Review — PACKAGE #1A
(Tapes 1-15)   Only $149   #PAC5
(Save $60 when ordering the set)

Tape 1: Cardiovascular/Respiratory Disorders (M/S Pt 1)
Myocardial infarction, congestive heart disease, COPD, TB, pneumonia, and drug and diagnostic procedures.

Tape 2: GI, Hepatic and Pancreatic Disorders (M/S Pt 2)
Ulcers, colostomies, GI tubes, hepatitis, cirrhosis, and cholecystitis.

Tape 3: Musculoskeletal Disorders (M/S Pt 3)
Arthritis, osteomyelitis, fractures, crutch walking, and complications of immobility.

Tape 4: Neurological Disorders (M/S Pt 4)
Neurological diagnostic tests, head and spinal cord injuries, increased intracranial pressure, seizures, and Parkinson's disease.

Tape 5: Endocrine and Renal (M/S Pt 5)
Diabetes, thyroid, acute and chronic renal failure, nephritis, dialysis.

Tape 6: Pharmacology
Vital information about the actions, side effects, and nursing implications associated with common drugs.

Tape 7: Math and Calculations
Presents concepts on how to calculate fractional dosages, IV drip rates, intake and output, and pediatric dosages.

Tape 8: Growth and Development
Human growth and development from the infant to the mature adult and reactions of the hospitalized client.

Tape 9: Pediatrics - Pt. 1 (PED Pt 1)
Communicable diseases such as meningitis, rheumatic fever, and chicken pox.

Tape 10: Pediatrics - Pt. 2 (PED Pt 2)
Congenital and surgical conditions such as Down's syndrome, spina bifida, tonsillectomy, and appendectomy.

Tape 11: Normal Pregnancy (OB Pt 1)
Basic info about normal pregnancy, prenatal care, labor and delivery, and postpartum.

Tape 12: Complications of Obstetrics (OB Pt 2)
Complications such as abortion, placenta previa, prolapsed cord, cesarean section, postpartum hemorrhaging, and infections. Includes the newborn.

Tape 13: Psycho-Social Component (PSY Pt 1)
Coping mechanisms, communication tools, crisis intervention, group therapy, and anxiety disorders.

Tape 14: Psychiatric Nursing (PSY Pt 2)
Depression, schizophrenia, substance abuse, organic brain disorders, eating disorders, and violence.

Tape 15: The Aging Client
Alzheimer's disease, physical changes of aging, osteoporosis, fractured hip, diabetes, dehydration and CHF. Also includes psychological changes such depression, anxiety, suicide, and drug management.

SPECIAL!
The Comprehensive NCLEX-PN Review
A $29.95 value FREE with any video package purchase.
Organize & Prioritize with this All-in-One Review!

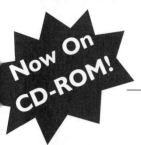

THE COMPREHENSIVE
NCLEX-RN REVIEW BOOK

HOW WILL THIS MULTIMEDIA TOOL GUARANTEE MY NCLEX SUCCESS?

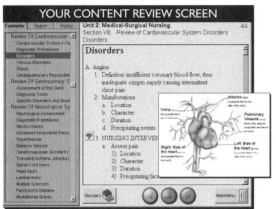

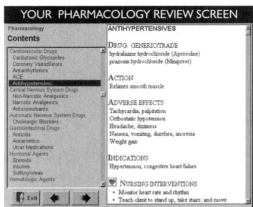

Customized Study Program

Search & Gather Essential NCLEX Information

Review at the Push of a Button:
- Medical/Surgical
- Psychiatrics
- Women's Health
- Pediatrics
- Pharmacology

Your Strengths Diagnosed
Our personal performance profile analyzes your strengths and weaknesses

Your Nursing Knowledge Strengthened

Your Test-Taking Skills Improved

Proven Features:
- Customized Study Program
- Hundreds of NCLEX-Style Questions
- Audio Glossary Learning Tool
- Full Color Illustrations
- Hundreds of Graphs and Tables
- Only Essential NCLEX Information
- Complete Pharmacology Section
- Quick Access Index

CD-ROM Updated for the April 1998 Test Changes!

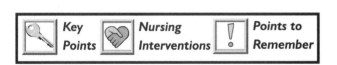

| Key Points | Nursing Interventions | Points to Remember |

ELIMINATE OVER-STUDYING
ORGANIZE & PRIORITIZE WITH THIS ALL-IN-ONE REVIEW

The Comprehensive NCLEX-RN Review Book with CD-ROM

The most complete & interactive NCLEX review available! The package includes MEDS Publishing's outstanding NCLEX-RN review book PLUS the entire book on CD-ROM with enhanced study aids. The CD-ROM features detailed illustrations, an audio glossary with over 800 terms, interactive test questions, and a unique NCLEX content review format.
1998, Windows Version 1.0
CD-ROM   ISBN# 1-56533-307-1 $69.95

The Comprehensive NCLEX-PN Review Book with CD-ROM
CD-ROM   ISBN# 1-56533-318-7 $69.95

Installation of the Comprehensive NCLEX-RN Review on CD-ROM

For Windows 95:
-Load CD into CD-ROM drive
-From the Start menu, click Run
-Type D:\setup.exe (or appropriate CD-ROM drive letter)
-Click "Full install all files"

From Windows 3.1
-Load CD into CD-ROM drive
-From the Program Manager, click Run
-Type D:\setup.exe (or appropriate CD-ROM drive letter)
-Click "Full install all files"